ENDOCRINOLOGY: PREMENOPAUSE AND POSTMENOPAUSE

Gabriel Duarte

ALLIED HEALTH PRESS

Endocrinology: Premenopause and Postmenopause

Author: **Gabriel Duarte**

Allied Health Press
4164 Lakeshore Road
Burlington ON L7L 1A4
Canada
www.alliedhealthpress.com
Email: orders@arclereducation.com

ISBN: 978-1-77956-265-4

ABOUT THE AUTHOR

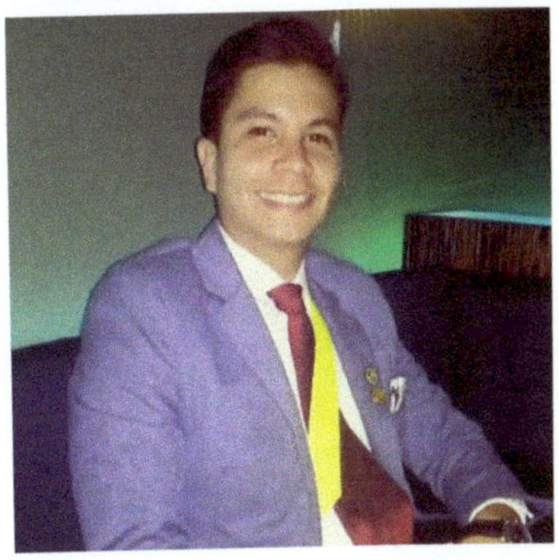

Gabriel is a doctor, passionate about radiology and diagnostic imaging with a solid clinical background. He completed his medical studies at the Universidad de Los Andes, Venezuela; and later he dedicated himself to the approach in anatomy, ultrasound, diagnosis and tomography studies. Besides, he has special training in teaching for undergraduate studies, human anatomy chairs and educational consulting. His passion for writing, editing and scientific research has led him to create experience as an author of many publications. Gabriel is a highly trained professional committed with teaching and high-quality professional medical practice.

Word Roots, Prefixes, and Suffixes by Chapter

Chapter 1 Introduction to Perimenopause and Postmenopause

Peri- Perinatal
Men/o- Menstrual
Post- Postpartum
Pre- Prenatal
Meta- Metamorphosis
-ology Endocrinology
-sis Menopause
Hyper- Hyperthyroidism

Chapter 2 Physiology of Menopause

mamm/o (breast)
mast/o (breast)
men/o (menstruation)
metr/o (uterus)
nat/i (birth)

Chapter 3 Clinical Manifestations and Diagnosis Process

Men/o – "menstruation"
Pause – "cessation" or "stop"
Pre- – "before"
Peri- – "around" or "about"
graphy – "process of recording"

Chapter 4 Hormone Replacement Therapy (HRT)

Hormone Chemical messengers in the body
Re- Replacement: Again, anew
Place To put or position
-ment Action or resulting state
Therap Treatment

Chapter 5 Bone Health and Osteoporosis

arthr/o joint
carp/o carpals, wrist
femor/o femur, upper leg bone
fibul/o fibula, lower leg bone
humer/o humerus, upper arm bone

Chapter 6 Cardiovascular Health

arteri/o artery
valv/o valve
coron/o crown or circle, heart
coron- pertaining to the heart

Chapter 7 Urogenital Health

-osis abnormal condition, increased number (blood)
-pathy disease
-uria urine, urination
ur- of or pertaining to urine, the urinary system
vagin- of or pertaining to the vagina

Chapter 8 Mental Health and Cognitive Function

aden- glands
adren- the adrenal glands
andro- male
cardi-, coron- the heart
cerebr- the brain
dendr- tree

Chapter 9 Sleep Disturbances

Somn-Somnambulism
Dys- Dysfunction
Insomn- Insomnia
-ation Meditation
Hypno- Hypnotherapy

Chapter 10 Weight Management and Metabolic Changes

abdomin/o abdomen
acanth/o thorny, spiny
acetabul/o acetabulum (hip socket)
acid/o acid
actin/o ray, radius

Table of Contents

LIST OF FIGURES

LIST OF TABLES

PREFACE

For many years, it was believed that the differences between males and females were minimal, and knowledge about men could be applied to women as well. However, an evolving understanding has led to the recognition that women's health encompasses more than just reproductive health and the absence of gynecological issues.

Changing lifestyles have led to smaller family sizes. The female-to-male sex ratio has declined, and instances of selective female foeticide present unique challenges to gynecologists, involving ethical, moral, and medical considerations. Additionally, there has been a rise in the number of divorced women and single mothers, leading to specific problems such as sexually transmitted diseases (STDs) and sexual dysfunction. The increased life expectancy means that women now spend a significant portion of their lives post-menopause, requiring gynecologists to effectively address their postmenopausal issues and expectations. The level of education attained by women in any society is correlated with their health, and today more women are literate than ever before. However, education also makes women more aware of their health issues, demanding a more responsive approach from physicians caring for women's health.

Careers have become increasingly important for women today, leading to later marriages and family planning at non-peak reproductive ages. This trend poses challenges such as subfertility, prompting patients to turn to assisted reproduction techniques. Advanced age itself is a risk factor for many pregnancy-related medical disorders, including gestational diabetes mellitus, gestational hypertension, and the need for operative interventions.

The rate of smoking among women is rising, with smoking having multifaceted effects including a higher incidence of heart disease and cancer. Smoking during pregnancy poses serious risks to the fetus, including low birth weight. Similarly, alcohol consumption not only causes psychological dependence but is also particularly harmful during pregnancy, leading to birth defects, developmental disorders, and fetal alcohol syndrome.

Drug abuse has increased among the young population, and while the percentage of pregnant women using illicit drugs is relatively low, the effects can be severe for both mother and fetus, including growth restriction, placental abruption, and fetal demise.

A woman's ability to control fertility is fundamental to her health. Although contraceptive acceptance has increased across all socioeconomic strata, it has not reached the desired levels. Emergency contraception has provided women with occasional exposure to greater freedom. Safe abortion services are now more accessible and well-utilized in cases of contraceptive failure, although some argue that it has led to increased promiscuity among women.

Women experience higher rates of psychological distress, depression, and physical morbidity compared to men. Increased workforce participation, rising divorce rates, single parenthood, and an aging population have significantly increased stress levels in women. Stress can impact neurohormonal and endocrinological pathways, leading to menstrual irregularities or altered reproductive behavior.

Changes in dietary habits and reduced physical activity have contributed to an obesity epidemic. When associated with obesity, polycystic ovarian syndrome poses specific challenges such as subfertility and hirsutism. Obesity is more prevalent among women of childbearing age than among older women. Obese patients have a higher incidence of heart disease, cardiac problems, endometrial cancer, and postmenopausal breast cancer. Overweight and obesity are serious concerns during pregnancy, increasing the risk of all pregnancy-related complications. Body image, or how a woman perceives her own body, is particularly important in the relational aspects of sexuality. Being overweight and obesity have significantly affected women's self-body image, leading many to adopt rigorous exercise routines, dietary regimens, and unnecessary cosmetic procedures.

This book on Obstetrics and Gynecology aims to provide a comprehensive text for scientists and clinical professionals working in the field. It covers topics related to obstetrics, maternal-fetal medicine, general gynecology, gynecologic oncology, urogynecology, reproductive medicine and infertility, reproductive endocrinology, and sexual medicine.

The aim of this book is to provide a comprehensive and up-to-date resource on the endocrinological aspects of perimenopause and postmenopause. It seeks to address the complex hormonal changes that occur during these stages of a woman's life and their impact on health and well-being. The book covers a wide range of topics, including the physiology of menopause, the role of hormones in menopausal symptoms, the management of endocrine disorders associated with menopause, and the latest advances in hormone replacement therapy and other treatment options.

This book is aimed at a broad population belonging to the health area, including endocrinologists, gynecologists, primary care physicians, nurse practitioners, researchers, and students in the field of endocrinology. It serves as a valuable resource for clinicians seeking to enhance their understanding of the endocrine changes that occur during perimenopause and postmenopause, enabling them to provide more effective care to their patients. Additionally, researchers will find the book to be a useful reference, providing a comprehensive overview of current knowledge and highlighting areas for further research. This book aims to advance the understanding and management of endocrine aspects of menopause, ultimately improving the quality of care for menopausal women.

Chapter 1

INTRODUCTION TO PERIMENOPAUSE AND POSTMENOPAUSE

Contents

Introduction

A woman's reproductive aging process has two distinct phases, perimenopause and postmenopause, each of which is marked by particular physiological changes. The time leading up to menopause when hormone fluctuations become more noticeable is called perimenopause, sometimes referred to as the menopausal transition. It usually starts in a woman's 40s but can occasionally occur earlier. This stage may extend for several months or even years. The ovaries' erratic production of estrogen and progesterone during perimenopause frequently causes mood swings, hot flashes, insomnia, and irregular menstrual cycles. Additional typical symptoms include changes in skin and hair texture, decreased libido, and dry vagina. Women may experience these symptoms at varying degrees of intensity and frequency.

Menstrual periods stop for 12 consecutive months at the end of perimenopause, indicating the start of menopause. After menopause, a woman experiences postmenopause, which lasts the rest of her life. This stage starts when a woman has not had a menstrual period for a year; this usually happens at age 51, though it can vary depending on genetics and personal health. The ovaries generate noticeably less progesterone and estrogen after menopause. Because of the waning protective effects of estrogen, the decline in these hormones may have long-term health implications, including an increased risk of osteoporosis and cardiovascular disease. Hot flashes and night sweats are two examples of perimenopausal symptoms that can last into the early postmenopausal years, but they usually get less severe with time. Additionally, because postmenopausal women have lower estrogen levels, which can impact the elasticity and health of the tissues in the vagina and the urine, they may continue to have vaginal dryness and urinary problems (Sherwin, 2001).

A woman's life undergoes major changes during perimenopause and postmenopause, which frequently call for dietary changes, lifestyle modifications, and occasionally medical interventions to control symptoms and preserve health. Some women think that hormone replacement therapy (HRT) is a good option for easing severe symptoms, but there are risks and benefits associated with it that should be carefully discussed with a healthcare professional. Additional strategies for managing the condition include dietary changes that support a healthy diet high in calcium and vitamin D, regular exercise to support cardiovascular and bone health, and stress-reduction techniques like yoga or meditation to enhance general wellbeing. By being aware of these stages and their effects, women can take charge of their health and well-being both during and after the menopausal transition.

Orientation and Directional Terms

Term	Definition	Illustration
Progesterone	Progesterone is an endogenous steroid hormone with effects on the female reproductive tract, mammary gland, central nervous system and pituitary gland. It is produced by the adrenal cortex and the ovary, and is released by the ovarian corpus luteum during the second part of the menstrual cycle, stopping the endometrial changes induced by estrogens and stimulating maturational changes, preparing it for embryo implantation, maintaining pregnancy and decreasing uterine contractility.	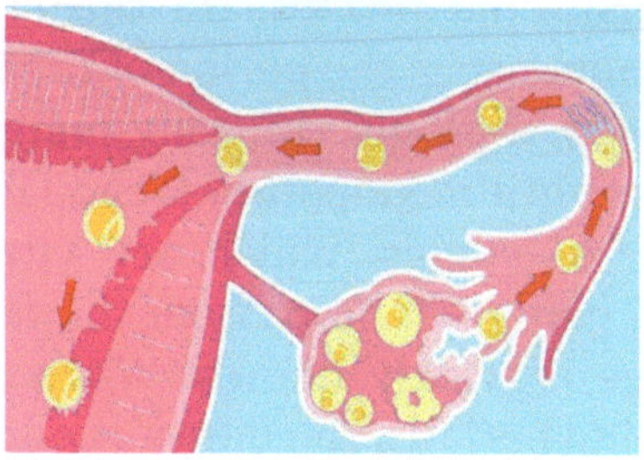
Menorrhagia	Menorrhagia is excessive menstrual bleeding for consecutive cycles in a woman of childbearing age, estimated at an amount greater than 80 ml per menstruation, a duration of menstrual bleeding greater than 7 days or the sum of both circumstances.	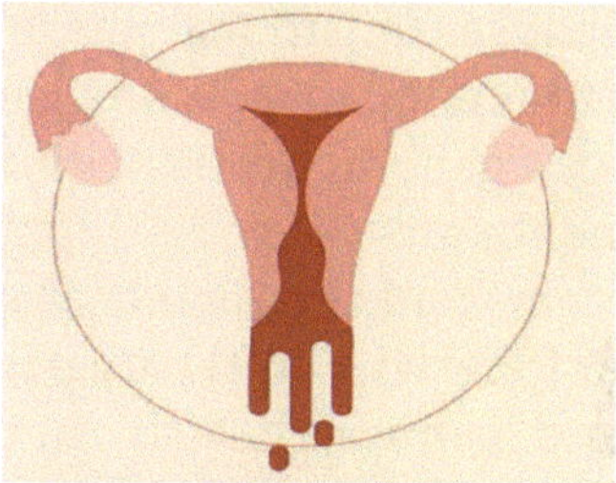
Urinary tract infections	Urinary tract infections (UTIs) are infectious processes that can affect any segment of the urinary system, where microorganisms overcome the body's defenses in the urinary system. They can cause discomfort and problems urinating.	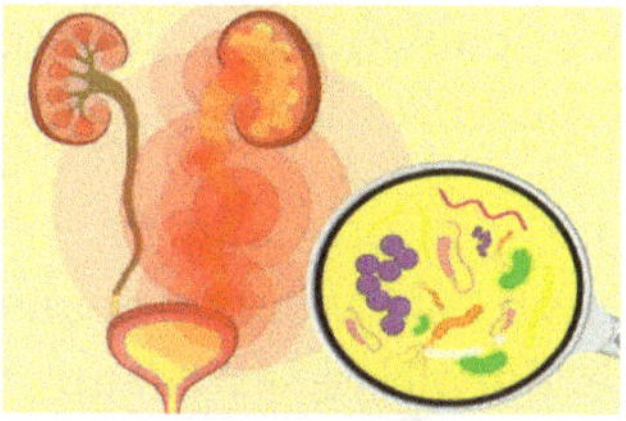
Cardiovascular health	The health and functioning of the heart and blood vessels, a critical aspect of overall well-being. The cardiovascular system is responsible for circulating blood throughout the body, delivering oxygen and nutrients to tissues, and removing waste products.	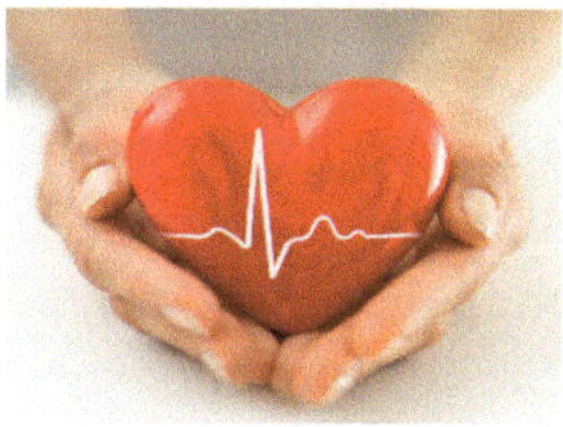
Lipoprotein	A biochemical assembly whose primary function is to transport hydrophobic lipid molecules in water, as in blood plasma or other extracellular fluids.	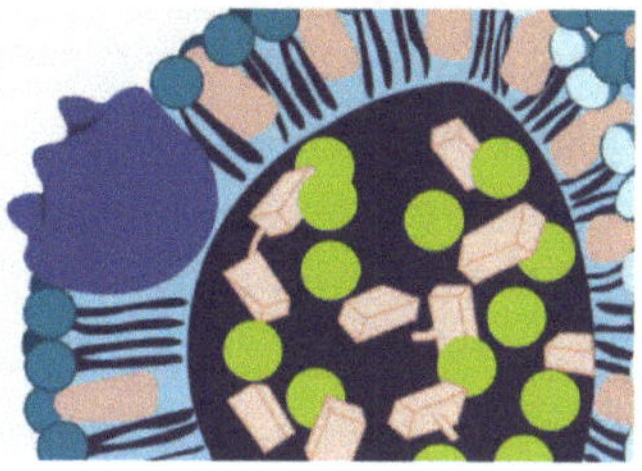

1.1. Perimenopause

A woman's reproductive years come to an end during the perimenopause and menopause, two transitional phases. On the other hand, pre-menopause is the period of time without any of these symptoms. Officially, female reproduction ends with menopause. Menopause actually has several stages, which are vital to recognize and comprehend despite the fact that this life stage is widely known. When a woman stops having periods, she officially enters menopause. However, perimenopause literally translates to "around menopause." It is also referred to as the menopause transitional phase because it occurs prior to menopause. While they both belong to the same general life transition, menopause and perimenopause are distinguished by distinct symptoms and treatments. The menstrual cycle phases (Sherwin, 2001) are periods of a woman's life and general health that are marked by transition; they are also known as menopause, perimenopause, and postmenopause. Decreases in female hormones, especially estrogen.

The period leading up to menopause is known as perimenopause. The essential female hormone, estrogen, begins to decline during perimenopause. Years may pass during perimenopause. In perimenopause, the ovaries begin to produce less hormones causing an unpredictable or irregular menstrual cycle. Perimenopause may begin in the mid-50s or early 30s. Some people spend very little time in perimenopause, but it lasts four to eight years for most women. The body may experience additional physical symptoms and changes as it adjusts to the altered hormone levels. Although fertility declines during perimenopause, pregnancy is still possible. Every woman experiences perimenopause differently, as do her symptoms, age of onset, and duration.

1.1.1. When Perimenopause Occurs

In perimenopause, estrogen decreases and its fluctuations may be more irregular than those seen in a standard 28-day cycle. Along with other symptoms, this can lead to irregular periods. The female body will progressively produce less estrogen as perimenopause nears its end. When the ovaries stop producing enough estrogen to release eggs, menopause officially begins (Spinelli, 2004). A woman may enter menopause earlier than normal if she:

- have a family history of early menopause
- are a smoker
- have had a hysterectomy or oophorectomy
- have undergone cancer treatments

1.1.2. Complications

Perimenopause is characterized by a variety of hormonal fluctuations that can cause various problems negatively affecting a woman's physical and mental health. Menstrual cycles that are irregular and can become unpredictable in terms of frequency, duration, and flow are among the most common complications. The ovaries' erratic production of progesterone and estrogen is the root cause of these abnormalities. Menorrhagia, or heavy menstrual bleeding, can also happen and can occasionally result in anemia, which is characterized by low red blood cell counts and weakness and exhaustion. The increased frequency and severity of vasomotor symptoms, such as night sweats and hot flashes, is another serious side effect. These symptoms can seriously interfere with daily activities and sleep cycles, which can lead to chronic fatigue and irritability. During perimenopause, emotional and psychological issues are also common. Women are prone to mood swings, anxiety, and depression; these symptoms are probably caused by hormonal fluctuations and the strain of dealing with erratic symptoms. These emotional disorders may necessitate psychological support or counseling since they can have an impact on one's personal and professional relationships. Cognitive abnormalities, which further impair everyday functioning and quality of life, are also reported during this stage. These abnormalities include problems focusing and memory lapses, commonly referred to as "brain fog."

During perimenopause, atrophy and dryness of the vagina caused by lowering estrogen levels can affect sexual health. These alterations can result in dyspareunia, which is pain and discomfort during sexual activity, and can lower sexual desire, which can strain close relationships. Lower estrogen levels can also result in problems related to the urine, like increased frequency, urgency, and a higher chance of urinary tract infections (UTIs), which can be difficult to treat and recurrent. Another crucial issue during the perimenopause is bone health. Estrogen deficiency can hasten bone loss, raising the risk of fractures and osteoporosis. To maintain bone health, it is crucial for women to keep an eye on their bone density and to think about making lifestyle or medical changes. Concerns about cardiovascular health also arise because of the potential negative effects of fluctuating and eventually falling estrogen levels on vascular function and cholesterol levels, which may raise the risk of heart disease. During perimenopause, weight gain and changes in fat distribution are common; these effects are frequently made worse by changes in metabolism and a decrease in muscle mass. This may result in a higher chance of type 2 diabetes, insulin resistance, and metabolic syndrome. During this time, maintaining a healthy weight with a balanced diet and frequent exercise becomes essential. Another major perimenopausal complication is sleep disturbances. Night sweats or elevated anxiety can cause insomnia and poo- quality sleep, which can lead to a vicious cycle of exhaustion and stress. Mitigating these issues can involve addressing sleep hygiene and seeking medical advice for severe sleep issues.

Irregular periods are a hallmark of perimenopause. Most of the time this is normal and nothing to be concerned about. Some warning signs are:

- Bleeding is extremely heavy—you're changing tampons or pads every hour or two for two or more hours
- Bleeding lasts longer than seven days
- Bleeding occurs between periods
- Periods regularly occur less than 21 days apart

1.1.3. Hormonal Changes During Perimenopause

The main factor causing the hormonal changes you go through during perimenopause is a decrease in estrogen. Estrogen is produced by your ovaries and is essential to the upkeep of the reproductive system. Your estrogen levels begin to drop as soon as you reach perimenopause. A different hormone, progesterone, is produced when estrogen levels fall, upsetting the equilibrium (Spinelli, 2004) by the ovaries. Together, these two hormones are in charge of menstruation and ovulation. Hormone fluctuations, resembling a rollercoaster ride, are typical during the perimenopause. Your ovaries stop releasing eggs when you enter menopause because your body produces so little estrogen at that point. You stop getting your period at this point. The main hormones controlling the menstrual cycle and reproductive system, estrogen and progesterone, start to decrease in the ovaries during the perimenopause, causing major hormonal changes. Hormone fluctuations can cause a range of physical and emotional symptoms that are typical of this transitional phase.

Unpredictable fluctuations in estrogen levels begin during the perimenopause, after having been relatively stable during a woman's reproductive years. In addition to supporting numerous bodily processes, such as bone density and cardiovascular health, this hormone is essential for controlling the menstrual cycle and preserving the reproductive system. Menstrual cycles often become irregular as estrogen levels drop, with periods that may be heavier, lighter, shorter, or longer than usual. Hot flashes and night sweats, which are unexpected sensations of warmth frequently accompanied by perspiration and flushing, are examples of vasomotor symptoms that can result from these variations. Perimenopause is also accompanied by a decrease in progesterone, which stabilizes the endometrium, the lining that lines the uterus, and controls the menstrual cycle. Inverse periods and heavy menstrual bleeding (menorrhagia) are symptoms of an imbalance between estrogen and progesterone that may result from this decrease. Estrogen dominance is the term for the relative decrease in progesterone relative to estrogen, which can worsen perimenopausal symptoms as well. Additional hormone-regulated systems within the body are impacted by the imbalance and general decrease in progesterone and estrogen. Decreased estrogen levels, for instance, can result in atrophy and dryness of the vagina, which hurts and hurts when you mate. Increased frequency, urgency, and a higher risk of urinary tract infections are among the symptoms of declining estrogen, which is also linked to the elasticity and health of the urinary tract (Siddle et al., 1987).

Estrogen also affects mood management and cognitive abilities. Many women experience mood swings, elevated anxiety, and depressive symptoms as their estrogen levels rise and fall. Known as "brain fog," cognitive abnormalities including memory loss and concentration problems are also frequent during this period. Estrogen has a major impact on bone health because it preserves bone density (Cummings, et al., 1998). Osteoporosis and fractures are more likely during the perimenopause because of the acceleration of bone loss caused by the decrease in estrogen. Hormonal fluctuations also affect cardiovascular health, since estrogen supports normal vascular function and cholesterol levels. A higher risk of heart disease may result from its decline. Furthermore, perimenopausal hormonal changes can impact metabolism, resulting in weight gain and alterations in the distribution of fat. This is frequently exacerbated by reductions in muscle mass and alterations in physical activity levels, raising the possibility of metabolic disorders like type 2 diabetes and insulin resistance (Soares and Taylor, 2007).

1.1.4. Symptoms and Causes

Throughout the menopausal transition, some subtle—and some not-so-subtle—changes in female body. Some are:

- **Irregular Periods:** The length of time between periods can vary, as can the intensity of flow; some periods may even be skipped as ovulation becomes more temperamental. Should the duration of menstrual cycle consistently fluctuate by seven days or more, you might be in the early stages of perimenopause. You probably are in late perimenopause if it takes you 60 days or longer to get the period.
- **Hot Flashes and Sleep Problems:** Perimenopause is a common time for hot flashes. The degree, duration, and regularity differ. Hot flashes and night sweats are frequently the cause of sleep issues, but they are not always the cause.
- **Mood Changes:** During the perimenopause, mood swings, irritability, or an increased risk

of depression may occur. These symptoms might be brought on by hot flashes interfering with sleep. Aside from hormone changes associated with the perimenopause, other factors can also contribute to mood swings.

- **Vaginal and Bladder Problems:** Sexual activity may become painful when estrogen levels drop because the vaginal tissues may become less supple and lubricating. Additionally, low estrogen may make more susceptible to vaginal or urinary infections. Urinary incontinence may be exacerbated by loss of tissue tone.
- **Decreasing Fertility:** As ovulation becomes irregular, capacity to conceive decreases. However, as long as the woman having periods, pregnancy is still possible.
- **Changes in Sexual Function:** During perimenopause, sexual arousal and desire may change. But if exist satisfactory sexual intimacy before menopause, this will likely continue through perimenopause and beyond.
- **Loss of Bone:** With declining estrogen levels, start to lose bone more quickly than you replace it, increasing risk of osteoporosis—a disease that causes fragile bones.
- **Changing Cholesterol Levels:** Reduced levels of estrogen can cause negative alterations in blood cholesterol, such as an elevation in low-density lipoprotein (LDL) cholesterol, or bad cholesterol, which raises the risk of heart disease. Simultaneously, as women age, their levels of HDL cholesterol, or good cholesterol, tend to decline, further raising their risk of heart disease.

1.1.5. Diagnosis and Tests

The perimenopause is a process, a slow shift. It takes more than one test or indicator to diagnose perimenopause. Should be considered several factors, such as age, menstrual history, and any symptoms or physical changes. To measure the hormone levels, Tests may be prescribed. However, hormone testing is rarely required or helpful to assess perimenopause, aside from examining thyroid function, which can impact hormone levels (Olofsson et al., 2000). A formal diagnosis is not necessary for the menopause, by perceiving the associated symptoms, the diagnosis is assumed by the patient.

Examining symptoms, medical history, and, occasionally, laboratory testing are used to diagnose perimenopause. The process of diagnosing perimenopause and the tests that may be required are summarized as follows: a comprehensive assessment of symptoms is the first step in the diagnosis of perimenopause. Inconsistent menstrual cycles, hot flashes, nocturnal sweats, sleep difficulties, mood fluctuations, dry vagina, and altered sexual function are typical symptoms. Both the patient and the healthcare professional may find it useful to monitor patterns and recognize trends over time by keeping a symptom journal. To rule out conditions other than perimenopausal symptoms that could mimic them, a thorough medical history is necessary. Discussing the patient's menstrual history, past surgeries or illnesses, family history of menopause onset, and any current medications or treatments are all included in this. Other factors taken into account are lifestyle, general health, and stress levels (Baram, 1997).

1.1.5.1. Physical Examination

Any physical symptoms that may be connected to the perimenopause can be found with the aid of a physical examination. This entails a general health examination to gauge general health and a pelvic exam to look for changes in the reproductive organs.

1.1.5.2. Laboratory Tests

While symptom evaluation and medical history are primary tools for diagnosing perimenopause, certain laboratory tests can help confirm the diagnosis and rule out other conditions:

1. **Follicle-Stimulating Hormone (FSH) Test**: The ovaries start to produce less estrogen during the perimenopause, which causes FSH levels to fluctuate and sometimes even rise. The menopausal transition can be identified by perimenopausal symptoms and consistently high FSH levels, usually greater than 30 mIU/mL. However, this test alone is not conclusive because FSH levels can fluctuate greatly during the perimenopause.
2. **Estrogen (Estradiol) Test**: Measuring estradiol levels can provide insight into how much estrogen the ovaries are producing. Lower levels of estradiol are common during perimenopause.
3. **Thyroid Function Tests**: To rule out thyroid disorders as the cause of symptoms, it can be helpful to measure the levels of thyroid hormones, including TSH, since they can resemble perimenopausal symptoms.
4. **Other Hormone Tests**: Levels of other hormones, such as progesterone, testosterone, and luteinizing hormone (LH), might also be measured to provide a more comprehensive hormonal profile.

1.1.5.3. Additional Diagnostic Tools

In some cases, additional diagnostic tools may be used to assess bone density and cardiovascular health, given the increased risks of osteoporosis and heart disease during perimenopause:

1. **Bone Density Test (DEXA Scan)**: This test measures bone mineral density and can help determine the risk of osteoporosis, which increases as estrogen levels decline.
2. **Lipid Profile**: Assessing cholesterol levels can help evaluate cardiovascular risk, which can be affected by the hormonal changes of perimenopause.

1.1.5.4. Personalized Approach

Diagnosis and treatment strategies are customized to each woman's unique symptoms and health profile because perimenopause is a highly individual experience. To track progress and make necessary adjustments to treatment plans, follow-up appointments are crucial. To sum up, the diagnosis of perimenopause is mainly based on the assessment of symptoms and medical history, with specific laboratory tests being used as needed for confirmation. By taking a comprehensive approach, it is possible to make sure that other conditions are ruled out and that women are given the right care and support during this transitional period.

1.1.5.5. What FSH Level Means Perimenopause?

The pituitary produces the hormone known as FSH, or follicle stimulating hormone. During ovulation, it stimulates the ovaries to release an egg. It is possible to confirm the onset of menopause by testing your FSH level. Menopause may be indicated by an FSH level that is consistently high. But because your hormones fluctuate wildly during the perimenopause, FSH testing can be deceiving. Hormone tests will not be accurate if certain medications, such as birth control pills or hormone therapy, interfere with hormone levels. High prolactin and an overactive thyroid can also affect those outcomes (Soules et al., 2001).

1.1.6. Management and Treatment

There isn't any treatment to stop perimenopause. Perimenopause is a natural part of life. The "cure" for perimenopause happens when periods stop and enter menopause.

Medications are often used to treat perimenopausal symptoms.

- **Hormone Therapy:** The most successful treatment for perimenopausal and menopausal hot flashes and night sweats is still systemic estrogen therapy, which is available as pills, skin patches, sprays, gels, or creams.
- **Vaginal Estrogen:** One can apply estrogen directly to the vagina with a vaginal ring, cream, or tablet. The vaginal tissue absorbs the tiny amount of estrogen released during this treatment. It can ease some urinary symptoms, discomfort during sexual activity, and dry vagina.
- **Antidepressants:** Menopausal hot flashes may be lessened by some antidepressants that belong to the class of medications known as selective serotonin reuptake inhibitors (SSRIs). For women who require an antidepressant for a mood disorder or who are unable to take estrogen due to health concerns, an antidepressant may be helpful in managing hot flashes.
- **Gabapentin (Neurontin):** Gabapentin is approved to treat seizures, but it has also been shown to help reduce hot flashes. This drug is useful for women who can't use estrogen therapy for health reasons and for those who also have migraines.
- **Fezolinetant (Veozah):** This medicine is a hormone-free option for treating menopause hot flashes. It works by blocking a pathway in the brain that helps regulate body temperature.

1.2. Measuring Postmenopausal Syndrome

The menstrual cycle permanently ending and ovarian follicle development being lost is known as menopause. Age at menarche, race, socioeconomic status, or number of previous ovulations do not appear to have an impact on the age at menopause, which appears to be genetically determined. Menopause frequently occurs earlier in life due to factors that are harmful to the ovaries; women who smoke, for example, menopause earlier in life. Women who have undergone ovarian surgery or who have undergone a hysterectomy but kept their ovaries may also go through an early menopause. Menopause occurring before the age of 40 is known as premature ovarian failure. It could be idiopathic or linked to an autoimmune disease, chromosomal abnormality, or toxic exposure.

Menopause is a primary ovarian failure rather than a central event, despite being linked to changes in the pituitary and hypothalamic hormones that control the menstrual cycle. There is a reduction in ovarian follicles at the ovarian level. Follicle-stimulating hormone (FSH) and luteinizing hormone (LH) are the pituitary hormones that the ovary can no longer respond to, and as a result, ovarian estrogen and progesterone production stops. Ovarian androgen production persists after the menopausal transition due to stromal compartment sparing. Because of peripheral aromatization of ovarian and adrenal androgens, menopausal women still have low levels of circulating estrogens. Since fat tissue is a key location for aromatization, obesity has an impact on numerous menopausal side effects. Because the ovarian-hypothalamic-pituitary axis is unbroken during the menopausal transition, ovarian failure and the lack of ovarian negative feedback cause an increase in FSH levels. A major indicator of menopause, atresia of the follicular apparatus, specifically the granulosa cells, causes decreased production of estrogen and inhibin, which lowers inhibin levels and raises FSH levels (Schiff et al., 1979).

Reproductive hormone fluctuations characterize the menopausal transition, also known as the "perimenopause," which is a defined period of time that starts with the onset of irregular menstrual cycles and ends with the last menstrual period. Menstrual irregularities, a prolonged and heavy menstrual cycle mixed with bouts of amenorrhea, decreased fertility, vasomotor symptoms, and insomnia are the hallmarks of this time. A few of these signs may appear four years before the menstrual cycle ends. Estrogen levels fall and FSH and LH levels rise during the menopausal transition. Variable cycle lengths and missed menses are signs of the menopausal transition, while amenorrhea indicates the postmenopausal phase. The final menstrual period marks the end of the menopausal transition, which is marked by fluctuations in the length of the menstrual cycle and an increase in FSH levels. Retroactively, the menopause is defined as the end of the last menstrual cycle, which is followed by a year and a half of amenorrhea. The time after the last menstrual cycle is referred to as the postmenopause. The ovary is a woman's exclusive source of oocytes and a major source of androgens as well as her main source of progesterone and estrogen. Infertility during menopause is caused by oocyte depletion. With the exception of the elevated risk of endometrial proliferation, hyperplasia, and cancer linked to continued endogenous estrogen production or the administration of unopposed estrogen therapy in menopausal women, ovarian cessation of progesterone production appears to have no clinical consequences.

The main effects of menopause are mostly caused by low estrogen levels. Because menopause and aging are closely related, it can be very challenging to distinguish between the effects of estrogen deficiency and aging. Vasomotor symptoms, urogenital atrophy, osteoporosis, cardiovascular disease, cancer, psychiatric symptoms, cognitive decline, and sexual issues are the main health issues that menopausal women face. It has proven challenging to differentiate symptoms resulting from ovarian function loss from those caused by aging or the socio-environmental stressors associated with midlife. Postmenopausal syndrome is characterized by a wide range of symptoms, including hot flashes, irritability, mood swings, insomnia, dry vagina, difficulty concentrating, mental confusion, urge incontinence, stress incontinence, depression, headaches, vasomotor symptoms, and insomnia.

1.2.1. Vasomotor Symptoms

Approximately 75% of women who are perimenopausal experience vasomotor symptoms. Most women experience symptoms for 1–2 years following menopause, but some may experience them for up to 10 years or longer. The main reason women seek medical attention during menopause is hot flashes. In addition to interfering with daily activities and disturbing women at work, hot flushes also cause sleep disturbances. During the menopausal transition, many women experience emotional instability and trouble focusing. If these mood and cognitive symptoms are brought on by sleep disturbance and the ensuing weariness during the day, treating the vasomotor symptoms should help. Given that thyroid disease is more common in older women, thyroid function tests ought to be carried out if vasomotor symptoms are unusual or treatment-resistant. We still don't fully understand the physiological mechanisms underlying hot flashes. An elevated core body temperature, metabolic rate, and skin temperature are caused by a central event that is most likely started in the hypothalamus. Some women experience peripheral vasodilation and sweating as a result of this reaction. Dopaminergic, serotoninergic, or noradrenergic activation may cause the central event. While an LH surge frequently coincides with a hot flush, it is not the cause because women who have had their pituitary glands removed also experience vasomotor symptoms. It's unclear exactly how estrogen affects these processes. Vasomotor symptoms are not just a result of low estrogen levels; they are also a result of estrogen withdrawal (Utian et al., 2001).

1.2.1.1. Treatment

The best treatment currently available for vasomotor symptoms and the resulting sleep disturbance is systemic estrogen therapy. Oral contraceptives may be helpful for healthy perimenopausal women who are still having menstrual periods but are having uncomfortable hot flashes. For many women, very-low-dose estrogen therapy is an effective treatment for hot flushes. Low-dose transdermal estradiol (0.025 mg weekly) or oral esterified and conjugated estrogens (0.3 mg daily) are frequently effective, have few side effects, and stimulate the endometrium. If a woman has not had a hysterectomy, progestin therapy needs to be administered concurrently; however, intermittent progestin therapy may be possible with low-dose estrogen therapy.

There are alternatives when using estrogen is not advised. For certain women, progestin therapy alone may be an option. Vasomotor symptoms can be effectively treated with megestrol acetate (20 mg twice a day) and medroxyprogesterone acetate (MPA) (20 mg/day). Several medications that modify central neurotransmitter pathways are also beneficial. Hot flushes are relieved by drugs that lower central noradrenergic tone, such as clonidine. Randomized, placebo-controlled trials have demonstrated a significant reduction in vasomotor symptoms with clonidine. It can be applied topically (0.1–2 mg/day) or topically (0.1–2 mg/week) as a transdermal patch. Drowsiness and orthostatic hypotension are possible side effects.

Moreover, hot flushes can be effectively relieved by selective serotonin reuptake inhibitors (SSRIs). Menopausal women with hot flashes saw a significant decrease in the frequency and intensity of episodes in a double-blind, randomized, placebo-controlled study using paroxetine controlled release (12:05 and 25 mg/day). In the paroxetine group, hot flush composite scores dropped by 62%, while in the placebo group, they dropped by 38%. The actual hot flush frequency decreased by 3.3 hot flushes per day with paroxetine versus 1.8 on placebo. There was no discernible improvement in mood or anxiety symptoms in conjunction with the improvement in vasomotor symptoms. Though the lower dose was better tolerated, both doses were equally effective. Headache, nausea, and sleeplessness were the most frequent side effects.

A randomized, double-blind, placebo-controlled crossover trial of fluoxetine (20 mg/day) also showed a slight improvement in symptoms. Not all research indicated that SSRIs reduced vasomotor symptoms. In a nine-month, double-blind, parallel-group study, neither citalopram (10–30 mg/day) nor fluoxetine significantly reduced hot flashes when compared to placebo.

Although there is a greater chance of negative effects, altering other central neurotransmitters with different antidepressants may also be beneficial. In a controlled trial, venlafaxine (75 mg/day) significantly decreased hot flashes. Scores for hot flushes dropped 61% in the venlafaxine group and 27% in the placebo group. Anorexia, nausea, and dry mouth were among the much more common side effects that the active treatment group encountered. In a placebo-controlled, randomized, crossover trial, vitamin E (800 IU/day) only slightly decreased hot flushes, despite being frequently advised. Compared to women of normal weight and nonsmokers, overweight and smoker women experience more severe vasomotor symptoms. These results offer more justification for encouraging women to give up smoking and lose weight.

1.2.2. Urogenital Atrophy

Urinary urgency, dyspareunia, dysuria, and vaginal dryness and pruritus are all caused by urogenital atrophy. Therapy is effective in treating these typical issues that menopausal women face. Systemic estrogen therapy is useful in treating dyspareunia, vaginal dryness, and urinary symptoms. Topical application is an additional choice. Endometrial stimulation is minimal because systemic absorption is low. Only one to three times a week is sufficient for the effectiveness of low-dose estrogen cream (0.05 g). A vaginal tablet containing 25 μg of estradiol, inserted twice a week, could be a less complicated and less messy option than estrogen cream. Any vaginal bleeding should be reported by women undergoing vaginal estrogen therapy, and any such bleeding should be carefully assessed. Women taking low-dose vaginal estrogen are generally not prescribed systemic progestin therapy. When urogenital atrophy is present, lubricants provide a non-hormonal alternative for minimizing discomfort during sexual activity. Vaginal estrogen therapy has been demonstrated to lower the risk of recurrent urinary tract infections in postmenopausal women and appears to reduce symptoms related to urination, including frequency and urgency. It is unclear how estrogen treatment affects urine incontinence. While the results of some studies indicate that estrogen therapy improves incontinence, those of other studies indicate that the symptoms worsen (Genant et al., 1997).

1.2.3. Osteoporosis

Osteoporosis frequently results in musculoskeletal symptoms such as back pain, fractures from minor trauma, reduced height, and decreased mobility. When choosing a course of treatment, it's critical to take into account a woman's osteoporosis risk factors and to take high-risk women's bone mineral density screening into account. Age, Asian or Caucasian ancestry, family history, small stature, history of a previous fracture, early menopause, and previous oophorectomy are examples of non-modifiable risk factors. Risk factors that can be changed include smoking, leading a sedentary lifestyle, and consuming less calcium and vitamin D. Osteoporosis is linked to certain medical conditions, such as anovulation during the reproductive years (e.g., as a result of overtraining or an eating disorder), hyperparathyroidism, hyperthyroidism, chronic kidney disease, and conditions necessitating systemic corticosteroid administration.

It is crucial to provide women with counseling regarding the modification of modifiable risk factors to prevent and treat osteoporosis. Many women would benefit from dietary adjustments and supplementation because their diets are low in calcium and vitamin D. 400–800 IU of vitamin D and 1000–1500 mg of calcium should be taken daily by women. Supplementing with vitamins and minerals or changing one's diet can help achieve this. One of the many health advantages of regular exercise and quitting smoking is a decreased risk of osteoporosis. All women with osteoporosis and those with osteopenia and other risk factors should receive treatment. Anti-resorptive medications, which lessen bone loss, and anabolic agents, which promote the formation of new bone, are the main types of drug therapies used to treat and prevent osteoporosis (Weiss et al., 1999).

Osteoporosis can be effectively prevented and treated with hormone therapy (HT). Long-term use of estrogen therapy, initiated soon after menopause, has been demonstrated in observational studies to reduce fractures related to osteoporosis by about 50%. It also considerably lowers fracture rates in female patients who already have a diagnosis. After an average follow-up of five years, the Women's Health Initiative (WHI) randomized controlled trial verified a significant (34 percent) decrease in hip fractures in healthy women receiving HT (conjugated equine estrogen 0.625 mg with MPA 5 mg). When combined with calcium and vitamin D, even very-low-dose estrogen therapy (transdermal estradiol 0.025 mg/day; conjugated equine estrogen 0.3 mg/day with MPA 1.5 mg/day; estradiol 0.25 mg/day) significantly increases bone mineral density when compared to placebo, according to recent studies. Bisphosphonates are very effective in treating and preventing osteoporosis because they specifically block bone resorption. Examples of these drugs are ibandronate (150 mg monthly), risedronate (35 mg weekly), and alendronate (35–70 mg weekly). Certain compounds, known as selective estrogen receptor modulators or SERMs, function as estrogen agonists or antagonists, contingent upon the tissue in question. One SERM that has been approved for the treatment and prevention of osteoporosis is raloxifene (60 mg). An additional authorized treatment for established osteoporosis is calcitonin nasal spray (200 IU).

1.2.4. Depression

While the majority of women go through menopause without any mental health issues, 20% of them experience depression at some point during the menopausal period. Research on menopausal mood has generally shown that there is a higher risk of depression during the perimenopause and a lower risk during the postmenopausal years. Cohort research, the Penn Ovarian Aging Study, revealed that depression symptoms peaked during the menopausal transition and declined following menopause. Previous history of depression and variations in reproductive hormone levels linked to depression were the best indicators of depressed mood. A cross-sectional population survey conducted in the Netherlands asked 2103 women to rate their depression symptoms both before and during the menopausal transition, which occurred 3–5 years later. The majority of the women's depressive symptoms appeared during the menopausal transition. An increase in depressive symptoms during the perimenopause was also shown in a study conducted in the United States on a community sample of women going through natural menopause. Premenopausal women between the ages of 36 and 44 who had never experienced a major depressive episode were chosen by researchers from the Harvard Study of Moods and Cycles, and they were followed up on for nine years to look for any new major depressive episodes. Clinically significant depressive symptoms were twice as common in women who entered perimenopause compared to those who had not yet transitioned into menopause.

1.2.4.1. Pathophysiology

Part of the reason for depression during perimenopause is probably the fluctuating and decreasing levels of estrogen. There are several ways that steroid hormones, like estrogen, influence the central nervous system (CNS). For example, they affect membrane permeability and promote the expression of receptors and the synthesis of neurotransmitters. Serotonin and norepinephrine are believed to be the neurotransmitters most closely linked to the physiological basis of depression, and estrogen amplifies their effects. Estrogen inhibits the breakdown of serotonin and norepinephrine in the central nervous system (CNS) by reducing monoamine oxidase (MAO) activity, among other mechanisms. Furthermore, estrogen upregulates 5-hydroxytryptamine (5-HT1) receptors and downregulates 5-HT2 receptors, while also increasing serotonin synthesis. Additionally, estrogen raises norepinephrine activity in the brain, possibly through inhibiting the enzymes MAO and catechol-O-methyltransferase, which reduces reuptake and degradation. Estrogen levels can alter the way serotonin and norepinephrine are regulated, which can lead to depression even though the exact mechanisms are still unclear. Estrogen helps serotonin and norepinephrine function, so a drop in estrogen levels may also result in a drop in these hormone levels. In certain women going through the menopausal transition, depression symptoms may be connected to changes in estrogen levels, possibly as a result of processes involving these neurotransmitters.

1.2.4.2. Hormonal Changes

Hormonal fluctuations in women appear to have a substantial correlation with depression. This theory is supported by several observations and study data. For instance, puberty is when the difference in depression rates between men and women first appears. Additionally, it is believed that hormonal changes play a significant role in premenstrual dysphoric disorder, postpartum mood swings, and the menopausal transition. Furthermore, serotonin and norepinephrine—the two neurotransmitters most strongly linked to depression—are both impacted by estrogen. Notably, gonadal hormone levels in their absolute form do not correlate with depression. The levels of progesterone and estrogen do not differentiate between women with and without depression. Hormone levels were normal in perimenopausal or postmenopausal women with depression who had their levels measured. Instead, it appears that some women are more likely than others to experience mood disorders brought on by changes in hormone levels. Women in this subgroup have a history of mood disorders or symptoms related to mood that occur before or after menstruation. When hormone levels are fluctuating during the perimenopause, as opposed to when they are low but stable during the postmenopause, there seems to be a greater chance of depression (Schiff et al., 1980).

1.2.4.3. Life Stressors

Societal roles and expectations may contribute to the heightened rate of depression in women. Women with particular types of stressors seem to be at increased risk for perimenopausal depression. Such stressors include the following:

- Lack of social support
- Unemployment
- Surgical menopause
- Poor overall health status.

The dysphoric mood during the early perimenopausal transition is most common in women with relatively low educational status. Therefore, low levels of education may be a marker for other stressors, such as ongoing low socioeconomic status.

An Australian study of women transitioning to menopause revealed more depression in women with the following states:

- Negative mood before menopause
- Negative attitude toward menopause and aging
- Smoking
- Little or no exercise
- No partner
- Poor self-perceived health
- Negative feelings toward partner
- Several perceived problems
- Interpersonal stress.

Other stressors that tend to correspond with perimenopause and that are postulated to relate to depression include the following:

- Onset of illness in self or others
- Care of aging parents
- Changes in employment.

1.2.4.4. Psychological or Social Conditions

Numerous psychological and social theories have been proffered to explain why women may become depressed during perimenopause. Some of these are related to the following factors:

- Change in the childbearing role
- Loss of fertility, which may be associated with a loss of an essential meaning of life
- Empty nest syndrome
- The societal value of youth (in societies where age is valued, women tend to report having fewer symptoms at the menopause transition).
- **Pre-Existing Tendency to Develop Depression:** A personal or family history of major depression, postpartum depression, or premenstrual dysphoric disorder seems to be a major risk factor for depression in the perimenopausal period. However, the perimenopausal depressive syndrome is a risk even in women without a history of depression.

1.2.4.5. Treatment

Standard antidepressants are first-line treatments for major depression. When treating perimenopausal depression, SSRIs are the antidepressants that are most frequently prescribed. SSRIs are generally regarded as safe and beneficial. Four to six weeks is when the action starts. They do carry a risk of serotonin syndrome, along with several common side effects that include jitteriness, dizziness, sedation or activation, insomnia, akathisia, excessive sweating, decreased libido and/or anorgasmia, headaches, and gastrointestinal effects (nausea, diarrhea, and anorexia). Hormone treatments for depression have been shown to be effective in managing depressive symptoms during the perimenopause, but not in the postmenopausal stage. However, the results of these studies have been inconsistent. Hormone replacement therapy (HRT) on its own may be suitable for treating mild depression. When standard antidepressants are ineffective, patients refuse psychotropic drugs, or patients exhibit other clinically significant vasomotor symptoms, estrogen (0.45–0.625 mg conjugated estrogen QD, 1.5–5 mg medroxyprogesterone QD) may be used. According to data from multiple studies, estrogen replacement therapy either improved the antidepressant effects of antidepressant treatment in perimenopausal women or had its own antidepressant effects.

Other research did not support the idea that estrogen amplifies the benefits of SSRIs. Whether estrogen's antidepressant effects are related to how it affects vasomotor symptoms is a topic of debate. Only in women with vasomotor symptoms does estrogen appear to have antidepressant benefits, according to some studies. Other studies' findings point to a separate antidepressant effect. Research has examined the potential benefits of estrogen therapy on mood and quality of life in perimenopausal women who do not have depression. Small-scale study findings point to a marginally beneficial effect on mood. Nonetheless, the majority of research indicates that estrogen has no positive impact on mood or quality of life in healthy women who are not depressed. Menopause symptoms that are physical seem to be linked to higher rates of depression and negative menopausal anticipation. Anxiety, depression, and irritability are reduced in women who attend educational groups that teach them about menopause. This effect is seen both immediately following group therapy and a year later (Freedman et al., 1990).

1.2.5. Cognitive Functions

Perimenopausal and recently postmenopausal women frequently complain of memory issues. The higher incidence of cognitive complaints in women going through menopause implies that memory issues in this group are more closely linked to the menopause transition than to aging. The etiologic role of estrogen in the cognitive difficulties experienced by perimenopausal and recently postmenopausal women is supported by clinical trials that describe the improvement of cognition with hormone replacement therapy. Particular cognitive areas (e.g., learning ability, verbal memory, and attention) that could be impacted by the menopause transition have not been thoroughly studied. The correlation observed in certain women between cognitive challenges and the menopausal transition implies that the hormonal shifts associated with the menopause could potentially be linked to this type of cognitive disruption. Cognitive problems may arise from altered hormone levels in brain regions that control thought processes, or they may be the result of sleep disturbance brought on by hot flashes at night.

Compared to men, women are more likely to develop Alzheimer's disease. According to several observational studies and small trials, using HT may lower the risk of Alzheimer's disease. However, a year-long estrogen treatment did not slow the progression of the disease or improve cognition in women with mild to moderate Alzheimer's disease, according to a randomized, controlled study. Women 65 years of age or older who were enrolled in the WHI trial participated in the WHI Memory Study (WHIMS), a randomized, double-blind, placebo-controlled trial, to examine the impact of HT on cognitive function in women without dementia. Women randomized to HT in WHIMS had a significant twofold increased risk of dementia, most commonly Alzheimer disease, in contrast to the results of observational studies. Furthermore, using HT was linked to a negative impact on cognition. Women in the HT group had significantly lower Modified Mini-Mental State Examination scores than women receiving a placebo. It is plausible that the HT group experienced a higher risk of dementia due to the possibility of small, undetected cerebrovascular events, given the higher incidence of stroke found in HT users in the WHI trial.

1.2.6. Sexual Dysfunction

During menopause, many women experience sexual dysfunction; however, the precise incidence and etiology remain unknown. Reduced arousal or the inability to experience an orgasm during sexual relations are two signs of sexual dysfunction, as can diminish interest in or desire to initiate activity. The causes of sexual dysfunction are frequently complex and include psychological disorders like depression or anxiety, relationship conflict, problems related to past physical or sexual abuse, use of medications, and physical conditions like endometriosis or atrophic vaginitis that cause discomfort during sexual activity. The complex issue of female sexual dysfunction following menopause has numerous etiologies. To maximize therapy, a thorough assessment of the relationship, lifestyle, psychological, and physiological variables is needed. Enhancing sexual function may involve relationship counseling, antidepressant medication adjustments, and treatment for anxiety and depression. For many women and couples suffering from sexual dysfunction, specific exercises and activities—often carried out under the supervision of a sex therapist—are helpful. Dyspareunia is successfully reduced and sexual arousal and response may be enhanced by the specific treatment of genitourinary atrophy with systemic or local vaginal estrogen therapy or vaginal lubricants. A large-scale randomized, double-blind, placebo-controlled study of women with sexual dysfunction showed no benefit from sildenafil citrate (Ursic-Vrscaj et al., 2001).

Menopausal women with low testosterone levels and no other known cause for their sexual dysfunction may benefit from androgen therapy. Surpassologous intramuscular testosterone doses produced significantly higher scores of sexual desire, fantasy, and arousal than either placebo or estradiol alone in a double-blind crossover study of postmenopausal women undergoing surgery. When oral methyltestosterone (1.25 mg/day) plus esterified estrogens (0.625 mg/day) were given to women randomly assigned to treatment, their libido improved significantly more than that of women treated with estrogen alone. This was observed in a double-blind, randomized study. Transdermal testosterone therapy, administered physiologically via a transdermal patch, significantly increased sexual pleasure and activity in randomized, double-blind, placebo-controlled studies of sexually dysfunctional, estrogen-treated women without ovaries. Harrowed voice, acne, hirsutism, and unfavorable changes to lipid levels and liver function are among the possible side effects of androgen therapy. As most androgens aromatize into estrogens, there may be similar risks associated with androgen therapy as with estrogen therapy.

1.2.7. Problems with Sleep

During the menopausal transition, 40–50% of women experience insomnia. Sleep issues may or may not be linked to mood disorders. Compared to other women, those who suffer from insomnia are more likely to report issues like anxiety, tension, stress, and depressive symptoms. Exogenous estrogen has been demonstrated to improve both subjective and objective sleep, which has been linked to a decrease in hot flashes. As a result, sleep disturbances during menopause have been linked to estrogen deficiency. A recent study suggested that high core body temperatures are caused by elevated LH levels during late menopause, which in turn leads to poor sleep quality through a thermoregulatory mechanism. Whether hormonal fluctuations, age-related alterations in the architecture of sleep, or other menopausal symptoms (e.g., vasomotor symptoms) is unclear. Age-related increases in sleep apnea rates are observed, with rates going from 6.5% in women aged 30–39 to 16% in women aged 50–60. Although the exact pathophysiology is unknown, theories point to a link between postmenopausal weight gain and low progesterone levels, which are thought to stimulate breathing. Postmenopausal women experience a decrease in melatonin and growth hormone levels, which both have an impact on sleep, in addition to changes in estrogen and progesterone levels. Vasomotor symptoms that interfere with sleep or that may directly affect sleep itself may be lessened by estrogen. The study involved postmenopausal women who experienced hot flashes, night sweats, insomnia, anxiety, and/or mood swings. The results showed that low-dose progesterone and estrogen enhanced sleep more than the reduction in vasomotor symptoms could account for (Stearns et al., 2003).

1.2.8. Course of Some Important Psychiatric Disorders During Menopause

- **Schizophrenia:** Schizophrenia typically first appears in young adults, and after early adulthood, the number of new cases in both males and females decreases. There is a second peak in the incidence of schizophrenia among women between the ages of 45 and 50; men do not exhibit this second peak. A worsening of the course of schizophrenia in women during the menopausal transition has been noted by some researchers. These findings could imply that estrogen regulates some aspects of the pathophysiology of schizophrenia.
- **Bipolar Disorder:** In women who already have bipolar disorder, menopause has been observed to exacerbate mood symptoms. Studies have indicated that during the menopausal transition, women with bipolar disorder experience more depressive episodes. Compared to the premenopausal years, this population seems to experience depressive episodes more frequently. Previous research revealed that the menopausal transition was associated with an increase in rapid cycling; however, this finding has not been replicated.
- **Panic Disorder:** Perimenopause is a common time for panic disorder. Menopause can bring on the onset of a new panic disorder or exacerbate an existing one. Women who have many of the physical signs of menopause may be more susceptible to panic disorder. Women in the menopausal transition were most likely to experience panic attacks, according to a cross-sectional survey of 3369 postmenopausal women aged 50–79. Negative life events, functional impairment, and medical comorbidity have all been linked to panic attacks.
- **Obsessive-Compulsive Disorder:** New-onset obsessive-compulsive disorder (OCD), a relapse of OCD, or a change in OCD symptoms may occur during menopause. Fluctuations in OCD have been correlated with the menstrual cycle and with pregnancy, suggesting that hormone levels may contribute to the disorder.

1.2.9. Status of Hormone Replacement Therapy

For doctors, weighing the advantages and hazards of HRT has become a difficult task. Lately, there has been controversy regarding postmenopausal women's use of hormone replacement therapy.

The short-term risks and long-term benefits of hormone replacement therapy have been called into question by several randomized controlled trials that offer conflicting data. The Heart and Estrogen/Progestin Replacement Study (HERS) trial and the WHI both produced data against the use of HRT in preventing cardiovascular disease. Examined is the relationship between hormone replacement therapy (HRT) and gallbladder disease, osteoporosis, cardiovascular disease, stroke, cancer, and cognitive decline. The most recent contentious outcomes of randomized controlled trials have presented doctors with additional difficulties when it comes to prescribing HRT to postmenopausal women. In recent years, the topic of HRT for postmenopausal women has been surrounded by controversial issues. Numerous recent evidence-based studies have demonstrated that using HRT did not significantly increase the risk of breast cancer, but rather reduced the risk of osteoporosis fractures and atherosclerosis. According to a study, using HRT was associated with low risks of Alzheimer's disease and colon cancer. In 1994, additional analysis showed that the advantages of estrogen replacement therapy outweighed the risks. Another decision analysis suggested longer life expectancy and lower morbidity in 99% of US postmenopausal women. Among the suggested advantages of hormone replacement therapy (HRT) were the reduction of menopausal symptoms, enhancement of life quality, and defense against osteoporosis and cardiovascular disease. But over the past few years, evidence-based medicine has presented the findings of multiple randomized double-blind placebo-controlled trials, particularly the WHI study's results, which have had a significant impact on the standard practice of prescribing HRT in clinics. The results of the randomized controlled trials are incongruous, casting doubt on the long-term advantages and short-term hazards of hormone replacement therapy (Olofsson et al., 2000).

Some of the risks are mentioned below: An increase in the risk of venous thromboembolism was reported in both WHI and HERS, with the highest risk in the 1st year of use. Studies on the effects of hormone replacement therapy (HRT) on the incidence of stroke have yielded inconsistent results. While some studies reported a protective effect, the WHI study showed an increased risk. In laboratory animals, estrogen has been linked to the development of tumors. A higher risk of breast cancer has been revealed by a meta-analysis of the available data. In 52,000 women using hormone replacement therapy, the Collaborative Group on Hormonal Factors in Breast Cancer found no statistically significant increase in breast cancer risk. <5 years, however, in women in estrogen replacement therapy, for > Five years later, there was a higher risk. In several trials, the use of combined estrogen and progestin has been linked to a slightly higher risk of breast cancer than the use of estrogen alone. Endometrial hyperplasia has been linked to higher dosages and longer unopposed estrogen use, which raises the risk of endometrial cancer. Results regarding the use of HRT in relation to colorectal and ovarian cancer have been contradictory. It has been established that hormone replacement therapy (HRT) directly causes cancer by causing ovarian cells to proliferate. The results of the WHI study, which suggested that estrogen may reduce the risk of colorectal cancer, contradicted the findings of the HERS study, which examined evidence-based research and found no reduction in the risk of colorectal cancer in women. In short-term HRT users, the Nurses Health Study found a positive correlation between HRT and cholecystitis.

1.3. Postmenopause: Diagnosis and Interventions

The third and final stage of menopause is known as postmenopause. Postmenopause is associated with various health complications related to changes in the hormonal levels of the female body, which are the cause of the symptoms.

Menopause is considered to be a three-stage process:

- **Perimenopause** refers to the 8–10 years before menopause when your ovaries slowly produce less estrogen.
- **Menopause** refers to the time when your menstrual periods have stopped for at least a year
- **Postmenopause** is the stage of life after you have not had a period for 12 months or longer

The menopause typically occurs at age 51. Menopause can strike at any point during your 40s, 50s, or even 60s. The body will change at a time that is specific for the woman. Menopause is typically a very normal stage of a woman's life. A hysterectomy or other type of surgery may cause you to enter menopause earlier than expected. The postmenopausal hormone levels won't change once you reach this stage. Both monthly menstrual cycles and the ability to become pregnant will cease to exist for this patients.

May be at increased risk for the following conditions after menopause:

- Osteoporosis
- Cardiovascular disease (Langrish et al., 2009)
- Depression and other mental health conditions
- Changes in vaginal health, such as vaginal dryness

Adopting healthy lifestyle habits and checking in with your doctor regularly will help you manage your risk factors for these conditions.

1.3.1. Interventions

The goals of postmenopausal interventions are to treat health risks and manage symptoms related to other hormonal changes and the decline in estrogen. These interventions aim to improve quality of life and lower the risk of chronic illnesses like osteoporosis and cardiovascular disease. They also include medication treatments and lifestyle changes (Langrish et al., 2009).

1.3.1.1. Lifestyle Modifications

- **Diet and Nutrition:** Bone health requires a well-balanced diet high in calcium and vitamin D. Women who have gone through menopause should eat foods like dairy, leafy greens, and fortified foods. A diet high in fiber and low in saturated fats helps control cholesterol levels, while an adequate protein intake promotes the health of muscles.
- **Exercise:** Frequent exercise, especially weight-bearing activities like resistance training and walking, lowers the risk of osteoporosis, strengthens bones and muscles, and enhances cardiovascular health. Aerobic exercises improve general fitness and assist with weight management.
- **Healthy Habits:** Reducing alcohol intake and quitting smoking are essential for lowering the risk of cardiovascular disease and other illnesses. A healthy weight can be maintained through diet and exercise, which helps reduce the symptoms and conditions associated with postmenopause.

1.3.1.2. Medical Treatments

- **Hormone Replacement Therapy (HRT):** In addition to preventing osteoporosis, hormone replacement therapy (HRT) can be useful in reducing severe vasomotor symptoms like night sweats and hot flashes. It involves giving progesterone and/or estrogen either on their own or in combination. HRT should be discussed individually with a healthcare professional due to its risks, which include an increased risk of blood clots, stroke, and breast cancer.
- **Non-Hormonal Medications:** Other medications can help manage symptoms for women who cannot take HRT or do not want to use it. Hot flashes and mood swings can be effectively treated with selective serotonin reuptake inhibitors (SSRIs) and serotonin-norepinephrine reuptake inhibitors (SNRIs). Osteoporosis can be prevented and treated with the aid of bisphosphonates, calcitonin, and selective estrogen receptor modulators (SERMs), such as raloxifene.
- **Vaginal Estrogen:** For vaginal dryness and atrophy, localized estrogen therapy in the form of creams, tablets, or rings can be effective. These treatments deliver estrogen directly to the vaginal tissue, minimizing systemic absorption and associated risks.

1.3.1.3. Preventive Health Measures

- **Bone Health:** Regular bone density screenings (DEXA scans) are recommended to monitor bone health and detect osteoporosis early. Calcium and vitamin D supplements may be prescribed if dietary intake is insufficient.
- **Cardiovascular Health:** Regular monitoring of blood pressure, cholesterol levels, and other cardiovascular risk factors is essential. Lifestyle changes, along with medications like statins, may be recommended to manage high cholesterol and reduce cardiovascular risk.
- **Cancer Screenings:** Continued screening for breast, cervical, and colorectal cancer is important. Mammograms, Pap smears, and colonoscopies should be done according to recommended guidelines based on age and risk factors.

1.3.1.4. Psychosocial Support

- **Mental Health:** Addressing mental health is crucial during postmenopause. Women may experience mood swings, anxiety, and depression. Counselling, support groups, and sometimes medication can help manage these issues.
- **Sexual Health:** Open communication with healthcare providers about sexual health is important. Treatments for vaginal dryness, counseling, and addressing libido changes can improve sexual well-being.

1.3.1.5. Regular Medical Check-Ups

Regular visits to healthcare providers for comprehensive evaluations help monitor and manage the diverse aspects of health affected by postmenopause. These check-ups ensure that any emerging health issues are detected early and addressed promptly.

1.3.2. Etiology

The main cause of postmenopausal symptoms is the lower amount of circulating estrogen. Menopause-related complex changes include hot flashes, vulvovaginal atrophy, and sexual dysfunction. The number of ovarian follicles, particularly the granulosa cells, is decreasing at the ovarian level. As a result, the ovary can no longer react to pituitary hormones. Due to a lack of feedback inhibition, luteinizing hormone (LH) and follicle-stimulating hormone (FSH) levels rise, and the production of ovarian estrogen, progesterone, and inhibin stops. Nonetheless, the remaining adrenal gland and ovarian theca cells continue to produce androgen, which is then transformed into estrogen by peripheral aromatization.

- **Hot Flashes:** The cause of hot flashes is a complicated one. The loss of estrogen production is thought to be the secondary cause of the thermoregulatory system's narrowing and reset. It has also been suggested that changes in FSH and estrogen levels cause hot flashes. It might also be connected to the hypothalamus's over-expression of the 5-hydroxytryptamine receptor (5-HT2A) in reaction to a drop in serotonin levels. It is believed that the decrease is the result of lower estrogen levels.
- **Vulvovaginal Atrophy:** The tissues of the uterus are extremely sensitive to estrogen, and a deficiency in this hormone can result in vaginal atrophy and shortening, uterine prolapse, and dyspareunia. Many people experience urinary incontinence as a result of decreased estrogen levels, which have an impact on the bladder and urethra. When left untreated, vulvovaginal atrophy does not get better over time like vasomotor symptoms do.
- **Sexual Dysfunction:** In contrast to hot flashes and vulvovaginal atrophy, sexual dysfunction is not associated with hormonal fluctuations in its etiology. In addition, vasomotor symptoms, sleep disturbances, and mood swings in postmenopausal women may be responsible for the decreased libido.

1.3.3. Effect of Osteoporosis

Bone thinning is a symptom of the disease osteoporosis. After menopause, this change in bone density intensifies, especially in the first few years after the period ends. This is a result of losing estrogen in the woman's body (Grady et al., 2001). After menopause, could lose up to 25% of bone density until you're 60 years old. The predisposition to fractures is favored, especially in the wrists, spine, and hips. Bone tissue thins and loses density due to the disease osteoporosis. This results in bones that are weaker and more prone to breaking. Very few symptoms are present in advanced stages of osteoporosis, and the condition can advance without causing any issues. Therefore, it's frequently not noticed until your weakening bones break or fracture.

The weaker bones are typically not noticed until after a severe fall that breaks hip or back. The woman could be experience weeks or months of restricted or nonexistent mobility as a result of these injuries. Treatment may also include surgery.

Treating osteoporosis can be as simple as making lifestyle adjustments:

- Consume foods that contain calcium or take calcium supplements

- Add vitamin D supplements to your daily routine
- Exercise, incorporating both aerobic and strength-building activities into your routine
- Limit alcohol intake
- Quit smoking

1.3.3.1. Understanding Risks

The following are additional risk factors for osteoporosis:

- **Age:** Up to around age 30, your body creates more bone than you lose. After that, bone deterioration occurs more rapidly than bone creation. The net effect is a gradual loss of bone mass.
- **Smoking:** Smoking has been shown to increase your risk for osteoporosis. It also seems to cause earlier onset of menopause, meaning there's less time that your bones are protected by estrogen.

People who smoke also have a harder time healing after a fracture compared to nonsmokers.

- **Body Composition:** Women who are petite or thin have a greater risk of developing osteoporosis compared to women who are heavier or have a larger frame. This is because thinner women have less bone mass overall compared to larger women. The same is true for men.
- **Existing Bone Density:** The lower your risk of developing osteoporosis after menopause, the higher your bone density.
- **Gender:** Women are up to four times more likely to develop osteoporosis than men. This is because women tend to be smaller and usually weigh less than men. Women over the age of 50 have the greatest risk for developing the bone disease.
- **Race and Ethnicity:** In global terms, individuals of northern European and Caucasian descent face the highest risk of osteoporosis-related fractures. However, the incidence of osteoporosis is actually declining within this demographic. Conversely, the Women's Health Initiative Observational Study revealed that African American, Native American, Asian, and Hispanic women experienced more osteoporosis-related fractures than cases of invasive breast cancer, stroke, and heart attack deaths combined within their respective populations.

1.3.3.2. Treatment Options

A variety of treatments can help stop the development of osteoporosis. Here are some steps you can take to prevent bone deterioration:

- **Take Calcium and Vitamin D Supplements:** Strong bones can be developed and maintained as you age with the aid of calcium. People between the ages of 19 and 50 should consume 1,000 mg of calcium daily, according to the National Institutes of Health (NIH). A minimum of 1,200 mg of calcium should be consumed daily by women over 50 and by all adults over 70. Good forms of calcium are supplied to your body by both calcium carbonate and calcium citrate. Your body needs vitamin D to properly absorb calcium, which is essential for strong bones. Good dietary sources of vitamin D include milk and cereals that have been fortified with the vitamin, as well as fatty fish like salmon and mackerel. The body naturally produces vitamin D when exposed to sunlight. However, the amount of time that a person spends in the sun varies depending on the time of day, the weather, where they live, and the natural pigmentation of their skin. Supplements are available for those who are worried about skin cancer or who want to get their vitamin D from other sources. The NIH recommends that individuals between the ages of 19 and 70 receive 600 international units (IU) or more of vitamin D daily. A person over 70 should take 800 IU of vitamin D daily (Rossouw et al., 2002).

- **Bisphosphonates are a Class of Medications that Help Stop Bone Loss:** These medications have been demonstrated to decrease the risk of bone fractures, slow the loss of bone, and increase bone density over time. Bisphosphonates can lower the incidence of osteoporosis-related fractures by up to 60%, according to a 2017 study. Another option for halting bone loss is to employ monoclonal antibodies. Among these medications are romosozumab (Evenity) and denosumab. Drugs with estrogen-like characteristics are referred to as selective estrogen receptor modulators, or SERMs. They are occasionally used to treat and prevent osteoporosis. According to a 2016 study, SERMS frequently has the greatest benefit in lowering the risk of spinal fractures by up to 42%.
- **For the Purpose of Establishing and Preserving Strong Bones, Exercise Frequently Outperforms Medication:** It strengthens bones, aids in preventing bone loss, and expedites the healing process in the event of a bone break. Weight-bearing exercises such as walking, jogging, dancing, and aerobics are all beneficial. Swimming and other water-based exercises help to strengthen bones, but not as much as weight-bearing exercises, according to a 2017 study.

The lower estrogen levels that accompany perimenopause and menopause can contribute to bone loss; hormone replacement therapy (HRT) can help prevent this from happening. For bone health, experts currently advise against using HRT until after other options have been exhausted (Ursic-Vrscaj et al., 2001). HRT may be useful in the treatment of mood swings, night sweats, and hot flashes, among other menopausal symptoms. Not everyone can benefit from this therapy, though.

It may not be the correct treatment option if you have a personal history of or are at an increased risk for:

- Heart attack
- Stroke
- Blood clots
- Breast cancer

There are also other medical conditions where HRT isn't the best choice.

1.3.4. Symptoms and Causes

Most people in postmenopause feel lingering symptoms from menopause. The symptoms are less intense. In some cases, they almost disappear. Lingering symptoms are caused by low levels of reproductive hormones.

People in postmenopause can feel symptoms such as:

- Hot flashes and night sweats.
- Vaginal dryness and sexual discomfort.
- Depression.
- Changes in sex drive.
- Insomnia.
- Dry skin.
- Weight changes.
- Hair loss.
- Urinary incontinence.

If the symptoms become more intense or interfere with daily life, patient would be talk with healthcare provider. They may want to rule out any underlying condition causing these symptoms.

- **What Causes Postmenopausal Bleeding?:** Reduced hormone levels during the postmenopausal period do not normally result in vaginal bleeding. The vagina may occasionally become dry and cause mild bleeding or spotting after sex. In other situations, it might be a sign of cancer, an infection like endometritis, or a condition like endometrial hyperplasia or uterine fibroids.
- **Will My Hot Flashes Stop After Menopause?:** After menopause, some people continue to have hot flashes. Reduced estrogen levels are the cause of postmenopausal hot flashes. Hot flashes that occur at random for years after menopause are not unusual.

1.3.5. Diagnosis and Tests

A postmenopausal diagnosis is made after the woman has not had a menstrual period for a full year and considers the health risks that come with going through this stage of life. Postmenopause is distinguished by persistently low levels of progesterone and estrogen, in contrast to perimenopause, which is characterized by fluctuating hormone levels (Prestwood et al., 2003). The absence of menstruation for a full year is the main diagnostic criterion for postmenopause. This usually happens around the age of 51, though it can vary depending on genetics and personal health. To verify postmenopause, its necessary examining the patient's menstrual history. They'll inquire about the length of time since the last menstrual cycle as well as any additional symptoms, like mood swings, vaginal dryness, hot flashes, and insomnia. To rule out additional causes of amenorrhea (absence of menstruation), such as thyroid conditions or hyperprolactinemia, a thorough medical history is also obtained. To validate the diagnosis and evaluate the health hazards linked to postmenopause, a physical examination and laboratory tests are imperative. To look for changes in the reproductive organs, such as vaginal atrophy and dryness, which are frequently caused by low estrogen levels, a pelvic exam may be done. A general health assessment is also carried out to determine any conditions that might need to be attended to and to assess general well-being (Lindsay et al., 2002).

When it comes to identifying postmenopause and comprehending its consequences, blood tests are essential. Follicle-stimulating hormone (FSH) levels are a crucial diagnostic tool because they are a reliable indicator of postmenopause because they are usually high (above 30 mIU/mL). This is because less estrogen produced by the ovaries means that the pituitary gland receives less negative feedback, which raises FSH secretion. Low levels of this primary form of estrogen, which is also measured, further support the postmenopausal state. Thyroid function tests and a complete blood count (CBC) may also be performed to rule out other illnesses like anemia or thyroid problems that can resemble postmenopausal symptoms. More testing is frequently advised due to the long-term health risks connected to postmenopause. To determine the risk of osteoporosis, which is a common concern because decreased estrogen levels affect bone strength, a bone density test, also known as a DEXA scan, measures bone mineral density. Because heart disease is more likely to occur when estrogen levels decline, cardiovascular health is another important factor to keep an eye on. A lipid profile test assesses cholesterol levels, guiding preventive care and offering insight into cardiovascular risk.

Maintaining postmenopausal health requires routine monitoring and follow-up.

1.3.6. Management and Treatment

Hormone therapy is an option, though doctors usually advise against using it in people under 60 years old or for a brief period of time. Hormone therapy carries certain health risks, including the possibility of stroke and blood clots (Ettinger et al., 2004).

Some medications your healthcare provider may consider helping with postmenopausal symptoms are:

- Antidepressants for mood swings or depression.
- Vaginal creams for pain related to sexual intercourse and vaginal dryness.
- Gabapentin (Neurontin®) to relieve hot flashes.

A Closer Look

First Aid for Fracture

Hormone Replacement Therapy (HRT) is a medical treatment used to alleviate symptoms associated with the decrease in estrogen and progesterone levels that occur during menopause and perimenopause. HRT involves the administration of estrogen alone or in combination with progesterone to compensate for the body's declining hormone levels. This therapy is particularly effective in managing common menopausal symptoms such as hot flashes, night sweats, vaginal dryness, mood swings, and sleep disturbances. By restoring hormonal balance, HRT can significantly improve the quality of life for many women during and after the menopausal transition.

Estrogen therapy (ET) is typically prescribed for women who have undergone a hysterectomy, as they no longer require progesterone to protect against endometrial hyperplasia, a condition that can lead to uterine cancer. For women with an intact uterus, combined estrogen-progesterone therapy (EPT) is recommended to mitigate the risk of endometrial cancer by balancing the proliferative effects of estrogen on the endometrium. HRT can be administered in various forms, including oral tablets, transdermal patches, gels, creams, and vaginal rings, allowing for personalized treatment plans based on individual preferences and medical histories (Cummings et al., 1998).

The benefits of HRT extend beyond symptom relief. Estrogen has protective effects on bone density, making HRT a valuable intervention for preventing osteoporosis and reducing the risk of fractures in postmenopausal women. Additionally, HRT can have positive effects on cardiovascular health by improving lipid profiles and maintaining the elasticity of blood vessels. However, the decision to use HRT is complex and must consider potential risks, including an increased risk of breast cancer, blood clots, stroke, and heart disease, particularly with long-term use.

The timing of HRT initiation, known as the "timing hypothesis," plays a critical role in its safety and efficacy. Research suggests that starting HRT near the onset of menopause may offer cardiovascular benefits and reduce risks compared to starting therapy later in postmenopause. Nonetheless, individual risk factors such as age, family history of cancer or cardiovascular disease, and personal health history must be carefully evaluated. HRT is not a one-size-fits-all solution, and its appropriateness varies from woman to woman. For those who cannot or choose not to use HRT, alternative treatments are available. Non-hormonal medications, such as selective serotonin reuptake inhibitors (SSRIs) and serotonin-norepinephrine reuptake inhibitors (SNRIs), can effectively manage hot flashes and mood changes. Additionally, lifestyle modifications, including regular exercise, a healthy diet, stress management techniques, and the use of vaginal lubricants and moisturizers, can help alleviate some menopausal symptoms. Regular follow-up with healthcare providers is essential for women on HRT to monitor its effects and adjust the treatment plan as necessary. This ongoing assessment helps optimize the benefits of HRT while minimizing potential risks. Women are encouraged to discuss their symptoms, medical history, and concerns with their healthcare providers to make informed decisions about the use of HRT.

Summary

- Perimenopause and postmenopause are distinct phases in a woman's reproductive aging process, each characterized by unique physiological changes. Perimenopause, also known as the menopausal transition, is the period leading up to menopause when hormonal fluctuations become more pronounced, typically beginning in a woman's 40s but sometimes earlier.
- Perimenopause and menopause are both transitional phases that indicate an end to your reproductive years. Premenopause, on the other hand, is when there are no symptoms of either. Menopause officially marks the end of female reproduction.
- Perimenopause is marked by a drop in estrogen, the main female hormone produced by the ovaries. The estrogen levels can also go up and down more sporadically than they do in a typical 28-day cycle. This can cause irregular periods and other symptoms.
- Perimenopause, the transitional phase leading up to menopause, is marked by a range of hormonal fluctuations that can lead to various complications affecting a woman's physical and emotional well-being.
- Perimenopause is a process—a gradual transition. No one test or sign is enough to determine if a woman entered perimenopause. The doctor takes many things into consideration, including age, menstrual history, and what symptoms or body changes.
- A physical examination can help identify any physical signs that might be associated with perimenopause. This includes a pelvic exam to check for changes in the reproductive organs and a general health assessment to evaluate overall well-being.
- Menopause is the permanent cessation of menstruation resulting in the loss of ovarian follicle development. The age at menopause appears to be genetically determined and is unaffected by race, socioeconomic status, age at menarche, or number of prior ovulations.

References

1. Adena, M. A., & Gallagher, H. G. (1982). Cigarette smoking and the age at menopause. *Annals of Human Biology, 9*, 121–130.
2. Baram, D. (1997). Physiology and symptoms of menopause. In D. E. Steward & G. E. Robinson (Eds.), *A Clinician's Guide to Menopause* (pp. 9–28). Health Press International.
3. Cauley, J. A., Zmuda, J. M., Ensrud, K. E., Bauer, D. C., & Ettinger, B. (2001). Timing of estrogen replacement therapy for optimal osteoporosis prevention. *Journal of Clinical Endocrinology and Metabolism, 86*, 5700–5705.
4. Cummings, S. R., Black, D. M., Thompson, D. E., Applegate, W. B., Barrett-Connor, E., Musliner, T. A., et al. (1998). Effect of alendronate on risk of fracture in women with low bone density but without vertebral fractures: Results from the Fracture Intervention Trial. *JAMA, 280*, 2077–2082.
5. Ettinger, B., Ensrud, K. E., Wallace, R., Johnson, K. C., Cummings, S. R., Yankov, V., et al. (2004). Effects of ultralow-dose transdermal estradiol on bone mineral density: A randomized clinical trial. *Obstetrics & Gynecology, 104*, 443–451.

6. Freedman, R. R., Woodward, S., & Sabharwal, S. C. (1990). Alpha 2-adrenergic mechanism in menopausal hot flushes. *Obstetrics & Gynecology, 76*, 573–578.

7. Genant, H. K., Lucas, J., Weiss, S., Akin, M., Emkey, R., McNaney-Flint, H., & Estratab/Osteoporosis Study Group. (1997). Low-dose esterified estrogen therapy: Effects on bone, plasma estradiol concentrations, endometrium, and lipid levels. *Archives of Internal Medicine, 157*, 2609–2615.

8. Grady, D., Brown, J. S., Vittinghoff, E., Applegate, W., Varner, E., Snyder, T., & Heart and Estrogen/Progestin Replacement Study. (2001). Postmenopausal hormones and incontinence: The Heart and Estrogen/Progestin Replacement Study. *Obstetrics & Gynecology, 97*, 116–120.

9. Langrish, J. P., Mills, N. L., Bath, L. E., Warner, P., Webb, D. J., Kelnar, C. J., Critchley, H. O., Newby, D. E., & Wallace, W. H. (2009). Cardiovascular effects of physiological and standard sex steroid replacement regimens in premature ovarian failure. *Hypertension, 53*, 805–811.

10. Lindsay, R., Gallagher, J. C., Kleerekoper, M., & Pickar, J. H. (2002). Effect of lower doses of conjugated equine estrogens with and without medroxyprogesterone acetate on bone in early postmenopausal women. *JAMA, 287*, 2668–2676.

11. Olofsson, A. S., & Collins, A. (2000). Psychological factors, attitude to menopause and symptoms in Swedish perimenopausal women. *Climacteric, 3*(1), 33–42.

12. Prestwood, K. M., Kenny, A. M., Kleppinger, A., & Kulldorff, M. (2003). Ultralow-dose micronized 17beta-estradiol and bone density and bone metabolism in older women: A randomized controlled trial. *JAMA, 290*, 1042–1048.

13. Rossouw, J. E., Anderson, G. L., Prentice, R. L., LaCroix, A. Z., Kooperberg, C., Stefanick, M. L., & Women's Health Initiative Research Group. (2002). Risks and benefits of estrogen plus progestin in healthy postmenopausal women: Principal results from the Women's Health Initiative randomized controlled trial. *JAMA, 288*, 321–333.

14. Schiff, I., Regestein, Q., Tulchinsky, D., & Ryan, K. J. (1979). Effects of estrogens on sleep and psychological state of hypogonadal women. *JAMA, 242*, 2405–2404.

15. Schiff, I., Tulchinsky, D., Cramer, D., & Ryan, K. J. (1980). Oral medroxyprogesterone in the treatment of postmenopausal symptoms. *JAMA, 244*, 1443–1445.

16. Sherwin, B. (2001). Menopause: Myths and realities. In N. L. Stotland & D. E. Stewart (Eds.), *The Interface Between Psychiatry and Obstetrics and Gynecology* (pp. 241–259). American Psychiatric Publishing.

17. Siddle, N., Sarrel, P., & Whitehead, M. (1987). The effect of hysterectomy on the age at ovarian failure: Identification of a subgroup of women with premature loss of ovarian function and literature review. *Fertility and Sterility, 47*, 94–100.

18. Soares, C. N., & Taylor, V. (2007). Effects and management of the menopausal transition in women with depression and bipolar disorder. *Journal of Clinical Psychiatry, 68*(Suppl. 9), 16–21.

19. Soules, M. R., Sherman, S., Parrott, E., Rebar, R., Santoro, N., Utian, W., & STRAW Group. (2001). Executive summary: Stages of Reproductive Aging Workshop (STRAW). *Fertility and Sterility, 76*, 874–878.

20. Spinelli, M. G. (2004). Depression and hormone therapy. *Clinical Obstetrics and Gynecology, 47*, 428–436.

21. Stearns, V., Beebe, K. L., Iyengar, M., & Dube, E. (2003). Paroxetine controlled release in the treatment of menopausal hot flashes: A randomized controlled trial. *JAMA, 289*, 2827–2834.

22. Ursic-Vrscaj, M., Bebar, S., & Zakelj, M. P. (2001). Hormone replacement therapy after invasive ovarian serous cystadenocarcinoma treatment: The effect on survival. *Menopause, 8*(1), 70–75.

23. Utian, W. H., Shoupe, D., Bachmann, G., Pinkerton, J. V., & Pickar, J. H. (2001). Relief of vasomotor symptoms and vaginal atrophy with lower doses of conjugated equine estrogens and medroxyprogesterone acetate. *Fertility and Sterility, 75*, 1065–1079.

24. Weiss, S. R., Ellman, H., & Dolker, M. (1999). A randomized controlled trial of four doses of transdermal estradiol for preventing postmenopausal bone loss. *Obstetrics & Gynecology, 94*, 330–336.

Chapter 2

PHYSIOLOGY OF MENOPAUSE

Contents

Introduction

The menstrual cycle permanently ends at menopause, also referred to as the climacteric, signifying the end of reproduction. It usually happens between 45 and 55 years of age, though the precise time can change. Usually, menopause is a natural transition. In tobacco smokers, it may happen sooner. Additional causes include certain forms of chemotherapy and ovarian cancer surgery. Menopause is physiologically caused by a reduction in the ovaries' ability to produce progesterone and estrogen. Menopause can be diagnosed by blood or urine hormone levels, although this is usually not necessary. Menarche, or the beginning of a girl's menstrual cycle, is the opposite of menopause (Agosta et al., 2011).

A woman's periods usually become irregular in the years leading up to menopause; this means that the length of her periods can vary, as can the amount of flow. Women frequently have hot flashes during this time; they usually last between thirty seconds and ten minutes and can be accompanied by shivering, nocturnal sweats, and skin reddening. For four to five years, hot flashes can recur. Mood swings, difficulty sleeping, and vaginal dryness are possible additional symptoms (American-Psychiatric-Association, 2000). Women's symptoms differ in intensity. Menopause occurring before the age of forty-five is referred to as early menopause, and ovarian failure or surgical ovarian excision occurring before the age of forty-five is referred to as premature ovarian insufficiency. A woman's bone density, central abdominal fat, vascular function, and cholesterol profile can all be negatively impacted by menopause, in addition to the symptoms (hot flushes/flashes, arthralgia, mood swings, and dry vagina). Postmenopausal women are more susceptible to osteoporosis, bone fractures, and cardio-metabolic diseases (diabetes and cardiovascular disease) as a result of these changes.

Orientation and Directional Terms

Terms	Definition	Illustration
Menstruation	Menstruation is the regular discharge of blood and mucosal tissue from the inner lining of the uterus through the vagina.	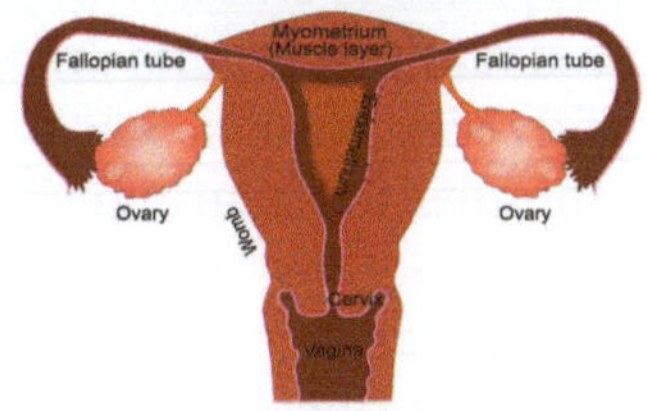
Vaginal dryness	Vaginal dryness may be a problem for women at any age, although it occurs more frequently in older women, particularly after menopause.	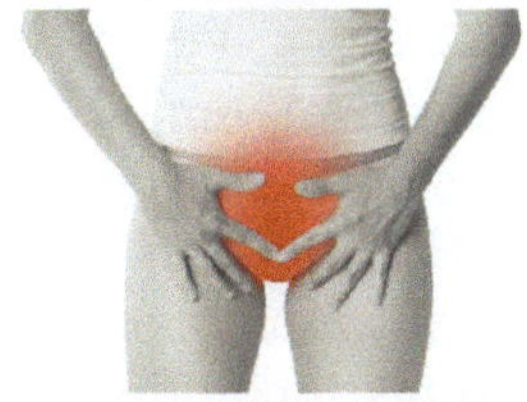
Luteinizing hormone	Luteinizing hormone (LH) is a glycoprotein hormone that is co-secreted along with follicle-stimulating hormone by the gonadotrophin cells in the adenohypophysis (anterior pituitary).	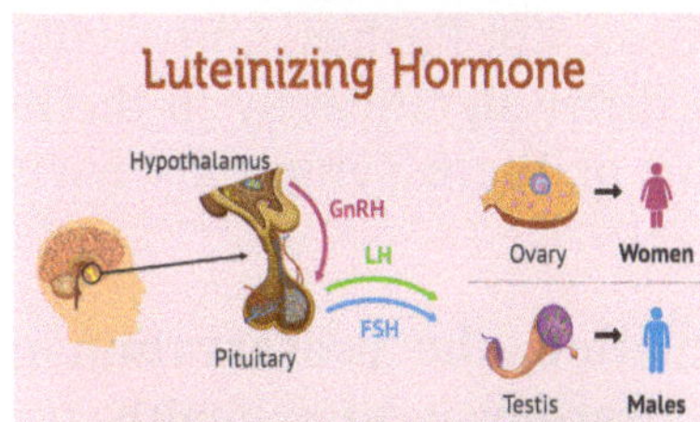
Pregnancy	Pregnancy (or gestation) is calculated as 40 weeks and starts from the first day of your last menstrual period. Pregnancy is classified into 3 stages known as trimesters.	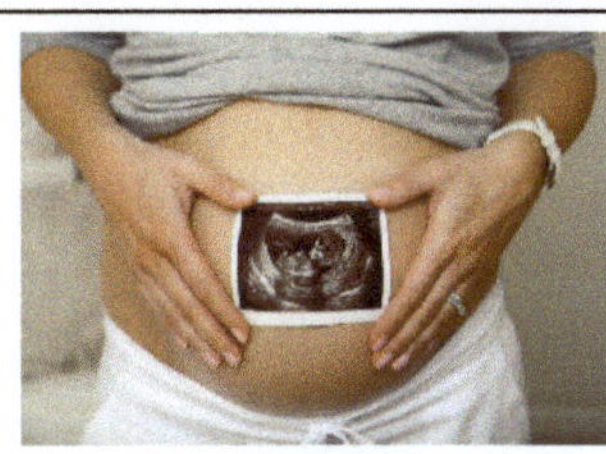
Tachycardia	Tachycardia is an increased heart rate for any reason. If a fast heart rate is caused by exercise or stress, it's called sinus tachycardia.	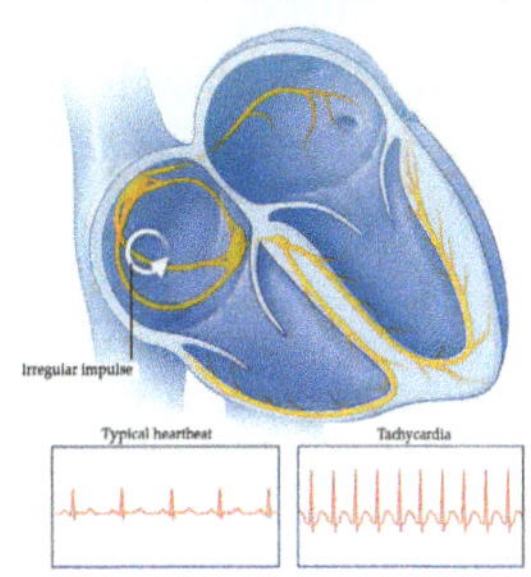

2.1. Overview of Physiology of Menopause

A woman's menopause is a major physiological milestone that usually happens between the ages of 45 and 55, though each woman's experience is unique. It is characterized by the end of reproductive potential and the reversal of menstrual cycles as a result of hormonal changes, specifically a decrease in the ovaries' production of estrogen. Perimenopause, or period leading up to menopause, frequently starts several years before the actual end of the menstrual cycle. Hormone fluctuations occur during this time, causing irregular periods and a range of symptoms including mood swings, vaginal dryness, hot flashes, and night sweats. Women can differ significantly in the intensity and duration of these symptoms (Avis et al., 2001).

Menstruation, the preservation of bone density, and cardiovascular health are just a few of the physiological processes in the female body that estrogen is crucial in controlling. Women may see changes in these areas during menopause as their estrogen levels drop. For instance, a reduction in estrogen may cause bone loss, raising the risk of fractures and osteoporosis. Furthermore, variations in blood vessel function and cholesterol levels may raise the risk of cardiovascular disease (Baeza et al., 2010).

Beyond just physical symptoms, menopause also has an impact on one's psychological and emotional health. Many women report struggling with issues related to body image and sexuality, as well as feeling a sense of loss or mourning for their reproductive years. Mood disorders, including anxiety and depression, are also prevalent at this time and are probably influenced by both psychosocial and hormonal changes. Menopause is a normal and inevitable stage of a woman's life, though each woman experiences it in a very unique way. Some women may experience minimal disruption to their daily lives during the menopause transition, while others may find the symptoms extremely difficult and seek medical assistance to manage them (Baksu et al., 2005).

One such treatment is hormone replacement therapy (HRT), which supplements progesterone and sometimes estrogen to treat menopausal symptoms. HRT is not risk-free, though, and its suitability should be carefully considered in light of each person's unique health circumstances and medical background. A woman's menopause is the result of a complex interaction between her social, psychological, and physiological aspects of her life. A comprehensive strategy that takes into account the various needs and experiences of women as they move through this important life stage is necessary to comprehend and manage this transition successfully. With the right information, encouragement, and individualized medical care, women can accept menopause as a normal aspect of aging and move into this new stage of life with dignity and fortitude (Bromberger et al., 2003).

2.1.1. Menopause

Menopause: the end of a woman's reproductive life marked by a permanent cessation of menstruation brought on by the loss of ovarian function. The ovaries have shrunk in size and are primarily made up of fibrous tissue, some interstitial cells, and atretic (shrunken) follicles at the menopausal stage. Follicle loss and an 80% or greater reduction in estrogen production cause luteinizing hormone (LH) and follicle-stimulating hormone (FSH) to be secreted in markedly higher amounts. Menstrual cycles may end suddenly or may continue irregularly for about a year before stopping. Similarly, menopausal symptoms can come on suddenly or gradually. Menopausal symptoms are more likely to start after a woman's menstruation stops, though they can start while she is still having periods (Bromberger et al., 2013).

An analogous aging-related decline in testicular function that causes testosterone deficiency in men is sometimes referred to as "male menopause." Another name for this process is andropause or late-onset hypogonadism. It may start at age 40 and affects roughly 2% of men. In contrast to women experiencing menopause, men experiencing late-onset hypogonadism experience a gradual decline in testosterone levels over an extended period of time. Reduced libido, exhaustion, depression, and erectile dysfunction are among the symptoms. The illness may go years undiagnosed because the symptoms are often mild at first (Bryant et al., 2012).

2.1.1.1. Menopause and Ovarian Function

Most women go through menopause between the ages of 45 and 55, though it can start as early as 40 or happen later, in their late 50s. The individual's ancestry seems to play a significant role in determining the age of onset. Indeed, genes linked to age differences in a typical menopause have been found on several chromosomes. However, the age of onset can also be influenced by health behaviors and nutrition. About 8% of women experience premature menopause, which is the spontaneous onset of menopause before the age of 40. Early menopause is the term used to describe the spontaneous onset of menopause before the age of forty-five. If the ovaries are surgically removed (during a hysterectomy or as part of the treatment for ovarian cancer, for example) or inadvertently damaged or destroyed (as a side effect of radiation therapy or chemotherapy), early or premature menopause may result (Canonico et al., 2007).

Since the ovaries have a natural life span of approximately 35 years, the aging process naturally causes an ovarian function decline, though this decline accelerates as menopause gets closer. Under hypothalamic-pituitary stimulation, follicles in the ovaries mature and periodically release their mature eggs, or ova, during the reproductive years. However, some follicles fail to rupture and release their ova in the years just before menopause, a transitional phase known as perimenopause that can start as early as 10 years before menopause. Eventually, all follicles fail to rupture and release their ova. Estrogen levels drop rapidly in the final year or two of perimenopause (Carretti et al., 2007).

Prolonged periods or irregular bleeding episodes may result from the ongoing decrease in ovarian activity. The intervals could be shorter or longer, and the flow could get thinner or thicker. In a tiny percentage of cases, the periods end suddenly.

2.1.1.2. Symptoms of Menopause

Smaller and smaller amounts of the hormone estrogen are produced by the ovaries as they become less functional, which causes the hormone activity of the glands that regulate reproduction to shift subtly. A lack of estrogen during menopause and beyond results in smaller uteri and breasts as well as dry, atrophic vaginal mucosa. Furthermore, having sex frequently results in pain (dyspareunia).

Hot flashes, a common symptom of decreased estrogen levels during menopause, present with a sensation of warmth in the face and upper body, flushing of the skin, sweating, accelerated heart rate, irritability, and headache. Lasting a few minutes, hot flashes may be followed by feelings of cold and shivering, affecting about 75% of women at menopausal age and around 30% for up to five years. The frequency of hot flashes can range from one or two per day to one per hour, potentially causing embarrassment and sleep disturbances.

These episodes are believed to be triggered by sudden autonomic nerve activation that dilates blood vessels supplying the skin, resulting in increased skin temperature (Charoenphandhu et al., 2011).

Menopause can cause physiological symptoms including decreased libido, dry skin, and changes in hormonal activity of the adrenal and thyroid glands. Some women may also experience weight gain due to decreased thyroid function, but menopause does not necessarily lead to significant changes in physical appearance or fitness. Psychological symptoms, such as mood swings, depression, and feelings of anxiety, are common among menopausal women. Fear of aging or changes in lifestyle may contribute to these feelings (Chen et al., 2014).

2.1.2. Ovarian Aging and Hormonal Decline

As women age, their ovaries naturally decline in function, leading to a decrease in reproductive capacity and the beginning of menopause. The ovaries are crucial for producing hormones like estrogen and progesterone, which are essential for regulating the menstrual cycle and supporting fertility. However, with age, the ovaries undergo changes that affect their structure, function, and hormone production.

A reduction in the number and quality of ovarian follicles—tiny sacs inside the ovaries that hold immature eggs—is one of the main signs of ovarian aging. Women are born with a limited number of follicles, and over time, this ovarian reserve gradually decreases due to a condition called follicular atresia. The pool of remaining follicles is drastically reduced by the time a woman reaches her late 30s or early 40s, which lowers her potential for reproduction and raises her risk of infertility (Chung-Park. et al., 2005).

The main female sex hormone, estrogen, is produced less often when ovarian follicles are being destroyed. In addition to affecting bone health, cardiovascular health, mood regulation, and other physiological processes, estrogen has a complex role in the female body. Hot flashes, vaginal dryness, and mood swings are among the symptoms of menopause that are caused by a decrease in estrogen production that occurs with aging ovarian function.

As ovaries age, progesterone levels also decline, albeit more slowly than estrogen's. Progesterone is another hormone that the ovaries produce. Progesterone primarily aids in early gestation and prepares the uterus for pregnancy. Changes in menstrual patterns and the eventual cessation of menstruation are linked to its decline in menopausal women. Hormonal alterations linked to ovarian aging affect not only the ovaries but also other endocrine glands like the pituitary and hypothalamus (Daendee et al., 2013).

Through the synthesis and secretion of luteinizing hormone (LH), follicle-stimulating hormone (FSH), and gonadotropin-releasing hormone (GnRH), these glands play critical roles in controlling the menstrual cycle. These hormonal signals are frequently dysregulated when ovarian function declines, leading to irregular menstrual cycles and ultimately the cessation of ovulation and menstruation.

Although hormonal decline and ovarian aging are normal processes that happen to women as they age, they can have a significant impact on several different aspects of health and wellbeing. Falling estrogen levels have consequences for reproduction as well as an increased risk of osteoporosis, cardiovascular disease, and cognitive decline. Therefore, creating plans to encourage healthy aging and lessen the negative effects of menopause requires an understanding of the mechanisms underlying ovarian aging and hormonal decline. Women can manage this change more easily and keep their best health and vitality as they age with hormone replacement therapy, lifestyle changes, and other interventions (De Jesús-Burgos et al., 2012).

2.1.3. Changes in the Hypothalamic-Pituitary-Ovarian Axis

The intricate neuroendocrine system known as the hypothalamic-pituitary-ovarian (HPO) axis is crucial for controlling female reproductive function. It orchestrates the menstrual cycle, ovulation, and the release of sex hormones by coordinating the actions of the hypothalamus, pituitary gland, and ovaries. The HPO axis significantly alters with age in women, which affects reproductive function and helps menopause begin. The brain region known as the hypothalamus, which integrates signals from the nervous system and regulates hormone secretion, is at the center of the hypothalamus-pituitary axis. A crucial regulator of the menstrual cycle, gonadotropin-releasing hormone (GnRH) is produced by specialized neurons in the hypothalamus. The pituitary gland secretes follicle-stimulating hormone (FSH) and luteinizing hormone (LH), two significant gonadotropin hormones, in response to the pulsatile release of GnRH into the bloodstream (Depypere et al., 2014).

The ovaries are influenced by FSH and LH to control ovulation, folliculogenesis, and the synthesis of progesterone and estrogen. The maturation of ovarian follicles, each of which contains an immature egg, is referred to as folliculogenesis. Many follicles within the ovary start to develop under the influence of FSH, but only one dominant follicle usually matures fully and releases its egg during ovulation, which is brought on by an increase in LH. Estrogen and progesterone levels change during the menstrual cycle in response to the growth of ovarian follicles and the creation of the corpus luteum, a transient endocrine structure that develops from the ruptured follicle following ovulation. The primary source of estrogen in developing follicles, estrogen acts as a positive feedback loop on the HPO axis, stimulating GnRH secretion and encouraging LH surges that lead to ovulation. When conception happens, progesterone, which is produced by the corpus luteum, helps to maintain a pregnancy by preparing the uterus for the possible implantation of a fertilized egg (Diz-Chaves. Et al., 2012).

The dynamics of the HPO axis are significantly altered as women age and approach menopause because of modifications in hormone feedback mechanisms and ovarian function. A reduction in ovarian follicular reserve and abnormalities in menstrual cycle length and ovulatory function are two of the main characteristics of perimenopause, the transitional period preceding menopause. Changes in the pituitary and hypothalamic glands' sensitivity to progesterone and estrogen, as well as modifications to the feedback regulation of the hypothalamus, accompany this decline (**Đoković** et al., 2015).

The feedback loops controlling GnRH, FSH, and LH secretion are altered when ovarian function declines because there is a corresponding drop in the production of estrogen and progesterone. In particular, the hypothalamus becomes less sensitive to progesterone and estrogen's negative feedback loop, which leads to elevated levels of FSH and LH and increased GnRH secretion. The perimenopausal symptoms, which include irregular menstrual cycles, hot flashes, and dry vagina, are partly brought on by these hormonal shifts. The HPO axis eventually experiences additional changes that lead to menopause, the permanent end of menstruation, as ovarian follicular reserve is exhausted and ovarian function completely ceases. At this point, the HPO axis enters a state of relative quiescence marked by decreased FSH and LH levels, decreased GnRH secretion, and consistently low estrogen and progesterone levels (Dornstauder et al., 2001).

Throughout a woman's life, the hypothalamic-pituitary-ovarian axis experiences substantial changes, especially as she approaches menopause. Modifications in neuroendocrine regulation, hormone feedback mechanisms, and ovarian function are responsible for these changes. Determining the physiological mechanisms behind this transition and creating strategies to manage the accompanying symptoms and enhance women's health and well-being require an understanding of the dynamics of the HPO axis during menopause (Eckel, 2001).

2.1.4. Impact on Other Endocrine Systems

The onset of menopause, which is characterized by the reduction of ovarian function and hormonal alterations, has a substantial impact on the reproductive endocrine system in addition to other endocrine systems within the body. The complex interactions between hormones and other physiological functions highlight the extensive effects of menopause on general health and wellbeing. The impact of menopause on bone health is one of the most significant effects on other endocrine systems. Because it inhibits bone resorption and promotes bone formation, estrogen is essential for maintaining bone density. An imbalance between bone resorption and formation occurs during menopause as a result of declining estrogen levels, which accelerates bone loss and raises the risk of osteoporosis. A systemic skeletal disorder called osteoporosis is characterized by a decrease in bone mass and an increased risk of fractures, especially those that occur in the wrist, hip, and spine. Because of this increased risk of osteoporosis and fractures, menopausal women should take extra precautions like taking calcium and vitamin D supplements, exercising with weights, and getting their bone density checked (Erekson et al., 2013).

Estrogen has cardioprotective effects on the heart and blood vessels, which is one way that menopause affects the cardiovascular system. In addition to controlling lipid metabolism and preventing atherosclerosis from developing, estrogen also aids in maintaining vascular tone. As a result, the decrease in estrogen levels that occurs during menopause is linked to detrimental modifications in cardiovascular risk factors, such as elevated levels of triglycerides, total cholesterol, and LDL cholesterol, as well as changes in endothelial integrity and vascular function. The increased incidence of cardiovascular disease seen in postmenopausal women relative to premenopausal women can be attributed in part to these alterations. Thus, controlling cardiovascular risk factors by changing one's lifestyle (e.g., a balanced diet, consistent exercise, and giving up smoking) and, when necessary, pharmaceutical interventions (e.g., statins, blood pressure-lowering drugs) is crucial for maintaining menopausal women's cardiovascular health (Espinosa et al., 2012).

Menopause can also have an impact on body composition and metabolic health, which puts women at risk for dyslipidemia, insulin resistance, and weight gain. The distribution of adipose tissue, insulin sensitivity, and energy metabolism are all influenced by estrogen, and changes in these processes are linked to the hormone's decline during menopause. Visceral adiposity is a known risk factor for metabolic syndrome, type 2 diabetes, and cardiovascular disease, and it frequently increases in postmenopausal women. Furthermore, insulin resistance and dyslipidemia may be exacerbated by menopause-related hormonal changes, which would further aggravate metabolic dysfunction. Thus, it is essential to adopt a healthy lifestyle that includes consistent exercise, a balanced diet, and weight control to minimize the metabolic effects of menopause and lower the chance of obesity-related comorbidities (Formoso et al., 2012).

Furthermore, menopause's effects on the neurotransmitter and hypothalamic-pituitary-adrenal (HPA) axis can affect mood, cognition, and mental health. There are many estrogen receptors in the brain, including areas related to stress response, mood regulation, and cognitive function. Neuroprotective and neurotrophic properties of estrogen support neurotransmitter synthesis, mood stability, and synaptic plasticity. As a result, the drop in estrogen levels that occurs during menopause is linked to a higher chance of mood disorders like anxiety and depression as well as memory loss and cognitive decline. Additionally, mood swings, irritability, and sleep disturbances may be caused by changes in hormone levels during perimenopause. Therefore, promoting mental health and quality of life in menopausal women requires addressing psychological and emotional well-being through counseling, support groups, and, when necessary, medication (Freeman et al., 2005).

Menopause has a significant impact on the body's endocrine systems, which include those responsible for bone metabolism, cardiovascular health, metabolic control, and neuroendocrine function. Comprehending the complex effects of menopause on endocrine health is essential to formulating all-encompassing approaches that promote women's health and welfare throughout this shift. Healthcare professionals can enable women to move through this stage of life with resilience and vitality by addressing the physiological, psychological, and metabolic changes related to menopause (Genazzani et al., 2015).

2.2. Anxiety in Natural and Surgical Menopause Physiologic and Therapeutic Bases

One of the most prevalent mental illnesses, generalized anxiety disorder affects a significant portion of the global population. There are notable gender differences in this emotional disorder, with women experiencing it at a 2:1 ratio more frequently than men. Significant variations in the concentrations of brain and plasma steroid hormones, such as progesterone, allopregnanolone, and estradiol, occur in tandem with women's reproductive cycles. These hormonal shifts are linked to the emergence of anxiety and mood swings during the premenstrual and postpartum periods, especially during the menopause, as well as to certain illnesses (Glickman-Simon and Lindsay, 2013; González-Jiménez et al., 2010; Hanisch et al., 2008).

Menopause is a term used to describe the natural or surgically induced cessation of a woman's reproductive ability. Natural menopause typically occurs in a woman's late 40s or early 50s, marked by hormonal changes and the end of the reproductive period. During this time, women may experience physical, emotional, and mental changes. Surgical menopause, on the other hand, occurs at a younger age and can result in more severe symptoms. In both cases, menopause can have a significant impact on a woman's mental health (Gong et al., 2014).

Low levels of steroid hormones are present during the premenstrual, post-partum, climacteric, or postmenopausal phases and are linked to irritability, anxiety, or depressive symptoms. The primary characteristic of either natural or surgical post-menopause is a decrease in both progesterone and estradiol due to declining ovarian function. Hormonal fluctuations are linked to a high frequency of vasomotor symptoms, dry vagina, osteoporosis, cognitive decline, and hot flashes that are accompanied by sweating, palpitations, restlessness, anxiety, and mood fluctuations. Regrettably, compared to women who underwent natural menopause, women who underwent surgical menopause experienced more severe emotional and affective changes linked to the long-term absence of ovarian hormones. Regrettably, young women in economically productive stages are experiencing surgical menopause at a higher rate. This has a negative impact on their quality of life, the economy, and, regrettably, their mental health (Gupta et al., 2013; Hickey et al., 2005).

Benzodiazepines (i.e., sleeping pills) are used to treat anxiety and depression symptoms that are brought on by the prolonged loss of ovarian hormones caused by surgical or natural menopause (i.e., diazepam), a few selective inhibitors of serotonin reuptake (i.e., paroxetine or fluoxetine), as well as hormone replacement treatment (i.e., progestagens, estrogens, or a mix of both), among other substances. Hormone replacement therapy has been used to treat post-menopausal women's physiological, behavioral, and emotional changes. For example, it has been shown to lessen mood swings, hot flashes, irritability, and bone loss. However, several side effects are linked to hormone replacement therapy, making it unsuitable for long-term use in women who are particularly vulnerable. Thus, studies looking for novel therapeutic options have looked into the effects of certain vegetables, like soy, which has high levels of the phyto-estrogens genistein, daidzein, glycitein, and their conjugate metabolites. There is evidence in certain reports that phyto-estrogens have physiological effects akin to those of endogenous estrogens. These effects seem to be caused by actions on the estradiol receptor-β, which has been implicated in the anxiolytic-like effect of synthetic and endogenous estrogens in experiments (Handley and Williams, 2015).

To investigate the impact of prolonged lack of ovarian hormones due to surgical menopause in women, researchers have utilized ovariectomy in rats as a preclinical model to examine changes in various organs and systems. Rats that undergo ovariectomy as a way to mimic the long-term absence of ovarian hormones are seen as an early representation of surgical menopause, enabling researchers to study alterations in cardiovascular, reproductive, motor, and skeletal systems, as well as changes in neurotransmitter receptor sensitivity in the brain. These brain changes have been linked to increased anxiety-like behavior and feelings of despair in the rats. This suggests that rats with chronic ovarian hormone deficiency through ovariectomy could provide insights into anxiety and mood disturbances observed in women who have undergone surgical menopause and may also aid in the development of new treatments to alleviate anxiety symptoms in this population.

Treatment for anxiety and depression symptoms related to the absence of ovarian hormones during menopause can include benzodiazepines, selective serotonin reuptake inhibitors, and hormone replacement therapy with estrogens or a combination of estrogens and progestagens. Hormone replacement therapy is commonly used to address various symptoms in post-menopausal women, such as bone loss, hot flashes, irritability, and mood swings. However, it is also associated with side effects that limit its long-term use in some individuals. Research has explored alternative therapeutic options, such as incorporating phyto-estrogens found in vegetables like soya, which contain compounds like genistein, daidzein, and glycitein. These phyto-estrogens have been found to have similar physiological effects to endogenous estrogens, potentially acting on estradiol receptor-β to produce anxiolytic-like effects similar to those seen with natural or synthetic estrogens (Iglesias et al., 2009).

Rats with ovariectomies have been employed preclinically to investigate changes in various organs and systems to investigate the impact of the prolonged lack of ovarian hormones linked to surgical menopause in women. An early model of surgical menopause, an ovariectomy-induced long-term loss of ovarian hormones in rats has made it possible to study alterations in the cardiovascular, reproductive, motor, and bone systems as well as changes in the sensitivity of neurotransmitter receptors in the brain (Ishiwata et al., 2009). The alterations in the brain have an adverse effect on the behavior of the rats, leading to an increase in markers of dejection and anxious behavior. These data lend credence to the theory that rats induced by ovarian excision to have a chronic lack of ovarian hormones may provide insight into the anxiety and mood fluctuations experienced by surgically menopausal women. They may also be used to identify novel drugs that may be effective in reducing the symptoms of anxiety experienced by this specific subset of women (Izumo et al., 2012).

2.2.1. Natural and Surgical Menopause

The term "menopause" refers to the clinical phenomenon wherein a woman's ability to reproduce ends. It can happen spontaneously or be surgically induced through uterine (hysterectomy), bilateral oophorectomy (removal of the ovaries), or salpingo-oophorectomy (removal of the Fallopian tubes with or without removal of the ovaries). Specific times (Figure 2.1) associated with the hormonal and physiological alterations brought on by ovarian failure are included in the natural menopause (Table 2.1). Menopause is typically a normal stage that happens to women naturally in their midlife, in their late 40s or early 50s, signifying the end of their reproductive years (Jafari et al., 2014). Women experience variations in ovarian hormone production and release during the menopause transition years, which results in notable adjustments to physiological and affective functions. Not all women have these effects to an unbearable degree; this varies widely from person to person and also depends on lifestyle. The majority of women notice that the frequency of their menstrual cycles is gradually decreasing and that the timing of the flow's onset is typically less predictable (Jin et al., 2005).

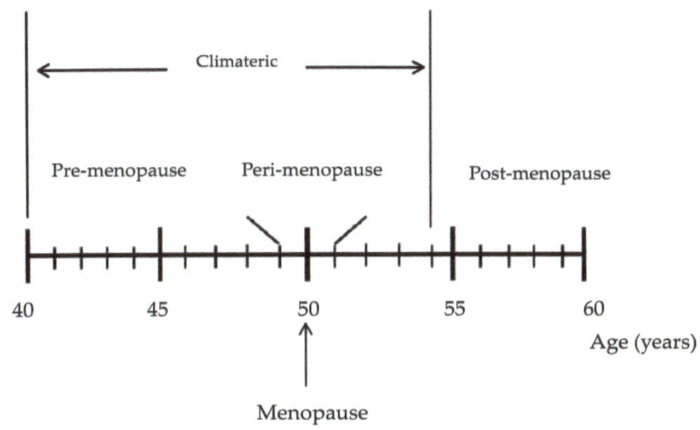

Figure 2.1. *Scheme illustrating the different phases that characterized the end of the reproductive period in women, under natural conditions.*

Source: Rodríguez-Landa, J. F., Puga-Olguín, A., Germán-Ponciano, L. J., García-Ríos, R.-I., & Soria-Fregozo, C. (2015). Anxiety in Natural and Surgical Menopause—Physiologic and Therapeutic Bases. InTech. doi: 10.5772/60621.

Menopause usually begins between the ages of 40 and 61, with the average age for the last period being around 51 years old. The average age for natural menopause is 51, but in countries like the Philippines and India, women may experience it earlier, around 44 years old. The World Health Organization states that menopause typically occurs between 45 and 55 worldwide (Lambrinoudaki et al., 2015).

Natural or surgical menopause leads to significant decreases in the levels of ovarian hormones, specifically estradiol, progesterone, and their byproducts. These hormonal changes contribute to the onset of menopausal symptoms such as decreased bone density, hot flashes, and emotional disturbances like irritability, anxiety, and depression in some cases. Natural menopause occurs due to follicular atresia, where ovarian follicles stop responding to gonadotrophins, causing the ovaries to lose function, halt ovulation, and mark the end of a woman's reproductive years. During this stage, estrogen levels decrease, while follicular stimulant hormone (FSH) and luteinizing hormone (LH) increase to a lesser extent (Leiblum et al., 2006).

Table 2.1. Terms Associated with Natural Menopause

Term	Description
Premenopause	Is a term used to mean the years leading up to the last menstrual period, when the concentrations of ovarian hormones are already becoming more variable and lower, and the effects of hormone withdrawal are present.
Perimenopause	It term refers to the menopause transition years, a span of time both before *and* after the date of the final menstrual period; which can last for four to eight years. It period may occur during six to ten year, ending approximately 12 months after the last menstrual period.
Menopause	Clinically, menopause is defined as the last menstrual flow period. It is necessary taken in count that this moment may only be identified retrospectively, once 12 months have gone without experiment any menstrual flow. Commonly, menopause is used to referrer to menopause transition years, but not the last menstrual period.
Postmenopause	This term include the period after 12 months without menstrual flow, assuming that women still have a uterus, and are not pregnant or lactating. Physiologically, this period is characterized by very high follicular stimulant hormone concentration (FSH) at plasma level. Thus postmenopause is all of the time that follows the point when her ovaries become inactive, evidenced by last menstrual period.

Source: Rodríguez-Landa, J. F., Puga-Olguín, A., Germán-Ponciano, L. J., García-Ríos, R.-I., & Soria-Fregozo, C. (2015). Anxiety in Natural and Surgical Menopause—Physiologic and Therapeutic Bases. InTech. doi: 10.5772/60621

Conversely, surgical menopause is linked to an abrupt and total decrease in plasma concentrations of testosterone, progesterone, and estradiol. This increases the risk of physiological and psychological changes that mimic those that happen during natural menopause, albeit more severely (Li et al., 2013).

2.2.2. Anxiety Disorders and Mood Swings Associated with Natural or Surgical Menopause in Women

A phase of a woman's biological development known as menopause is associated with social, psychological, and physiological changes. Women are susceptible to mental and physical disorders like anxiety and depression during menopause, in addition to physical impairment. A woman's quality of life can be negatively impacted by symptoms such as hot flushes, night sweats, dry skin and mucosa, even dry vagina, sleep disturbances, and behavioral and cognitive abnormalities. Premenopausal women frequently experience mild anxiety and stress vulnerability, whereas perimenopausal women experience more severe anxiety, depression, and irritability (Lipovac et al., 2010). When compared to mood disorders, anxiety disorders are typically more chronic (i.e., depression) in a woman experiencing menopausal symptoms. Notably, compared to natural menopause, emotional and affective disorders are more severe in surgical menopausal cases. This is likely because of the severe suppression of hormone production, the psychosocial context of the surgery, and the illness that goes along with it (McGregor et al., 2014).

In a naturally occurring menopause, ovarian hormone production (i.e., estrogens and androgens) gradually decreases, whereas surgical menopause is marked by a sharp reduction in hormone levels. This decrease in hormone levels affects neuronal functioning impairment that leads to mood swings and an increased risk of anxiety disorders, mostly in women with a history of mental health issues. Women with a history of psychiatric disorders may experience emotional and affective disorders more severely; conversely, women with a history of premenstrual syndrome or dysphoric premenstrual syndrome may experience menopause with a certain degree of liberty and comfort regarding their sexuality (McLaughlin et al., 2008).

Research indicates that women who experienced high levels of anxiety prior to menopause also continue to experience this during menopause between the ages of 42 and 52. Low anxiety premenopausal women may be more vulnerable to elevated anxiety during and after the menopause transition. In line with those conclusions, (Jafari et.al., 2014) discovered that premenopausal women, who are between the ages of 35 and 45, have lower levels of anxiety than postmenopausal women, who are between the ages of 45 and 55 (Mendoza et al., 2000).

According to some writers, the period leading up to menopause is the one where anxiety symptoms are most likely to appear or worsen. Anxiety disorders that do not change with the menopausal stages include panic disorder, social anxiety, and generalized anxiety. Nonetheless, research indicates that anxiety symptoms are more prevalent during the perimenopause than they are in the pre- and post-menopausal stages. Hot flushes are experienced by 74% of women going through natural menopause, and they are linked to the emergence of anxiety symptoms. It is still debatable whether anxiety appears prior to or after vascular symptoms (i.e., night sweats, and hot flashes) that were typical of menopause.

The symptoms of menopause vary significantly among different demographics. African-American women tend to experience more severe vascular motor symptoms compared to Asiatic women, including hot flashes, palpitations, and sweating. This difference is believed to be influenced by lifestyle, nutrition, metabolic activity, and neurotransmission systems in the brain. It is uncertain whether anxiety or vascular symptoms come first. Conversely, there is a strong correlation between the severity of anxiety and depression symptoms and overall quality of life. Post-menopausal women with a lower quality of life often report higher levels of anxiety and depression compared to pre-menopausal women with a better quality of life (Moilanen et al., 2010).

The most common reasons for perimenopausal women to seek medical advice are symptoms of anxiety, irritability, depression, bluntness, amnesic disease, impairment of general capacity, and sleep disorders. Women who report psychological discomfort to doctors throughout the menopause are frequently the ones who exhibit low self-esteem and a lack of personal fulfillment. Furthermore, there is a connection between menopausal women's hormone levels and psychological health. For instance, perimenopausal hormonal fluctuations appear to exacerbate depression, potentially due to an inability of estrogens to regulate serotonergic activity and other brain neurotransmission systems. Young post-menopausal women who experience mood disorders are linked to variations in circulating levels of androgens, demonstrating a direct correlation between androgen concentrations and post-menopausal symptoms of anxiety and depression (Nathorst-Böös et al., 2006).

One of the most prevalent anxiety disorders during menopause is panic disorder, which can arise at any point after menopause is fully established. A higher frequency of this disorder is seen in women who have noticeable physical symptoms during menopause. In three groups of women with varying age classifications (i.e., 50–59, 60–69, and 70–79 years old), women in the 50–59 age range experienced panic attacks more frequently. This group most likely went through perimenopause, which can lead to changes in the production of ovarian hormones, greater susceptibility to psychological stress, and more intense physical symptoms (Nissen et al., 2012). All of these factors can raise the risk of developing anxiety. Negative life experiences, overall physical impairment, and comorbidity with other illnesses are additional factors. For instance, 10% of women between the ages of 51 and 83 reported having at least one panic attack in the six months prior to having a cardiovascular condition. In postmenopausal women, anxiety appears to be a risk factor that raises the morbidity and mortality linked to cardiovascular disease.

A mental illness known as obsessive-compulsive disorder (OCD) is linked to various events in a woman's reproductive life. According to reports, the incidence of OCD is 47% among women going through menopause and drops to 9% in post-menopausal women. Despite research on the topic, the findings regarding menopause and OCD are incongruous. One study that examined the prevalence and comorbidity of OCD in women experiencing either a natural or surgical post-menopausal period found that the disorder was more common in obsessions with cleanliness than in compulsions with cleaning. The percentage of patients with co-occurring disorders was 63.2%, with generalized anxiety disorder and comorbidity being the most common (Pacchierotti et al., 2004). According to certain research, vascular abnormalities are associated with 18% of perimenopausal women who sought medical consultations having panic disorder (PD). These results must be carefully interpreted, though, as the research did not specify how menopause onset was determined. It appears that the researchers relied solely on verbal reports from patients (Pandaranandaka et al., 2006).

There is a dearth of research on anxiety attacks and surgical menopause in general. In one medical case, a woman who had her ovaries surgically removed experienced psychological and physiological changes that were comparable to those of a natural menopause. However, she also experienced acute anxiety symptoms right away, which negatively impacted her quality of life. Individual differences exist in the emotional and affective symptoms linked to surgical menopause; however, research has linked bilateral ovarian excision before natural menopause to an increased risk of anxiety disorders and cognitive impairment in comparison to women who go through natural menopause (Pandaranandaka et al., 2009).

2.2.3. Pharmacological Treatment of Anxiety Disorders in Menopausal Women: Benefits Versus Side-Effects

There are few controlled studies evaluating the effectiveness of pharmacological treatments in this particular population, despite the evidence that anxiety and depression disorders are highly prevalent in both surgical and natural menopause. Additionally, a concerningly high frequency of anxiolytic drug self-medication among menopausal women is concerning (Picazo et al., 2006). Menopausal women's symptoms can be controlled by choosing a treatment that strikes a balance between potential health risks and benefits for mood. It is crucial to take the patient's clinical history into account. For young women who underwent surgical menopause between the ages of 24 and 38, the effectiveness of the pharmacological response may differ from that of women who went through a natural menopause (Puga-Olguín et al., 2014).

The use of chemical compounds isolated from vegetables (i.e., hormone replacement therapy, antidepressants with anxiolytic activity, and certain other therapies) are among the therapeutic options for controlling symptoms of anxiety. (i.e., soy), which have demonstrated some promise as anxiolytics (Table 2.2).

Table 2.2. Pharmacological Treatment of Anxiety Disorders in Menopausal Women

Type of Therapy	Condition (Average Age)	Dosage	Therapeutic Effects	Side-Effects
Hormonal Ethinyl estradiol	Bilateral oophorectomy (24 year)	(3.9 mg/ week; td; 3 mouth)	Without Anxiolytic effects	Increased risk of endometrial hyperplasia and cancers other, venous thromboembolic events and stroke (Hickey et al., 2005).
	Bilateral oophorectomy (46 year)	(3.9 mg/ week; td; 3 month)	Anxiolytic	
	Hysterectomy and bilateral oophorectomy	(3.9 mg/ week; td; 6 mouth)	Anxiolytic	
Tibolone	Hysterectomy and bilateral oophorectomy (47 year)	(2.5 mg/ day; v. o.; 6 month)	Anxiolytic	Increased risk of stroke in women over 60 years (Cummings et al., 2008). Nausea, headache, breast tenderness, weight gain, bloating (Gupta et al., 2013).

	Hysterectomy and bilateral oophorectomy (50 year)	(2.5 mg/ day; v. o.; 12 month)	Anxiolytic	
	Natural menopause	(2.5 mg/ day; v. o.; 3 month)	Anxiolytic	
Estradiol valerianate-dehydroepiandrosterone enanthate (Gynodian Depo)	Hysterectomy with bilateral oophorectomy (35–45 year)	(4 mg/200 mg/ month; i.m.; 3 month)	Anxiolytic	Pruritus, eczema, urticaria, skin reactions at the site of injection, hair loss, erythema nodosum, acne (PLM, 2015).
17β-estradiol	Natural menopause	(50 mg/ day; t.d.; 3 month)	Anxiolytic	Increased risk of venous thromboembolic events (Canonico et al., 2007), cerebrovascular accidents and myocardial infarction (Welty, 2003).
	Hysterectomy and bilateral oophorectomy (48 year)	(2 mg/ day; v.o.; 6 month)	Anxiolytic	
	Hysterectomy and bilateral oophorectomy (50 year)	(50 mg/ day; t.d.; 12 month)	Anxiolytic	
Conjugated equine estrogen (Premarin)	Total abdominal hysterectomy/ bilateral salpingo-oophorectomy (48–51 year)	(0.625 mg/ day; v.o.; 12 month)	Anxiolytic	Increased risk of myocardial infarction, breast cancer and strokes, besides headache and nausea (Gupta et al., 2013).
Dehydroepiandrosterone (DHEA)	Total abdominal hysterectomy/ bilateral salpingo-oophorectomy (48–51 year)	(25 mg/ day; v.o.;12 month)	Anxiolytic	Acne and hair loss (Welty, 2003).
Testosterone (gel hidroalcoholyc TESTOGEL®)	Natural menopause (50–65 year)	(50 mg/ day; t.d.; 3 month)	Anxiolytic	Headache, weight gain, facial hair, increased appetite (Nathorst-Böös et al., 2006).
Antidepressant Venlafaxine	12 month of amenorrea (45–55 year)	(450 mg/ day; v.o.; 6 month)	Anxiolytic	Dry mouth, altered appetite, abdominal discomfort, decreased libido, insomnia, headache and nausea (Hickey et al., 2005; Iglesias et al., 2009; Handley et al., 2015).

Paroxetine	Natural menopause (62 year)	10 mg/day; 1 week and the subsequent dose of 20 mg/day; 6 months.	Anxiolytic	Decreased libido, insomnia, headache and nausea (Hickey et al., 2005; Handley et al., 2015).
Phytoestrogens Red clover extracts (MF11RCE, containing isoflavones)	>12 month of amenorrea (40 year)	(80 mg/ day; v.o.; 3 month)	Anxiolytic	Without effects.
Phytoestrogens PHYTO SOYA, capsules containing 17.5 mg isoflavones	Postmenopausal period	35 mg/ day; v.o.; 4 months	Anxiolytic	Without severe side effects.

Source: Rodríguez-Landa, J. F., Puga-Olguín, A., Germán-Ponciano, L. J., García-Ríos, R.-I., & Soria-Fregozo, C. (2015). Anxiety in Natural and Surgical Menopause—Physiologic and Therapeutic Bases. InTech. doi: 10.5772/60621.

2.2.4. Hormonal Replacement Therapy

The decrease in estrogen levels during menopause has a significant impact on various biological systems, including the central nervous system. Some of the most common psychiatric disorders experienced during this time include lack of motivation, difficulty concentrating, irritability, aggression, mood swings, mental tension, anxiety, and depression. Anxiety is especially prevalent in women who have a history of anxiety disorders. It is well-established that supplementing with exogenous estrogen or progesterone can not only alleviate menopausal symptoms but also improve mood, reduce anxiety, and enhance emotional well-being. Using estrogen to manage anxiety is preferred over psychopharmacological drugs (Rocca et al., 2008).

Research indicates that giving 17β-estradiol to women who are going through a surgical or natural menopause on a long-term basis can effectively lessen their anxiety symptoms. Nonetheless, certain research links the usage of 17β-estradiol to a higher chance of venous thromboembolism, strokes, and myocardial infarction in females with and without a family history of this condition; it seems that using an estrogen transdermal patch reduces side effects, but regrettably also reduces therapeutic benefits (Rodríguez-Landa et al., 2009).

Similar to the significant anxiolytic effects of dehydroepiandrosterone (DHEA) at a dose of 25 mg/day, equine conjugate estrogen therapy also produces significant reductions in genitourinary, vasomotor, psychological, and vaginal dryness symptoms, as well as improvements in libido. Regrettably, using estrogens by themselves or in conjunction with medroxyprogesterone acetate, a synthetic progestin, to treat menopausal symptoms comes with drawbacks and raises the risk of heart attacks, breast cancer, and strokes. Headaches, nausea, and (in the case of DHEA) androgenic side effects like acne and hair loss are additional symptoms (Rodríguez-Landa et al., 2012).

On the other hand, when estrogenic therapy is contraindicated, there are various other medications that can be used instead, such as gonadomimetics like Tibolone. This medicine is a synthetic steroid that breaks down into three metabolites: 3 beta-tibolone, which has estrogenic activity, 3 alpha-OH-tibolone, and the isomer tibolone, which has negligible effects on progestegenic and androgenic activity. Tibolone, 2.5 mg/day, helps women going through natural menopause as well as those who had bilateral oophorectomy or hysterectomy to lessen the symptoms of generalized anxiety. It appears that elevated levels of β-endorphin in the blood and pituitary gland may be linked to these anxiolytic effects (Rodríguez-Landa et al., 2014).

Vaginal bleeding in women who still have a uterus is one of the side effects of estrogenic therapy, and since Tibolone not only has anxiolytic properties but also reduces symptoms at the vegetative and cardiovascular levels, it may be necessary in certain situations. In addition, it raises levels of good cholesterol (HDL), lowers triglycerides, total cholesterol, and bad cholesterol (LDL), slows the loss of bone density, and boosts libido in postmenopausal women. According to data, long-term Tibolone use can lower the risk of breast and colon cancers, as well as bone fractures, but it also raises the risk of strokes in women over 60. Women who have a history of thrombovascular or cerebrovascular disease, breast or cervical cancer, hepatic or cardiovascular illness, or any combination of these conditions should not receive hormone replacement therapy (Rodríguez-Landa et al., 2014).

2.2.4.1. Antidepressants

Reduced serotonergic activity in women going through menopause is linked to low steroid hormone concentrations, which is linked to symptoms of anxiety and depression. Menopausal psychological symptoms may arise due to changes in the availability of cerebral tryptophan, which is involved in the synthesis of serotonin, caused by the reduction in estrogenic levels during menopause.

Consequently, menopausal women's anxiety and depressive symptoms can be managed with the help of selective serotonin reuptake inhibitors, or SSRIs. Hot flushes and vascular symptoms are primarily controlled by venlafaxine, paroxetine, fluoxetine, sertraline, citalopram, and other SSRIs. These medications are also used to treat anxiety and depression in menopausal women. These medications have a suitable tolerance and safety window, but there are some side effects as well, such as decreased libido, headaches, nausea, and insomnia (Russo and Corosu, 2003).

The most prevalent anxiety disorders associated with menopause, including social anxiety, panic attacks, and generalized anxiety, are treated with venlafaxine. Few studies assess the effects of antidepressants on women going through menopause who have been diagnosed with anxiety disorders because anxiety symptoms, like palpitations, irritability, and sweating, are often confused with emotional disturbances that are typical of menopause (Smoller et al., 2007).

A study conducted by Iglesias et al. (2009), which included women going through a natural menopause between the ages of 45 and 55, demonstrated the anxiolytic effect of venlafaxine (450 mg/day/six months). With the exception of mouth dryness, appetite changes, abdominal discomfort, headaches, and, in certain cases, sexual dysfunction, no potentially harmful side effects were reported, even when relatively high doses were used in comparison to the standard dose (150 mg/day).

2.2.4.2. Alternative Therapies

Research into new alternative therapies that control menopausal symptoms but have few or no unfavorable side effects has been spurred by the side effects of hormone replacement therapy and the dearth of controlled studies assessing the therapeutic effect of antidepressants in women going through menopause. The application of chemical substances derived from plants (i.e., due to their estrogenic activity over β-estrogen receptors in the osseous system, reproductive system, and central nervous system, phyto-estrogens) has been investigated as a possible therapeutic option (Smoller et al., 2003). While phyto-estrogens appear to be less effective than conventional estrogens, there is evidence from preclinical and clinical studies that suggest they may be useful in treating vascular disorders, anxiety, depression, and osteoporosis.

Isoflavones have been shown in some clinical studies to be beneficial in reducing the symptoms of classical menopause, such as anxiety and mood swings. With few adverse effects, the phyto-estrogens from magnolia bark extract dramatically lower the relevant psycho-affective symptoms in menopausal women, especially anxiety, irritability, and insomnia (Somunkiran et al., 2007).

The therapeutic effect of isoflavones synthesized from red clover (Trifolium pratense) extracts was investigated in women going through a natural menopause. In women going through a natural menopause, the administration of 80 mg/day of isoflavones for three months (MF11RCE capsule with 40 mg of isoflavones biochanin A, formonometin, genistein, and daidzein) reduced the symptoms of generalized anxiety by 76% when measured by the Hospital Anxiety and Depression Scale (HADS) and compared with basal measures. Similarly, there was a reduction of 80.6% of symptoms with respect to basal when using the Zung's Self Rating Depression Scale. It is important to note that women who received a placebo also experienced a significant reduction in anxiety symptoms, although the reduction was only 21.7% relative to basal. These authors propose that isoflavones extracted from red clover are effective in treating menopausal women's anxiety and depression symptoms (Taku et al., 2012).

190 post-menopausal women participated in a multicentric, open, prospective, observational, and nonrandomized clinical trial to examine the impact of an isoflavone-rich preparation (PHYTO SOYA, capsules containing 17.5 mg isoflavones) on symptoms associated with the absence of estrogens (i.e., hot flashes, insomnia, depression, anxiety, dry vagina, low libido, and bone pain). Over the course of four months of treatment, each patient received two doses of 35 mg of isoflavones per day. The majority of the women reported excellent tolerance, no severe side effects, and a statistically significant decrease in all evaluated parameters, including a significant reduction in anxiety and depression symptomatology (Tangen and Mykletun, 2008).

However, additional information from a double-blind, randomized study involving 50 women (average age 53.33 ± 3.11 years) exhibiting menopausal symptoms shows that giving the phyto-estrogens genistein and daidzein for three months only significantly reduced hot flashes—anxiety, insomnia, or vaginal dryness were not affected. Accordingly, several studies on menopausal women have found that phyto-estrogens are particularly useful in reducing vasomotor symptoms, primarily hot flashes. However, few studies have shown that phyto-estrogens are also useful in reducing anxiety and depressive symptoms. The widespread use of these drugs to treat anxiety and depressive disorders is actually restricted by the paucity of research on the clinical significance of phyto-estrogens in the management of emotional and affective disorders in menopausal women.

Given the debate surrounding the efficacy of phyto-estrogens in treating menopausal physiological and psychiatric disorders, more research is required to fully address the wide range of variables that may impact effectiveness, including dosage, isoflavone structure, the baseline of menopausal symptoms, and length of treatment. Only then will it be possible to remove the current obstacle to recommending the use of phyto-estrogens as a treatment option and acknowledge them as a safe and effective alternative for treating menopausal symptoms (Tominaga et al., 2001).

2.2.5. Ovariectomized Rats as an Animal Model for Surgical Menopause

Women who undergo surgical menopause undergo oophorectomy, or ablation of the ovaries, with or without the uterus. This procedure results in symptoms that are more intense than those of natural menopause (Uguz et al., 2010). This means that the surgical manipulation of rats is suggested as an experimental model to study the physiological and emotional changes that occur in women. Bilateral ovariectomy in rats has thus been proposed as a tool to reproduce physiological and emotional alterations related to the reduction of ovarian hormones (Table 2.3), as occurring in women subjected to surgical menopause.

Table 2.3. Cerebral and Anxiety-Like Behavior Changes Associated with Ovariectomy in the Rat

Weeks Post Ovariectomy	Effects
1	Reduced activation of glutamatergic receptors in the basolateral amygdala.
1–2	Reduced density of dendritic spines and synaptophysin in pyramidal neurons in the CA1 layer of the hippocampus.
3	Reduced density of dendritic spines in the CA1 layer of the hippocampus.
4	Reduced expression of mRNA of $\alpha2$ and $\alpha3$ subunits in the amygdala $GABA_A$ receptors.
4	Reduced expression of mRNA of the tryptophan hydroxylase enzyme and the serotonergic transporter (SERT) in the dorsal raphe nucleus.
4	Reduced concentration of serotonin in the hippocampus and nucleus accumbens.
5	Reduced thickness of the CA1 layer in the hippocampus and the cerebral prefrontal cortex.
6	Reduced concentration of dopamine in the central nucleus of the amygdala.
8	Reduced expression of mRNA of estrogen receptors (ERα y ERβ) in the hippocampus and cerebral cortex.
9	Reduced density of dendritic spines in the cerebral prefrontal cortex.
12	Anxiety-like behavior was higher in 12-weeks postovariectomized rats than 3-weeks postovariectomized rats in the burying behavioral test

12	Higher anxiety-like behavior in the elevated plus maze, which was reduced by phytoestrogen genistein treatment.
1–15	Anxiety-like behavior increase progressively after ovariectomy, it was higher from nine weeks post ovariectomy.
18	Reduced activity of the tryptophan-2-hydroxylase enzyme in the brain.

Source: Rodríguez-Landa, J. F., Puga-Olguín, A., Germán-Ponciano, L. J., García-Ríos, R.-I., & Soria-Fregozo, C. (2015). Anxiety in Natural and Surgical Menopause—Physiologic and Therapeutic Bases. InTech. doi: 10.5772/60621.

A decrease in bone density and an increase in body weight have been observed in some experimental studies using ovariectomized rats. This reduction is similar to the bone density seen in menopausal women due to the prolonged lack of ovarian hormones, specifically progesterone, and estradiol, and their reduced metabolites. Other physiological changes that result in atrophy of the skin and mucosa also happen in this state, including hair loss, a decline in the ability to focus and pay attention, a decrease in memory, and a decrease in libido. The immune, motor, and cardiovascular systems are all compromised by estrogen deficiency; additionally, elevated emotional (i.e., nervousness) and emotional (i.e., changes (such as depression) that have a detrimental effect on women's quality of life also happen. These changes have been linked to the long-term loss of ovarian hormones, which are crucial for controlling a variety of physiological processes in the gastrointestinal, metabolic, and bone systems as well as emotional and affective states. Since the rat's ovaries are ablationed to produce all those systemic changes at the experimental level, this surgical manipulation has been deemed a suitable model for studying the medical changes that occur in women undergoing surgical menopause (Velázquez-Zamora et al., 2012).

In rats, the long-term absence of ovarian hormones produced by ovariectomy reduces GABAergic neurotransmission in diverse brain structures. It also produces a reduced sensitivity of the $GABA_A$, possibly associated with a reduced expression of mRNA of α^2 and α^3 subunits of this receptor. As mentioned above, this is important because the $GABA_A$ receptor is the action site of clinically effective anxiolytic drugs such as benzodiazepines; those molecular modifications in the $GABA_A$ receptor could explain the reduced effectiveness of anxiolytic pharmacological therapies in menopausal women (Vulink et al., 2006).

However, ovariectomies in rats result in decreased estrogen receptor α and β density in the hippocampus as well as decreased glutamate receptor activity in the basolateral amygdala. These neurochemical alterations are accompanied by an increase in anxiety-like behavior. The administration of an agonist that binds to glutamate receptors causes anxiolytic-like effects in rats that have had their ovaries removed, but this effect is contingent upon the presence of estrogens in the basolateral amygdala (Wallacea et al., 2006).

Similarly, monoaminergic neurotransmission that influences the synthesis and release of norepinephrine, dopamine, and serotonin in the brain is decreased in rats after ovariectomies. The presence of anxiety-like behavior has been linked to reduced monoaminergic neurotransmission in the accumbens nucleus and the hippocampus, while the administration of estrogenic compounds in rats that have had their ovaries removed causes anxiolytic-like effects that may be related to the reactivation of brain neurotransmission. According to some research, the reduced estrogen concentration in the brain linked to ovariectomy lowers tryptophan hydroxylase-2 activity, which in turn lowers serotonin availability and transportation in the dorsal raphe nucleus. On the other hand, giving estrogenic drugs to ovariectomized rats results in effects that resemble anxiety (Welty, 2003).

The rats that undergo ovariectomy and consequently lack ovarian hormones over an extended period of time are more susceptible to environmental stressors. In the elevated plus-maze, rats with long-term ovariectomies exposed to mild chronic stress exhibit more anxiety-like behavior than rats with short-term ovariectomy, suggesting that the frame time in the absence of ovarian hormones is a critical factor in stress response. Reduced cellular proliferation in the dentate gyrus and a decreased density of dendritic spines in CA1 pyramidal neurons are linked to ovariectomized rats' susceptibility to stress. These alterations in brain structure are hypothesized to be a component of the neurobiological basis for the modified stress response and increased susceptibility to emotional (i.e., nervousness) and emotional (i.e., disorders such as depression in women going through either surgical or natural menopause (Xu and Zhang, 2006).

The same emotional and affective changes that occur in women after surgical menopause have been studied in rats with a long-term absence of ovarian hormones induced by ovariectomy. Rats that undergo a 12-week ovariectomy exhibit more anxiety-like behavior than rats that undergo a 3-week ovariectomy. It is interesting to note that anxiolytic medications (i.e., diazepam), a few naturally occurring substances (i.e., phytosterols), or a plant extract (Montanoa tomentosa). The effects of four consecutive days of varying doses of isoflavone genistein (0.25, 0.5, and 1.0 mg/kg) were investigated in rats with long-term absence of ovarian hormones produced by ovariectomy. In the light/dark test, this treatment plan results in more explorations of an illuminated compartment and more explorations overall, indicating that it is a reliable model for screening medications for possible anxiolytic effects. These behavioral alterations in rats are suggestive of decreased anxiety-like behavior, which is seen in this experimental model during the evaluation of anxiolytic medications like diazepam. Fascinatingly, tamoxifen, a non-selective antagonist of the β-estradiol receptors, counteracts the anxiolytic-like effect caused by the isoflavone genistein (Yang et al., 2013). The previously mentioned information lends credence to the theory that isoflavones stimulate the β-estrogen receptor, which is crucial for the anxiolytic effects of synthetic estradiol and natural estradiol. Thus, these findings lend credence to the theory that phyto-estrogen may offer a therapeutic option for the natural treatment of anxiety disorders in women going through menopause. In support, clinical research has demonstrated that a daily dose of 34–100 mg of soy-derived isoflavones lowers the typical menopausal woman's symptomatology, which primarily consists of vasomotor issues. In additional research, menopausal women who receive isoflavones report fewer symptoms of anxiety and depression.

An early study examined the impact of an aqueous extract of Montanoa tomentosa on rats lacking ovarian hormones long-term. The results showed that acute administration of the extract significantly reduced anxiety-like behavior in rats tested using the elevated plus maze. These findings are particularly intriguing as the traditional use of this plant extract has been documented in ancient Mexican traditional medicine, as described in the Badianus Codex or Libellus de Medicinalibus Indorum Herbis (1552). This suggests the potential future use of this extract as a natural alternative to alleviate anxiety symptoms associated with hormonal changes.

According to the previously mentioned data, ovariectomy in rats results in long-term behavioral and physiological alterations that resemble the symptoms experienced by women who have undergone surgical menopause. This allows for the investigation of potential therapeutic options to be tested in an experimental setting to treat emotional and affective disorders linked to the long-term lack of ovarian hormones (Yazici et al., 2003).

A Closer Look

Luteinizing Hormone

Luteinizing hormone (LH) is a crucial component of the hypothalamic-pituitary-ovarian (HPO) axis, playing a central role in regulating the menstrual cycle and ovulation in women. Produced by the anterior pituitary gland, LH levels surge mid-cycle, triggering the release of a mature egg from the ovary (ovulation). This surge in LH is preceded by a rise in estrogen levels, which exert positive feedback on the hypothalamus, leading to increased secretion of gonadotropin-releasing hormone (GnRH) and subsequent LH release (Zhou et al., 2014).

Beyond its role in ovulation, LH also promotes the formation of the corpus luteum, a temporary endocrine structure that develops from the ruptured follicle after ovulation. The corpus luteum secretes progesterone, which helps prepare the uterine lining for implantation and supports early pregnancy. Therefore, LH plays a critical role in the menstrual cycle, fertility, and reproductive health. In addition to its effects on the ovaries, LH also influences hormone production in men. In males, LH stimulates the Leydig cells in the testes to produce testosterone, the primary male sex hormone, which is essential for spermatogenesis, libido, and overall reproductive function. Thus, LH is integral to the regulation of reproductive physiology and plays a pivotal role in maintaining fertility and hormonal balance in both men and women.

Summary

- Menopause, also known as the climacteric, is the time when menstrual periods permanently stop, marking the end of reproduction. It typically occurs between the ages of 45 and 55, although the exact timing can vary.
- It signifies the end of reproductive capacity and is characterized by the cessation of menstrual cycles due to hormonal changes, particularly a decline in estrogen production by the ovaries.
- Ovarian aging and hormonal decline are intrinsic components of the natural aging process in women, marking the gradual cessation of reproductive capacity and the onset of menopause.
- The hypothalamic-pituitary-ovarian (HPO) axis is a complex neuroendocrine system that plays a central role in regulating female reproductive function.
- Generalized anxiety disorder is one of the most common psychiatric disorders, affecting a high percentage of human beings around the world.
- Menopause is a stage of biological development in women that implies physiological, psychological, and social changes. During menopause, women are vulnerable to cognitive and physical impairment as well as psychiatric illnesses such as anxiety and depression.
- Reduced estrogen concentrations during menopause impact different biological systems, including the central nervous system. The psychiatric disorders most common during menopause include loss of motivation, lack of mental concentration, irritability, aggression, mood swings, mental tension, anxiety, and depression disorders.
- Surgical menopause in women is produced by ablation of the ovaries (oophorectomy) with or without the uterus, which produces a similar symptomatology to that observed in natural menopause, but with an increase in intensity.

References

1. Agosta, C., Atlante, M., & Benvenuti, C. (2011). Randomized controlled study on clinical efficacy of isoflavones plus *Lactobacillus sporogenes*, associated or not with a natural anxiolytic agent in menopause. *Minerva Ginecologica, 63*(1), 11–17.
2. American Psychiatric Association. (2000). *Diagnostic and Statistical Manual of Mental Disorders* (4th ed.). American Psychiatric Press.
3. Avis, N., Stellato, R., Crawford, S., Bromberger, J., Ganz, P., Cain, V., & Kagawa-Singer, M. (2001). Is there a menopausal syndrome? Menopausal status and symptoms across racial/ethnic groups. *Social Science & Medicine, 52*, 345–356.
4. Baeza, I., De Castro, N. M., Giménez-Llort, L., & De la Fuente, M. (2010). Ovariectomy, a model of menopause in rodents, causes a premature aging of the nervous and immune systems. *Journal of Neuroimmunology, 219*, 90–99.
5. Baksu, A., Ayas, B., Citak, S., Kalan, A., Baksu, B., & Goker, N. (2005). Efficacy of tibolone and transdermal estrogen therapy on psychological symptoms in women following surgical menopause. *International Journal of Gynecology & Obstetrics, 91*(1), 58–62.

6. Bromberger, J. T., Assmann, S. F., Avis, N. E., Schocken, M., Kravitz, H. M., & Cordal, A. (2003). Persistent mood symptoms in a multiethnic community cohort of pre- and perimenopausal women. *American Journal of Epidemiology, 158*(4), 347–356.

7. Bromberger, J. T., Kravitz, H. M., Chang, Y., Randolph, J. F., Jr., Avis, N. E., Gold, E. B., & Matthews, K. A. (2013). Does risk for anxiety increase during the menopausal transition? Study of Women's Health Across the Nation. *Menopause, 20*(5), 488–495.

8. Bryant, C., Judd, F. K., & Hickey, M. (2012). Anxiety during the menopausal transition: A systematic review. *Journal of Affective Disorders, 139*, 141–148.

9. Canonico, M., Oger, E., Plu-Bureau, G., Conard, J., Meyer, G., Lévesque, H., Trillot, N., Barrellier, M. T., Wahl, D., Emmerich, J., & Scarabin, P. Y. (2007). Hormone therapy and venous thromboembolism among postmenopausal women: Impact of the route of estrogen administration and progestogens: The ESTHER study. *Circulation, 115*(7), 840–845.

10. Carretti, N., Florio, P., Reis, F. M., Comai, S., Petraglia, F., & Costa, C. V. (2007). Menopause alters the metabolism of serum serotonin precursors and their correlation with gonadotropins and estradiol. *Climacteric, 10*(5), 393–399.

11. Charoenphandhu, J., Teerapornpuntakit, J., Nuntapornsak, A., Krishnamra, N., & Charoenphandhu, N. (2011). Anxiety-like behaviors and expression of SERT and TPH in the dorsal raphe of estrogen- and fluoxetine-treated ovariectomized rats. *Pharmacology, Biochemistry and Behavior, 98*, 503–510.

12. Chen, M. N., Lin, C. C., & Liu, C. F. (2014). Efficacy of phytoestrogens for menopausal symptoms: A meta-analysis and systematic review. *Climacteric, 1*, 1–10.

13. Chung-Park, M. (2005). Anxiety attacks following surgical menopause: A case report. *Holistic Nursing Practice, 5*, 236–240.

14. Daendee, S., Thongsong, B., & Kalandakanond-Thongsong, S. (2013). Effects of time of estrogen deprivation on anxiety-like behavior and GABAA receptor plasticity in ovariectomized rats. *Behavioral Brain Research, 246*, 86–93.

15. De Jesús-Burgos, M., Torres-Llenza, V., & Pérez-Acevedo, N. L. (2012). Activation of amygdalar metabotropic glutamate receptors modulates anxiety, and risk assessment behaviors in ovariectomized estradiol-treated female rats. *Pharmacology, Biochemistry and Behavior, 101*(3), 369–378.

16. Depypere, H. T., & Comhaire, F. H. (2014). Herbal preparations for the menopause: Beyond isoflavones and black cohosh. *Maturitas, 77*(2), 191–194.

17. Diz-Chaves, Y., Kwiatkowska-Naqvi, A., Von Hülst, P., Pernía, O., Carrero, P., & Garcia-Segura, L. M. (2012). Behavioral effects of estradiol therapy in ovariectomized rats depend on the age when the treatment is initiated. *Experimental Gerontology, 47*, 93–99.

18. Đoković, D. D., Jović, J. J., Đoković, J. D., Knežević, M. Ž., Djukić-Dejanović, S., & Ristić-Ignjatović, D. I. (2015). Effects of hormone replacement therapy on depressive and anxiety symptoms after oophorectomy. *Medicinski Glasnik (Zenica), 12*(1), 79–85.

19. Dornstauder, E., Jisa, E., Unterrieder, I., Krenn, L., Kubelka, W., & Jungbauer, A. (2001). Estrogenic activity of two standardized red clover extracts (Menoflavon) intended for large-scale use in hormone replacement therapy. *Journal of Steroid Biochemistry and Molecular Biology, 78*, 67–75.

20. Eckel, L. (2001). The ovarian hormone estradiol plays a crucial role in the control of food intake in female. *Physiology & Behavior, 105*, 517–524.

21. Erekson, E. A., Martin, D. K., & Ratner, E. S. (2013). Oophorectomy: The debate between ovarian conservation and elective oophorectomy. *Menopause, 20*(1), 110–114.

22. Espinosa, J., Neri, T., Orozco, S., Campos, M., & Guerra, C. (2012). Chronic administration of tibolone modulates anxiety-like behavior and enhances cognitive performance in ovariectomized rats. *Hormones and Behavior, 61*, 76–83.

23. Formoso, G., Perrone, E., Maltoni, S., Balduzzi, S., D'Amico, R., Bassi, C., Basevi, V., Marata, A. M., Magrini, N., & Maestri, E. (2012). Short and long-term effects of tibolone in postmenopausal women. *Cochrane Database of Systematic Reviews*, (2), CD008536.

24. Freeman, E. W., Sammel, M. D., Lin, H., Gracia, C. R., Kapoor, S., & Ferdousi, T. (2005). The role of anxiety and hormonal changes in menopausal hot flashes. *Menopause, 3*, 258–266.

25. Genazzani, A. R., Komm, B. S., & Pickar, J. H. (2015). Emerging hormonal treatments for menopausal symptoms. *Expert Opinion on Emerging Drugs, 5*, 1–16.

26. Glickman-Simon, R., & Lindsay, T. (2013). Yoga for back pain, cranberry for cystitis prevention, soy isoflavones for hot flashes, curcumin for pre-diabetes, and breathing retraining for asthma. *Explore (NY), 9*(4), 251–254.

27. Gong, P., Madak-Erdogan, Z., Li, J., Cheng, J., Greenlief, C. M., Helferich, W., Katzenellenbogen, J. A., & Katzenellenbogen, B. S. (2014). Transcriptomic analysis identifies gene networks regulated by estrogen receptor α (ERα) and ERβ that control distinct effects of different botanical estrogens. *Nuclear Receptor Signaling, 12*, e001.

28. González-Jiménez, E., Cañadas de la Fuente, G. A., Fernández-Castillo, R., Álvarez-Ferre, J., & González-Antón, C. (2010). Phytoestrogens and their effects on osteoporosis in postmenopausal women. *Revista Clínica de Medicina de Familia, 3*(3), 201–205.

29. Gupta, B., Mittal, P., Khuteta, R., & Bhargava, A. (2013). A comparative study of CEE, tibolone, and DHEA as hormone replacement therapy for surgical menopause. *Journal of Obstetrics and Gynaecology of India, 63*(3), 194–198.

30. Handley, A. P., & Williams, M. (2015). The efficacy and tolerability of SSRI/SNRIs in the treatment of vasomotor symptoms in menopausal women: A systematic review. *Journal of the American Association of Nurse Practitioners, 27*(1), 54–61.

31. Hanisch, L., Hantsoo, L., Freeman, E., Sullivan, G., & Coyne, J. (2008). Hot flashes and panic attacks: A comparison of symptomatology, neurobiology, treatment, and a role for cognition. *Psychological Bulletin, 134*, 247–269.

32. Hickey, M., Davis, S. R., & Sturdee, D. W. (2005). Treatment of menopausal symptoms: What shall we do now? *Lancet, 366*, 409–421.

33. Iglesias, C., Pato, E., Ocio, S., Ortigosa, J. C., Santamarina, S., Merino, M. J., Alonso, M. J., Fernández, L., Alonso, J. L., & Rodríguez, L. (2009). Treatment with venlafaxine extended release for climacteric women with depression or anxiety diagnosis: An open-label study. *Actas Españolas de Psiquiatria, 37*(3), 137–142.

34. Ishiwata, N., Melby, M. K., Mizuno, S., & Watanabe, S. (2009). New equal supplement for relieving menopausal symptoms: A randomized, placebo-controlled trial of Japanese women. *Menopause, 16*(1), 141–148.

35. Izumo, N., Ishibashi, Y., Ohba, M., Morikawa, T., & Manabe, T. (2012). Decreased voluntary activity and amygdala levels of serotonin and dopamine in ovariectomized rats. *Brain Research, 227*(1), 1–6.

36. Jafari, F., Hadizadeh, M. H., Zabihi, R., & Ganji, K. (2014). Comparison of depression, anxiety, quality of life, vitality, and mental health between premenopausal and postmenopausal women. *Climacteric, 17*(6), 660–665.

37. Jin, M., Jin, F., Zhang, L., Chen, Z., & Huang, H. (2005). Two estrogen replacement therapies differentially regulate expression of estrogen receptors alpha and beta in the hippocampus and cortex of ovariectomized rats. *Molecular Brain Research, 142*, 107–114.

38. Lambrinoudaki, I., Bouziou, G., Armeni, E., Spyropoulou, A., Koundi, K., Rizos, D., Augoulea, A., Alexandrou, A., Creatsa, M., Panoulis, C., Dendrinos, S., Leonadrou, A. A., & Zervas, I. M. (2015). Circulating androgens are associated with mood disturbances in young postmenopausal women. *Climacteric, 7*, 1–9.

39. Leiblum, S. R., Koochaki, P. E., Rodenberg, C. A., Barton, I. P., & Rosen, R. C. (2006). Hypoactive sexual desire disorder in postmenopausal women: US results from the Women's International Study of Health and Sexuality (WISHeS). *Menopause, 13*, 46–56.

40. Li, F., Yang, X., Yang, Y., Guo, C., Zhang, C., Zhonglin, Y., & Li, P. (2013). Antiosteoporotic activity of echinacoside in ovariectomized rats. *Phytomedicine, 20*, 549–557.

41. Lipovac, M., Chedraui, P., Gruenhut, C., Gocan, A., Stammler, M., & Imhof, M. (2010). Improvement of postmenopausal depressive and anxiety symptoms after treatment with isoflavones derived from red clover extracts. *Maturitas, 65*(3), 258–261.

42. McGregor, C., Sau, A., Ruddy, S. C., Leung, D., Webb, M., Durst, T., Wright, J. S., Lagace, D., & Pratt, C. (2014). Novel ligands balance estrogen receptor β and α agonism for safe and effective suppression of vasomotor response in the ovariectomized female rat of menopause. *Endocrinology, 155*, 2480–2491.

43. McLaughlin, K. J., Bimonte-Nelson, H., Neisewander, J. L., & Conrad, C. D. (2008). Assessment of estradiol influence on spatial tasks and hippocampal CA1 spines: Evidence that the duration of hormone deprivation after ovariectomy compromises 17β-estradiol effectiveness in altering CA1 spines. *Hormones and Behavior, 54*, 386–395.

44. Mendoza, N., Suárez, A. M., Álamo, F., Bartual, E., Vergara, F., & Herruzo, A. (2000). Lipid effects, effectiveness and acceptability of tibolone versus transdermic 17β-estradiol for hormonal replacement therapy in women with surgical menopause. *Maturitas, 37*, 37–43.

45. Moilanen, J., Aalto, A., Hemminki, E., Aro, A., Raitanen, J., & Luoto, R. (2010). Prevalence of menopause symptoms and their association with lifestyle among Finnish middle-aged women. *Maturitas, 67*, 358–374.

46. Nathorst-Böös, J., Flöter, A., Jarkander-Rolff, M., Carlström, K., & Schoultz, B. v. (2006). Treatment with percutaneous testosterone gel in postmenopausal women with decreased libido: Effects on sexuality and psychological general well-being. *Maturitas, 53*(1), 11–18.

47. Nissen, I., Estrada, F. S., Nava-Kopp, A. T., Irles, C., de-la-Peña-Díaz, A., Fernández-G, J. M., & Govezensky, T. (2012). Prolame ameliorates anxiety and spatial learning and memory impairment induced by ovariectomy in rats. *Physiology and Behavior, 106*(2), 278–284.

48. Pacchierotti, C., Castrogiovanni, A., Cavicchioli, C., Luisi, S., Morgante, G., De Leo, V., Petraglia,

F., & Castrogiovanni, P. (2004). Panic disorder in menopause: A case control study. *Maturitas, 48*, 147–154.

49. Pandaranandaka, J., Poonyachoti, S., & Kalandakanond-Thongsong, S. (2006). Anxiolytic property of estrogen related to the changes of the monoamine levels in various brain regions of ovariectomized rats. *Physiology and Behavior, 87*, 828–835.

50. Pandaranandaka, J., Poonyachoti, S., & Kalandakanond-Thongsong, S. (2009). Differential effects of the exogenous and endogenous estrogen on anxiety as measured by elevated T-maze in relation to the serotonergic system. *Behavioral Brain Research, 198*, 142–148.

51. Picazo, O., Estrada-Camarena, E., & Hernandez-Aragon, A. (2006). Influence of the post-ovariectomy time frame on the experimental anxiety and the behavioral actions of some anxiolytic agents. *European Journal of Pharmacology, 530*, 88–94.

52. Puga-Olguín, A., Germán-Ponciano, L. J., Rodríguez-Landa, J. F., Rovirosa-Hernández, M. J., Rivadeneyra-Domínguez, E., & Bernal-Morales, B. (2014). Efecto de la ovariectomía sobre los indicadores de ansiedad en la rata Wistar. In G. V. Vázquez, A. Martínez-García, C. E. Solano-Sosa, & M. E. Sánchez (Eds.), *XI Encuentro Participación de la Mujer en la Ciencia* (pp. 1–5). León, Guanajuato: Centro de Investigaciones en Óptica A.C.

53. Rocca, W. A., Grossardt, B. R., Geda, Y. E., Gostout, B. S., Bower, J. H., Maraganore, D. M., de Andrade, M., & Melton, L. J., 3rd. (2008). Long-term risk of depressive and anxiety symptoms after early bilateral oophorectomy. *Menopause, 156*, 1050–1059.

54. Rodríguez-Landa, J. F., Hernández-Figueroa, J. D., Hernández-Calderón, B. C., & Saavedra, M. (2009). Anxiolytic-like effect of phytoestrogen genistein in rats with long-term absence of ovarian hormones in the black and white model. *Progress in Neuro-Psychopharmacology and Biological Psychiatry, 33*(2), 367–372.

55. Rodríguez-Landa, J. F., Hernández-López, F., & Saavedra, M. (2012). Involvement of estrogen receptors in the anxiolytic-like effect of phytoestrogen genistein in rats with 12-weeks postovariectomy. *Pharmacology and Pharmacy, 3*(4), 439–446.

56. Rodríguez-Landa, J. F., Rodríguez-Santiago, M. G., Rovirosa-Hernández, M. J., García-Orduña, F., & Carro-Juárez, M. (2014). Aqueous crude extract of *Montanoa tomentosa* exerts anxiolytic-like effects in female rats with long-term absence of ovarian hormones. *Journal of Chemical, Biological and Physical Sciences, 4*(5), 37–46.

57. Rodríguez-Landa, J. F., Vicente-Serna, J., Rodríguez-Blanco, L. A., Rovirosa-Hernández, M. J., García-Orduña, F., & Carro-Juárez, M. (2014). *Montanoa frutescens* and *Montanoa grandiflora* extracts reduce anxiety-like behavior during the metestrus-diestrus phase of the ovarian cycle in Wistar rats. *BioMed Research International*, Article ID 938060.

58. Russo, R., & Corosu, R. (2003). The clinical use of a preparation based on phyto-oestrogens in the treatment of menopausal disorders. *Acta Biomedica, 74*(3), 137–143.

59. Smoller, J. W., Pollack, M. H., Wassertheil-Smoller, S., Jackson, R., Oberman, A., Wong, N., & Sheps, D. (2007). Panic attacks and risk of incident cardiovascular events among postmenopausal women in the Women's Health Initiative Observational Study. *Archives of General Psychiatry, 64*, 1153–1160.

60. Smoller, J. W., Pollack, M. H., Wassertheil-Smoller, S., Barton, B., Hendrix, S. L., Jackson, R. D., Dicken, T., Oberman, A., & Sheps, D. S. (2003). Prevalence and correlates of panic attacks in

postmenopausal women. *Archives of Internal Medicine, 163*, 2041–2047.

61. Somunkiran, A., Erel, C. T., Demirci, F., & Senturk, M. L. (2007). The effect of tibolone versus 17β-estradiol on climacteric symptoms in women with surgical menopause: A randomized, cross-over study. *Maturitas, 56*(1), 61–68.

62. Taku, K., Melby, M. K., Kronenberg, F., Kurzer, M. S., & Messina, M. (2012). Extracted or synthesized soybean isoflavones reduce menopausal hot flash frequency and severity: Systematic review and meta-analysis of randomized controlled trials. *Menopause, 19*(7), 776–790.

63. Tangen, T., & Mykletun, A. (2008). Depression and anxiety through the climacteric period: An epidemiological study (HUNT II). *Journal of Psychosomatic Obstetrics & Gynecology, 29*, 125–131.

64. Tominaga, K., Yamauchi, A., Shuto, H., Niizeki, M., Makino, K., Oishi, R., & Kataoka, Y. (2001). Ovariectomy aggravates convulsions and hippocampal gamma-aminobutyric acid inhibition induced by cyclosporin A in rats. *European Journal of Pharmacology, 430*, 243–249.

65. Uguz, F., Sahingoz, M., Gezginc, K., & Karatayli, R. (2010). Obsessive-compulsive disorder in postmenopausal women: Prevalence, clinical features, and comorbidity. *Australian and New Zealand Journal of Psychiatry, 44*(2), 183–187.

66. Velázquez-Zamora, D. A., González-Tapia, D., González-Ramírez, M. M., Flores-Soto, M. E., Vázquez-Valls, E., Cervantes, M., & González-Burgos, I. (2012). Plastic changes in dendritic spines of hippocampal CA1 pyramidal neurons from ovariectomized rats after estradiol treatment. *Brain Research, 1470*, 1–10.

67. Vulink, N. C., Denys, D., Bus, L., & Westenberg, H. G. (2006). Female hormones affect symptom severity in obsessive-compulsive disorder. *International Clinical Psychopharmacology, 21*, 171–177.

68. Wallace, M., Luine, V., Arellanos, A., & Frankfurt, A. (2006). Ovariectomized rats show decreased recognition memory and spine density in the hippocampus and prefrontal cortex. *Brain Research, 1126*, 176–182.

69. Welty, F. K. (2003). Alternative hormone replacement regimens: Is there a need for further clinical trials? *Current Opinion in Lipidology, 14*(6), 585–591.

70. Wittchen, H. U., Kessler, R. C., Beesdo, K., Krause, P., Höfler, M., & Hoyer, J. (2002). Generalized anxiety and depression in primary care: Prevalence, recognition, and management. *The Journal of Clinical Psychiatry, 63*(8), 24–34.

71. Xu, X., & Zhang, Z. (2006). Effects of estradiol benzoate on learning-memory behavior and synaptic structure in ovariectomized mice. *Life Sciences, 79*, 1553–1560.

72. Yang, S. G., Mlcek, M., & Kittnar, O. (2013). Estrogen can modulate menopausal women's heart rate variability. *Physiology Research, 62*, 165–171.

73. Yazici, K., Pata, O., Yazici, A., Aklas, A., Tot, S., & Kanik, A. (2003). The effects of hormone replacement therapy in menopause on symptoms of anxiety and depression. *Turk Psikiyatri Dergisi, 14*(2), 101–105.

74. Zhou, B., Xie, S., Hu, J., Sun, X., Guan, H., & Deng, Y. (2014). Paroxetine increased the serum estrogen in postmenopausal women with depressive and anxiety symptoms. *Open Journal of Depression, 3*, 184–194.

Chapter 3

CLINICAL MANIFESTATIONS AND DIAGNOSIS PROCESS

Contents

Introduction

Menopause presents with a spectrum of symptoms that vary in severity and duration among women. Vasomotor symptoms, including hot flashes and night sweats, are among the most common and distressing complaints reported during the perimenopausal and postmenopausal periods. These sudden, transient episodes of heat and sweating can disrupt sleep, affect mood, and interfere with daily activities. Diagnosing menopause relies primarily on clinical criteria and does not always necessitate laboratory testing (Adler et al., 1993). The diagnosis is established based on a woman's medical history, symptoms, and the absence of menstrual periods for 12 consecutive months. A thorough medical history includes inquiries about menstrual patterns, reproductive history, and the presence of menopausal symptoms. Physical examination may reveal signs of estrogen deficiency, such as vaginal atrophy, skin changes, and decreased bone density. Laboratory tests, including hormone levels (e.g., follicle-stimulating hormone and estradiol), may be performed to support the diagnosis, although they are not always necessary (Alexander et al., 2010).

Orientation and Directional Terms

Term	Definition	Illustration
Vasomotor	Vasomotor refers to actions upon a blood vessel which alter its diameter. More specifically, it can refer to vasodilator action and vasoconstrictor action.	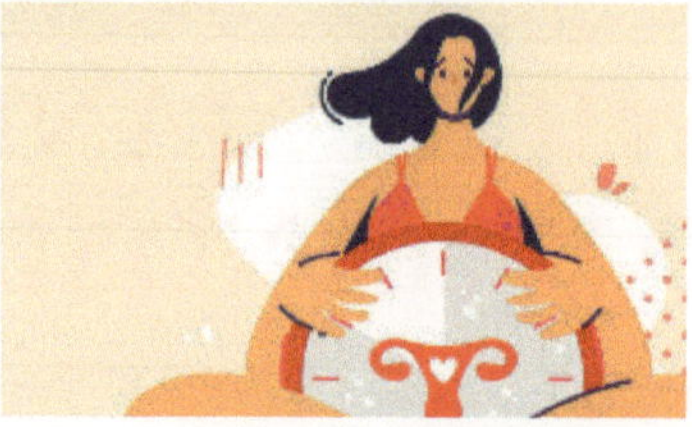
Sex Hormone Binding Globulin (SHBG)	Sex hormone binding globulin (SHBG) is a protein in your blood that binds certain hormones. It's produced in the liver and—in smaller amounts—in the testes.	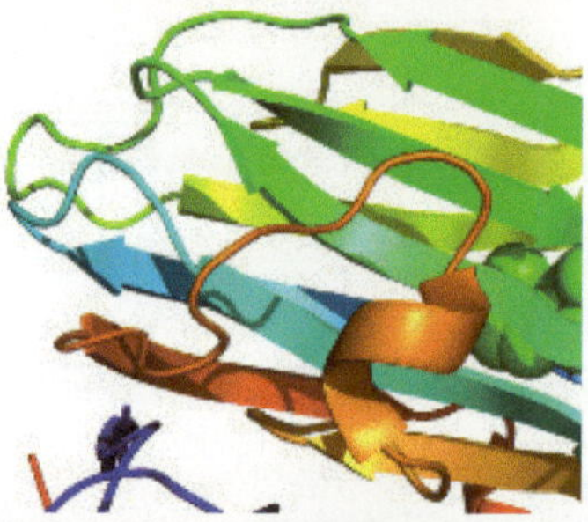
Adipose Tissue	Adipose tissue (also known as body fat or simply fat) is a loose connective tissue composed mostly of adipocytes. It also contains the stromal vascular fraction (SVF) of cells including preadipocytes, fibroblasts, vascular endothelial cells and a variety of immune cells such as adipose tissue macrophages.	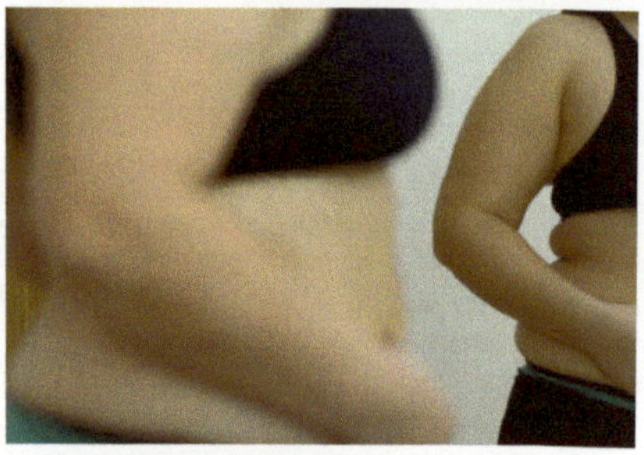
Polysomnogram (PSG)	A polysomnogram (PSG) is a procedure that utilizes electroencephalogram, electro-oculogram, electromyogram, electrocardiogram, and pulse oximetry, as well as airflow and respiratory effort, to evaluate for underlying causes of sleep disturbances.	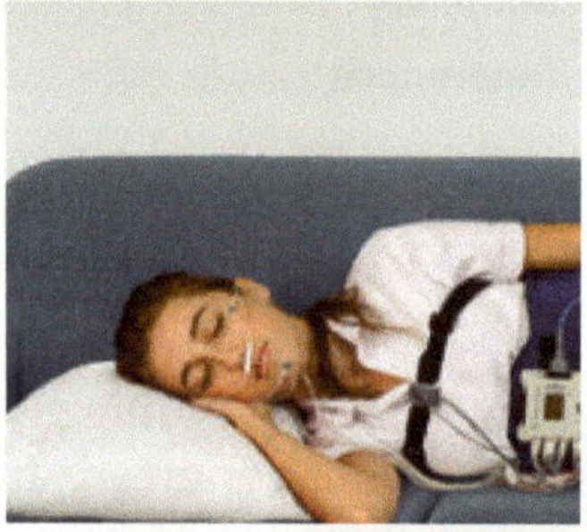
Vaginal Atrophy	Vaginal atrophy (atrophic vaginitis) is thinning, drying and inflammation of the vaginal walls that may occur when your body has less estrogen. Vaginal atrophy occurs most often after menopause.	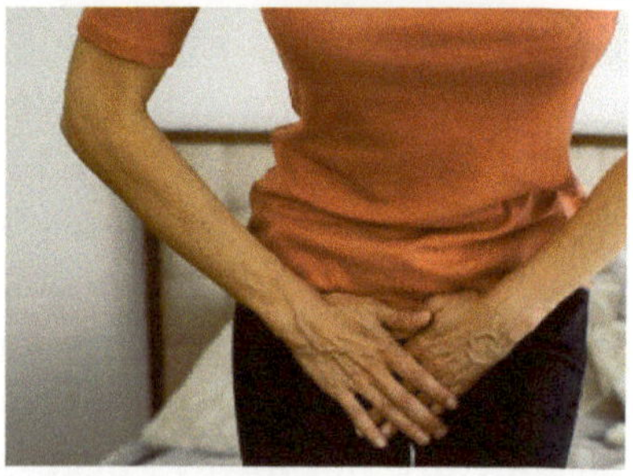

3.1. Vasomotor Symptoms

Vasomotor symptoms are common in women during or shortly after menopause. Primary menopausal symptoms, such as hot flashes and night sweats, can also be linked to mood and sleep disorders, reduced cognitive function, and other issues (Anderson, 1999). A substantial reduction in overall quality of life can result from social impairment and work-related challenges caused by any of these symptoms. The frequency and intensity of hot flashes in women have been found to vary widely. Hot flashes can linger for several months in some women and over a decade in others. Night sweats in particular, however, typically start in perimenopause. Traditionally, vasomotor symptoms were reported to start 5 to 10 years before the end of the last menstrual cycle, corresponding with the first decline in circulating gonadal hormones. Although the exact cause of hot flushes is still unknown, it is believed that altered homeostatic thermoregulatory mechanisms involving estrogen and neurotransmitters—specifically, norepinephrine and serotonin—play a significant role in the pathogenesis of these events (Archer, 2010).

Vasomotor symptoms related to menopause have substantial direct and indirect costs. The entire cost of using conventional medication or complementary and alternative medicine modalities, such as over-the-counter medications and dietary supplements, to treat vasomotor symptoms associated with menopause is high and includes both the initial and follow-up doctor visits as well as phone calls. Laboratory testing, handling unfavorable events, lost productivity at work, and other personal and incidental expenses are additional expenses (Avis et al., 2009). Hormonal therapy for menopause-associated vasomotor symptoms is generally considered to be cost-effective, as pharmacoeconomic analyzes, including those that take into account the risks identified by the Women's Health Initiative, have been the mainstay for the management of these symptoms for more than 50 years. However, there is a need for more targeted therapies that are safe, effective, affordable, and well-tolerated by symptomatic menopausal women, as many women today prefer to avoid hormone therapy. These needs have been validated by the findings of controlled clinical trials (Barnabei et al., 2005).

3.1.1. Definition and Epidemiology of VMS

Hot flashes and night sweats, or VMS, are frequently regarded as the hallmark signs of menopause. Episodes of intense heat, along with perspiration and flushing, are known as VMS, and they usually affect the head, neck, chest, and upper back. Most women go through VMS when going through the menopausal transition (Barnabei et al., 2002). In SWAN, prevalence rates of VMS vary by racial/ethnic group and affect 60–80% of women at some point during the menopausal transition. The late perimenopause and early postmenopausal years, or the years following the last menstrual period, are when the incidence and frequency of VMS peak, according to SWAN research. Nonetheless, a considerable minority of women report VMS well into their 60s and 70s, decades after the menopause transition, and earlier in midlife, before the onset of menstrual cycle changes, according to research from a variety of studies (Beerepoot et al., 2013). Given the frequency and duration of VMS in women in their midlife, it is imperative to comprehend the biology underlying this symptom, the degree to which VMS may degrade quality of life, and whether or not VMS may act as a marker for other significant health issues (Gold et al., 2006).

3.1.2. Physiology of VMS

3.1.2.1. Reproductive Hormones

Although the exact physiology of hot flashes is unknown, it is most likely the result of interactions between several central and peripheral physiologic systems. The fact that the onset of VMS coincides with the significant changes in reproductive hormones associated with the menopausal transition and that exogenous estrogen plays a therapeutic role in treating them suggests that reproductive hormones are probably important. Endogenous hormone levels are linked to VMS, according to SWAN analyzes. Every year, SWAN participants (N=3,302) gave a blood sample for the measurement of estradiol (E2), follicle stimulating hormone (FSH), testosterone (T), dehydroepiandrosterone sulfate (DHEAS), and sex hormone binding globulin (SHBG) (Bolanos et al., 2010). They also reported on their experience with VMS during the previous two weeks. When both hormones were taken into account separately, only higher FSH levels were linked to VMS, but when both hormones were taken into account together, higher FSH and lower E2 were associated with a greater likelihood of reporting VMS (over a 5-year period) (Randolph et al., 2005).

A subgroup of SWAN women (N=742) also took part in the SWAN Daily Hormone Study, which involved yearly urine collection for the measurement of urinary FSH, luteinizing hormone (LH), the progesterone metabolite pregnanediol glucuronide (PdG), and estrone conjugates (E1C) for a menstrual cycle (or a comparable period of time for women without menstrual cycles). During this period, women additionally finished a daily VMS diary (Brown et al., 1999). The results of this analysis, which included women with evidence of impaired ovulatory activity, were comparable to those found in the full cohort. A higher FSH and a lower E1C were linked to a higher probability of reporting VMS. Higher PdG levels were the only hormone linked to VMS in women who seemed to be ovulatory, and they did not exhibit this pattern. When combined, these results suggest that VMS reporting is linked to lower levels of estrogen and higher levels of FSH, especially in women who have anovulatory cycles. Not all perimenopausal women have VMS, despite the fact that all of them undergo these hormonal changes. Thus, other physiological systems besides the reproductive axis must be involved (Brown et al., 2001).

3.1.2.2. Thermoregulatory

Prominent models describe VMS as thermoregulatory heat dissipation events, at least partially. The thermoneutral zone, or the range in which core body temperature is maintained without inducing thermoregulatory homeostatic mechanisms like sweating or shivering, may have shrunk in some symptomatic postmenopausal women. Therefore, in women who experience symptoms, even slight changes in core body temperature have the potential to rise above this range and set off heat-dissipating processes like perspiration and peripheral vasodilation (i.e., a blazing flash). This model is strengthened by research showing that the administration of E2 decreases VMS and expands the thermoneutral zone (Casper and Yen, 1985). More research is required, even though this model is supported by some empirical data. The central serotonergic, noradrenergic, opioid, adrenal, and autonomic systems, as well as vascular processes, are other systems linked to the genesis of hot flashes; however, there is insufficient data to definitively explain their involvement (Chae et al., 2014).

3.1.2.3. Genetics

The goal of SWAN and other research has been to define the relationships between genetic polymorphisms and VMS. Thus far, variations in the estrogen receptor (ER) and specific single nucleotide polymorphisms (SNPs) of genes related to the synthesis and metabolism of various estrogens (i.e., estriol, E2, and estrone) have been investigated (Chen et al., 2013). In the various racial/ethnic groups examined in SWAN (n=1,538), it has been discovered that variations in genes encoding for ER alpha and in enzymes involved in the synthesis of and conversion between more and less potent estrogens predict the likelihood of VMS. Similar results have been observed in other studies examining SNPs involved in the synthesis and metabolism of estrogens as well as ER alpha, despite some discrepancies between the findings (Cody et al., 2012). After controlling for other significant contributing factors, such as levels of reproductive hormones, these associations typically remain. Because a large number of women from various racial/ethnic minority groups were included in the SWAN analysis, the results add significantly to our understanding of gene/VMS associations, given the established variability in genetic polymorphisms between race/ethnic groups. When combined, these findings imply that polymorphisms that change the activity of sex steroid hormones may be the cause of the association between VMS and genetic polymorphisms. It is unclear, nevertheless, if these genetic factors have a central effect on the brain or a peripheral one on the vasculature, autonomic nervous system, or other systems that might be involved in the development of VMS (Malacara et al., 2004).

3.1.3. Risk Factors for VMS

3.1.3.1. Race/Ethnicity

There are noticeable racial/ethnic differences in VMS. The majority of VMS reports came from African American women, out of the five racial/ethnic groups examined in SWAN. Even after accounting for the higher-than-average number of VMS reports from African American women, all women continued to describe their VMS as bothersome (Constantine et al., 2015). The rates of VMS reporting among SWAN's Caucasian and Hispanic female participants are relatively comparable. SWAN has observed significant variation among the various ethnic groups of Hispanic women, with women from Central America reporting the highest rates of VMS and women from Cuba reporting the lowest rates. Japanese women in SWAN are the least likely to report VMS and to characterize them as bothersome, compared to Chinese women (Crandall et al., 2006).

There are probably many different and poorly understood causes for these racial and ethnic disparities. Racial/ethnic disparities in VMS in SWAN continue even after adjusting for major variables linked to VMS, such as BMI, E2 levels, smoking, hormone use, and socioeconomic status, which exhibit notable racial/ethnic variation (Crandall et al., 2010). Some have proposed that Asian women's relatively high soy intake accounts for their lower VMS levels compared to Caucasian women. This does not seem to be the case in SWAN, though, which is in line with findings from randomized controlled trials that have yielded conflicting or ambiguous results when it comes to the application of soy or isoflavones for the treatment of VMS. Furthermore, a variety of perceptual and reporting processes influence the experience and reporting of any physical symptom, including VMS, making them complex. It's possible that cultural differences in how women perceive, understand, categorize, and report VMS to others contribute to the observed racial/ethnic disparities in VMS (Crawford, 2007).

3.1.3.2. Obesity

Obesity is a major risk factor for VMS. Due to the fact that body fat contains androgens that are aromatized into estrogens, it was long believed that obesity offered protection against VMS. Because adipose tissue contains higher levels of estrogen, one would expect that women with more of it would have a lower risk of VMS. Obesity may be a risk factor for VMS during the perimenopause and early postmenopause rather than a protective factor, according to SWAN and other large observational studies (den Tonkelaar et al., 1996). In SWAN (N=3,302), for instance, women who reported no or infrequent VMS had an average BMI of 28 kg/m^2, while women who reported at least six VMS days in the previous two weeks had an average BMI of 31 kg/m^2. Even after accounting for associated risk variables, there was still a correlation between higher BMI and VMS. A thermoregulatory model of VMS, in which adipose tissue functions as an insulator, preventing the heat-dissipating action of VMS and so increasing their occurrence or severity, is more consistent with the findings of positive associations between BMI and VMS (Freedman et al., 2002). The exact mechanisms underlying the connections between obesity and VMS are unknown, but they could involve other physiological processes or even the potential involvement of adipose tissue's other endocrine functions. Furthermore, women who are earlier in the menopausal transition may benefit most from the positive associations found between obesity and VMS (e.g., during the early stages of the postmenopausal phase (Sabia et al., 2008).

The analytical methods employed to investigate the relationship between obesity and VMS mainly rely on calculated BMI, which includes both lean and fat mass. As a result, it is not possible to identify the relative contributions of lean and fat mass as VMS predictors (Freedman and Krell, 1999). It is critical to comprehend the precise relationship between adiposity and VMS, as the thermoregulatory characteristics or endocrine products of adipose tissue may contribute to VMS risk. SWAN analyzes have used three different methods to look at the relationship between adiposity and VMS. In the first of these studies, adiposity was assessed using bioelectrical impedance analysis (BIA) (N=1,776), which provides measurements of lean and fat mass (Freedman et al., 1992). Once confounding variables like reproductive hormones, smoking, race/ethnicity, education, and negative affect were taken into account, a higher overall percentage of body fat—but not lean mass—was linked to a higher risk of VMS. Abdominal adiposity measured by computed tomography (CT) was used in a second SWAN analysis (N=461). Subcutaneous adiposity, or the fat between the skin and the abdominal muscle wall, and visceral adiposity, or the fat behind the abdominal muscle wall and in the peritoneal space surrounding the organs, are two measures of total abdominal fat that can be obtained from CT scans. Notably, fat under the skin acts as an especially good insulator. The findings showed that there was a correlation between a higher risk of hot flashes and abdominal obesity, specifically subcutaneous adiposity. Neither confounding variables nor reproductive hormones (FSH and E2) could explain these associations. In the end, a third SWAN analysis made use of BIA measures over a four-year period to examine how adiposity changed over time in relation to VMS (N=1,659). Considering that weight gain is typical in midlife, this analysis is especially pertinent. The results showed that increases in body fat from one year to the next were linked to a higher risk of VMS at the follow-up visit, compared to women who maintained stable body fat. Confounding variables and variations in reproductive hormone levels had no effect on these associations. All of these results point to the possibility that obesity increased the risk of VMS in women who were perimenopausal or just entering the postmenopausal stage. This finding is in line with the theories of thermoregulatory VMS and endocrine VMS (Freeman et al., 2001).

3.1.3.3. Health Behaviors

Particular attention has been paid to the possible involvement of health behaviors in VMS. Smoking is one of the health behaviors linked to VMS that is most frequently observed. Over the course of a six-year follow-up period in SWAN, current smokers were more likely than nonsmokers to report VMS by over 60%, even after accounting for confounding variables like education, BMI, menopausal status, and race/ethnicity (Freeman et al., 2005). Actually, the SWAN results indicate that there is a higher chance of VMS in both active smoking and passive smoke exposure. It has been suggested that smoking's anti-estrogenic properties account for the link between smoking and VMS. Evidence from SWAN, however, contradicts this theory, showing that variations in endogenous E2 levels were not responsible for the correlation between smoking and VMS (Gold et al., 2004).

Significantly weaker correlations have been found between VMS and other noteworthy health behaviors, such as diet and physical activity. After adjusting for confounding variables like education, smoking, and BMI, dietary factors like total calories, fat, fiber, caffeine, alcohol intake, or specific vitamin intake have not been linked to VMS in SWAN (Gold et al., 2007). While early reports suggested that the isoflavone genistein was beneficial for VMS, subsequent longitudinal analyzes did not find this association. Physical activity is another behavior that is particularly relevant to health. In SWAN and other studies, physical activity has also not been consistently linked to VMS after controlling for confounding variables. It is noteworthy that physical activity may play two roles in relation to VMS: on the one hand, it may improve VMS by positively influencing body weight and mood, and on the other hand, it may increase VMS by acutely raising core body temperature. Taken as a whole, these SWAN studies indicate that smoking is the health behavior most obviously linked to VMS, while diet and exercise have considerably weaker or erratic relationships with VMS (Gold et al., 2000).

3.1.3.4. Negative Affect

Investigation after investigation has consistently linked VMS to affective state (negative mood). Higher levels of stress, anxiety, and depressive symptoms at study entry have been linked to a higher chance of VMS occurring over the next six years in SWAN (N=3302). In fact, studies like SWAN and others have shown that anxiety is the psychological factor most consistently linked to hot flashes (Green et al., 2010). Not only do women with higher negative affect experience more frequent and occurrences of VMS, but even after controlling for frequency, they also tend to perceive their VMS as more bothersome. The intricate interactions between physiological and psychological elements may play a role in the relationships between negative affect and VMS, which are not entirely understood. Negative affect has been shown to have an impact on symptom reporting, with an increased propensity to report symptoms when negative affect is present (Greendale and Gold et al., 2005). For instance, women may report VMS more frequently if they are generally more sensitive to physical symptoms. Studies utilizing physiological hot flash monitors have substantiated the significance of negative effects in hot flash reporting, indicating a higher probability of hot flash reporting when no physiological detection of the hot flash occurs. But since VMS also affects mood, there is a reciprocal relationship between negative affect and VMS (Thurston et al., 2005).

3.1.3.5. Other Social and Demographic Factors

There are numerous additional social and psychological factors that have been linked to a higher risk of VMS. The SWAN population has a high prevalence of child abuse and neglect, which is linked to several detrimental physical and mental health outcomes (Grimaldi et al., 2012). VMS is not an exemption. Even after adjusting for several variables, such as negative affect, sociodemographic characteristics, and health behaviors, women who acknowledged a history of child abuse or neglect (38% of the sample evaluated) were still more likely to report VMS during the menopausal transition. Low socioeconomic status is a significant sociodemographic risk factor for VMS. Compared to their counterparts in higher socioeconomic positions, women in lower socioeconomic positions are more likely to report VMS (Hendrix et al., 2005). These women may include those with lower incomes, educational attainments, or endorsements of difficulties paying for necessities. It is unclear why socioeconomic status and VMS are related, despite this association being seen in several research studies. A lower socioeconomic status is more prevalent in some minority racial/ethnic groups and is linked to smoking, a higher BMI, a higher perceived stress level, and a higher negative affect. Nevertheless, in SWAN, none of these potentially confounding factors could explain the association between low socioeconomic position and VMS. It is noteworthy that several social, psychological, and physiological processes are probably at play when it comes to the impact of early exposures, such as child abuse, or low socioeconomic status on health. This makes it difficult to explain these associations with a particular set of midlife assessments (Hong et al., 2012).

3.1.4. Associated Quality-of-Life Symptoms

SWAN has looked into the relationship between VMS and important quality-of-life outcomes that VMS presence may have an impact on. Sleep, mood, and cognitive function are a few of these. Menopause stage was not linked to HRQL, but VMS has been strongly associated in SWAN analyzes with lower health-related quality-of-life (HRQL) (Hyde et al., 2004). Those with more frequent VMS have a stronger negative correlation between HRQL and VMS.

3.1.4.1. Sleep

In cross-sectional analyzes, longitudinal studies that track women annually throughout the menopausal transition, and daily diary studies that capture a more detailed pattern of the close association between reported VMS and sleep problems, SWAN results have demonstrated strong associations between VMS and perceived sleep disturbance (Hyun et al., 2010). VMS has been linked to all aspects of perceived sleep disruption, such as difficulty falling asleep, difficulty staying asleep, and difficulty waking up early in the morning, that lead to poor sleep continuity and quality. Even after adjusting for other significant predictive variables, VMS reporting consistently appears to be a factor that leads to reports of poor sleep. These findings align with a plethora of other research studies that have reported a strong correlation between reported VMS and subjective sleep disturbance (Johnston et al., 2004). A large amount of data from the SWAN Sleep Study will be used to investigate the relationship between VMS and objectively measured sleep using polysomnography (PSG). Given the more contentious body of existing literature on the relationship between VMS and objectively measured sleep parameters, results of ongoing analyzes pertaining to the relationship between VMS and PSG-measured sleep are eagerly awaited (Kim et al., 2015).

3.1.4.2. Mood

VMS and mood seem to be connected in a variety of possibly intricate ways. Studies like SWAN, which demonstrate that high levels of depressive symptoms and clinically significant depression are most common during the perimenopause and early postmenopause, when VMS are most prevalent, provide preliminary evidence for links between VMS and depression (Kingsberg et al.,

2013). According to SWAN and other studies, perimenopausal women with VMS are also more likely than perimenopausal women without VMS to experience depression after the onset of VMS. However, these findings may be explained by other variables linked to depressive episodes, such as stressful life events and a history of anxiety disorders (Lethaby et al., 2007).

Research has revealed that VMS can occur concurrently with depression as well as before and after it, suggesting that there could be several distinct causal pathways explaining the relationship between VMS and depression. VMS can cause mood disturbance when depression co-occurs or follows, as it can disrupt sleep, a major risk factor for depression. On the other hand, VMS could be a preliminary symptom of brain system disruptions that also underpin depression (Levine et al., 2008). The possibility that central nervous system processes contribute to both VMS and depression vulnerability is raised by indirect evidence that suggests the etiology of VMS may involve the serotonergic and noradrenergic systems, neurotransmitter systems frequently associated with depression (Link et al., 1995).

But a lot of women with VMS don't have depression. It appears that neither condition is necessary for the other symptom to appear, as evidenced by the findings that depression occurs in midlife women without VMS and that VMS occurs in the absence of depression. To determine the causal relationship between these two prevalent midlife symptoms, more research is necessary (Lobo et al., 2009).

3.1.4.2. Cognitive Function

SWAN analyzes (n=2362) have demonstrated a transient decline in cognitive function during the perimenopause, characterized by a reduction in learning capacity that then disappears as postmenopausal women enter the stage (Luthje et al., 2014). It has been determined by additional SWAN analyzes (n=1903) that VMS is not responsible for this temporary decline. These results are in line with those of a few other, smaller studies (not all of them), which similarly found no correlation between verbal memory performance and VMS when VMS are assessed through self-report. Conversely, research that measures VMS objectively demonstrates an inverse relationship between VMS and cognitive function, indicating that the physiologic alterations that underlie VMS may be directly and centrally related to cognitive function (Michnovicz et al., 1986).

3.1.5. Emerging Links Between VMS and Disease Outcomes

Traditionally, VMS have not been thought to have any particular effects on physical health; instead, they have been seen as a significant quality of life concern during the menopausal transition. However, new findings from SWAN and other studies are starting to challenge this presumption (Mirkin and Komm, 2013).

3.1.5.1. Cardiovascular Risk

Th0ere may be a connection between VMS and the risk of cardiovascular disease (CVD), according to preliminary findings from several significant hormone therapy trials, such as the Women's Health Initiative (WHI) and the Heart and Estrogen Replacement Study (HERS). In both trials, women with moderate to severe VMS at study entry and older VMS-afflicted women in WHI had the highest increased risk of coronary heart disease events linked to hormone therapy use (Nappi et al., 2013). We have investigated possible connections between VMS and CVD in SWAN as a follow-up to these preliminary findings. The majority of this research has been carried out in the framework of the SWAN Heart Study (N=588), an ancillary study to SWAN that gathered data on multiple measures of subclinical CVD, such as carotid intima media thickness (IMT), a well-established marker of atherosclerosis, coronary artery and aortic calcification, measures of calcified plaques in these arterial beds, and brachial artery flow mediated dilation, a marker of endothelial dysfunction (Nappi et al., 2012). Since all three of these subclinical CVD measures have been prospectively linked to higher rates of cardiovascular events in people without clinical CVD, they are helpful in understanding the risk for CVD among those who do not have the disease. The results showed that women with hot flashes had worse endothelial function, more aortic calcification, and higher IMT than women without hot flashes. In the case of IMT, these findings were especially true for women who reported having hot flashes more frequently. Even after adjusting for confounding demographic variables, other established cardiovascular risk factors and E2 levels, these associations remained. The results for hot flashes and night sweats were comparable, albeit somewhat lessened. Significant correlations were found between IMT and hot flashes in women who were overweight or obese, as well as in those who had hot flashes during multiple annual visits. These findings suggest that persistent hot flashes and those who have other CVD risk factors, like obesity, may provide the most information about the risk of CVD. More research and explanation are needed to determine the exact causes and characteristics of the relationship between VMS and CVD risk. Nonetheless, one possible interpretation of these results is that a woman's vasculature may be adversely changing beneath the surface, causing her to experience hot flashes as a symptom (Nappi et al., 2010).

3.1.5.2. Bone Health

VMS and bone turnover as well as bone mineral density have been related in recent research from SWAN and other studies (Nappi et al., 2014). Women reporting VMS had lower bone mineral density in the first of these SWAN analyzes (N=2213). All of the sample's menopausal women showed this association, but postmenopausal women showed it most strongly. Specific bone site studies revealed different associations between VMS and bone mineral density; these were most noticeable in postmenopausal women at the lumbar spine and hip, and in women who were earlier in the menopausal transition at the femoral neck (Nelson et al., 2006). The incidence of VMS was further investigated in connection to urinary N-telopeptide, a highly sensitive indicator of bone turnover, in a second set of SWAN analyzes (N= 2283). According to these analyzes, women with VMS who were postmenopausal or perimenopausal had higher urinary N-telopeptide levels (a measure of bone turnover) than women without VMS. After adjusting for possible confounders, associations were found in both analyzes of bone turnover and density; however, some of these associations were still explained by E2 and FSH levels. Additional research is necessary to determine the possible causes of associations between VMS and bone health, including an examination of the sympathetic nervous system and the hypothalamic-pituitary-adrenal axis. These findings, however, imply that VMS might be a significant marker of a component of ovarian function decline that is not indicated by variations in the menstrual cycle or yearly levels of reproductive hormones (Crandall et al., 2010).

3.2. Urogenital Symptoms of Menopause

One of the most distressing sets of symptoms associated with menopause is urogenital symptoms, which affect the urinary and genital systems. These symptoms are largely attributed to the decline in estrogen levels and can lead to conditions such as vaginal atrophy, urinary incontinence, and recurrent urinary tract infections.

3.2.1. Anatomy and Physiology of the Urogenital Tract

To understand the urogenital symptoms of menopause, it is essential to have a basic understanding of the anatomy and physiology of the urogenital tract. The urogenital system includes the urinary and genital organs, which are closely linked anatomically and functionally (Pinkerton et al., 2014).

- **The Urinary Tract:** The urinary tract comprises the kidneys, ureters, bladder, and urethra. Estrogen receptors are present in the bladder and urethra, and estrogen plays a crucial role in maintaining the health and function of these tissues (Portman et al., 2013). It helps maintain the mucosal lining, supports blood flow, and influences the function of the smooth muscles in the bladder and urethra.
- **The Genital Tract:** The genital tract includes the vagina, cervix, uterus, and external genitalia. Estrogen is vital for maintaining the elasticity, thickness, and lubrication of the vaginal and vulvar tissues. It also helps maintain the acidic pH of the vagina, which protects against infections by maintaining a healthy balance of the vaginal microbiota (Portman et al., 2014).

3.2.2. Decline in Estrogen and Its Effects

The decline in estrogen levels during menopause leads to various structural and functional changes in the urogenital tract, contributing to the development of urogenital symptoms.

- **Vaginal Atrophy:** One of the most common urogenital symptoms of menopause is vaginal atrophy, also known as atrophic vaginitis. This condition is characterized by the thinning, drying, and inflammation of the vaginal walls due to the decreased levels of estrogen. Vaginal atrophy can cause a range of symptoms including:
  - **Vaginal Dryness**: Reduced estrogen leads to decreased vaginal secretions, resulting in dryness. This can cause discomfort and pain, especially during sexual intercourse.
  - **Itching and Irritation**: The thinning of the vaginal walls can lead to itching and irritation.
  - **Dyspareunia**: Pain during sexual intercourse is a common complaint among menopausal women with vaginal atrophy.
  - **Discharge**: Some women may experience a watery discharge due to the thinning and fragility of the vaginal walls.
- **Urinary Symptoms:** Menopause can also lead to several urinary symptoms collectively referred to as genitourinary syndrome of menopause (GSM). These symptoms include:
  - **Urinary Incontinence**: The decline in estrogen can weaken the tissues around the bladder and urethra, leading to stress urinary incontinence (leakage of urine during activities that increase abdominal pressure, such as coughing or lifting) and urge incontinence (a sudden, intense urge to urinate followed by involuntary loss of urine).
  - **Increased Frequency and Urgency**: Many menopausal women experience an increased frequency of urination and a strong, sudden urge to urinate.

- **Recurrent Urinary Tract Infections (UTIs)**: The decrease in estrogen can alter the vaginal and urethral flora, making women more susceptible to UTIs. The thinning of the urethral lining and decreased acidity in the vagina can facilitate the growth of uropathogenic bacteria.

3.2.3. Mechanisms Underlying Urogenital Symptoms

Understanding the mechanisms underlying these urogenital symptoms is crucial for developing effective treatments and management strategies (Rahn et al., 2014).

- **Role of Estrogen:** Estrogen plays a key role in maintaining the structure and function of the urogenital tract. Its decline during menopause leads to:
    - **Thinning of the Epithelium**: Estrogen helps maintain the thickness of the epithelial lining in the vagina and urethra. Its decline causes thinning and atrophy of these tissues.
    - **Decreased Blood Flow**: Estrogen promotes blood flow to the urogenital tissues. Reduced estrogen levels result in decreased vascularization, contributing to dryness and atrophy.
    - **Altered Collagen Synthesis**: Estrogen influences collagen synthesis and degradation, impacting the strength and elasticity of the urogenital tissues. Its decline can lead to the weakening of the pelvic floor muscles and connective tissues, contributing to urinary incontinence.
    - **Changes in Microbiota**: Estrogen helps maintain the acidic pH of the vagina, which supports the growth of beneficial lactobacilli. Reduced estrogen levels can lead to an overgrowth of pathogenic bacteria, increasing the risk of infections.
- **Neurovascular Changes:** Menopause is associated with neurovascular changes that can affect the urogenital tract. Decreased estrogen levels can impact the autonomic nervous system, leading to altered bladder function and urinary symptoms (Randolph et al., 2010).
- **Pelvic Floor Dysfunction:** The pelvic floor muscles support the bladder, uterus, and rectum. Estrogen deficiency can weaken these muscles, leading to pelvic organ prolapse and urinary incontinence. Aging and childbirth also contribute to pelvic floor dysfunction.

3.2.4. Diagnosis of Urogenital Symptoms

Accurate diagnosis is essential for the effective management of urogenital symptoms. Diagnosis typically involves:

- **Medical History**: A thorough medical history, including menstrual history, sexual history, and history of urinary symptoms, is essential.
- **Physical Examination**: A pelvic examination can help assess vaginal atrophy, pelvic organ prolapse, and signs of infection.
- **Urinalysis**: This test helps detect urinary tract infections and other urinary abnormalities.

- **Urodynamic Studies**: These tests evaluate bladder function and can help diagnose urinary incontinence.
- **Vaginal pH Testing**: An elevated vaginal pH can indicate estrogen deficiency.

3.2.5. Management and Treatment

The management of urogenital symptoms of menopause involves a combination of lifestyle modifications, non-hormonal treatments, and hormonal therapies (Raz, 2011).

- Lifestyle Modifications
  - Pelvic Floor Exercises: Kegel exercises can strengthen the pelvic floor muscles and improve urinary incontinence.
  - Hydration: Adequate hydration can help maintain urinary health.
  - Diet: A diet rich in phytoestrogens (found in soy products, flaxseeds, and other foods) may help alleviate some menopausal symptoms.
  - Regular Sexual Activity: Regular sexual activity can increase blood flow to the vaginal tissues and help maintain elasticity.
- Non-Hormonal Treatments
  - **Vaginal Moisturizers and Lubricants**: Over-the-counter vaginal moisturizers can help alleviate dryness, while lubricants can reduce discomfort during intercourse.
  - **Pelvic Floor Physical Therapy**: This therapy can help strengthen the pelvic floor muscles and improve urinary symptoms.
  - **Laser Therapy**: Vaginal laser therapy has been shown to improve vaginal atrophy and urinary incontinence by promoting collagen synthesis and tissue regeneration.
- Hormonal Treatments
  - **Topical Estrogen Therapy**: Topical estrogen treatments, such as creams, rings, or tablets, can be applied directly to the vaginal area to alleviate symptoms of vaginal atrophy and urinary symptoms. These treatments are often effective with minimal systemic absorption.
  - **Systemic Hormone Replacement Therapy (HRT)**: HRT involves the administration of estrogen (with or without progesterone) and can alleviate a wide range of menopausal symptoms, including urogenital symptoms. However, HRT may have systemic side effects and risks, and its use should be carefully considered and monitored by a healthcare provider.
  - **Selective Estrogen Receptor Modulators (SERMs)**: SERMs, such as ospemifene, can mimic the effects of estrogen in the vaginal tissues without the risks associated with systemic estrogen therapy. Ospemifene is approved for the treatment of moderate to severe dyspareunia due to vaginal atrophy (Rebbeck et al., 2010).

3.3. Genitourinary Syndrome

A recent term, "genitourinary syndrome of menopause" (GSM), refers to a range of menopausal symptoms and indicators linked to physical changes in the lower urinary tract, vagina, and vulva. In addition to sexual symptoms like lack of lubrication, pain or discomfort, and impaired function, as well as genital symptoms like dryness, burning, and irritation, the GSM also includes urinary symptoms like urgency, dysuria, and recurrent urinary tract infections (UTI) (Table 3.1).

Table 3.1. Genitourinary Syndrome of Menopause (GSM): Symptoms and Signs

Symptoms	Signs
Genital dryness	Decreased moisture
Decreased lubrication during sexual activity	Decreased elasticity
Discomfort or pain during sexual activity	Labia minora resorption
Post-coital bleeding	Pallor, erythema
Decreased arousal, orgasm, desire	Loss of vaginal rugae
Irritation, burning, or itching of the vulva or vagina	Tissue fragility, fissures, petechiae
Dysuria	Urethral eversion or prolapse
Urinary frequency and urgency	Loss of hymenal remnants
	Prominence of urethral meatus
	Introital retraction
	Recurrent urinary tract infections

Source: https://www.ncbi.nlm.nih.gov/pmc/articles/PMC4561742/#B18.

Supportive findings: vaginal pH > 5, increased parabasal cells on maturation index, and decreased superficial cells on wet mount or maturation index.

Although they were commonly used until recently, the terms "vulvovaginal atrophy" and "atrophic vaginitis" have been deemed insufficient to describe the array of symptoms and indicators linked to the genitourinary system after menopause (Ryan et al., 1999). The phrase "vulvovaginal atrophy" refers solely to the vulva and vagina, and it is not commonly used in speech or in the media. Although inflammation or infection are not the main cause of menopausal changes, they are implied by the term "atrophic vaginitis." The terms "vulvovaginal atrophy" and "atrophic vaginitis" are also limited in that they fail to consider lower urinary tract symptoms, which are some of the most significant menopausal symptoms.

3.3.1. Prevalence of GSM

3.3.1.1. Vulvovaginal Symptoms and Sexual Dysfunction

According to recent large cohort surveys conducted in Western populations, between 45 and 63% of postmenopausal women reported having experienced vulvovaginal symptoms, the most common of which was dryness of the vagina. Other symptoms included dyspareunia, irritation, itching, tenderness, and bleeding or spotting of the vagina during sexual activity. Similarly, vulvovaginal symptoms, such as dyspareunia and vaginal dryness, were reported by 49% of postmenopausal women in a Korean study (Schilling et al., 2007).

Once menopause, there is a direct correlation between lower levels of circulating estrogen and these symptoms. During reproductive life, estrogen receptors (ERs; both α and β) are found in the vagina, vulva, pelvic floor muscles, endopelvic fascia, urethra, and bladder trigone; their levels decrease with menopause and can be replenished with estrogen therapy. Following menopause, estrogen deficiency causes anatomic and histologic changes in the female genital tissues. These changes include a decrease in the levels of elastin, hyaluronic acid, and collagen as well as a thinning of the epithelium, changes in the way smooth muscle cells function, an increase in connective tissue density, and a reduction in the number of blood vessels. These modifications weaken lubrication, raise vaginal pH, alter vaginal flora, decrease vaginal elasticity, and make the vagina more susceptible to physical trauma and irritation (Simon et al., 2013).

For postmenopausal women, these vaginal discomforts have a negative impact on sexual function. Levine and associates. found that vulvovaginal symptoms were almost four times more common in postmenopausal sexually active women with sexual dysfunction than in women without sexual dysfunction. 40% of women with vulvovaginal symptoms also reported having problems with orgasm (19%), arousal difficulties (34%), lack of desire (24%), and overall sexual dysfunction (45%). Vaginal dryness was regarded by women with sexual dysfunction as a significant factor linked to masturbation, pain, arousal, physical pleasure, and emotional satisfaction, according to the USA's Study of Women's Health Across the Nation (SWAN).

3.3.1.2. Lower Urinary Tract Dysfunction

The urogenital sinus is the common cradle of both the female genital tract and the lower urinary tract. Lower urinary tract symptoms, including dysuria, urgency, frequency, nocturia, urinary incontinence (UI), and recurrent UTIs, are caused by estrogen deficiency following menopause because estrogen is crucial for the lower urinary tract's function during the premenopausal period (Robinson and Cardozo, 2003).

About 20% of postmenopausal women in a Robinson and Cardozo study experienced severe urgency, and nearly 50% experienced stress-related urinary incontinence (SUI). Specifically, urge UI is more common in women with estrogen deficiency after menopause than it is before, and its prevalence rises over time. Estrogen may raise the urethral closure pressure and bladder sensory threshold because ERs are found in the trigone of the bladder as well as in the squamous epithelium of the proximal and distal urethra. The research conducted by Hyun and colleagues. proposed that the primary cause of UI in postmenopausal women was intrinsic sphincteric dysfunction associated with changed connective tissue after estrogen deficiency, whereas the primary cause of UI in premenopausal women was anatomical change (Sinha and Ewies, 2013).

In older women, the incidence of UTI increases dramatically. According to studies, bacteriuria affects 15–20% of women in their 65–70 age range and 20–50% of women in their 80+ age range. Women who are premenopausal and postmenopausal may have distinct UTI risk factors. While sexual activity is the most common cause in younger women, in older women the risk factors for recurrent UTIs include UI, anatomic changes like a cystocele, increased residual urine, and diabetes (Sowers et al., 2006). Antimicrobial drug resistance patterns may be changed, multiple needless courses of antibiotic therapy, and antibiotic prophylaxis may ensue from a lack of knowledge regarding the link between GSM and recurrent UTIs.

3.3.2. GSM and Quality of Life (QOL)

In 2000, there were 5.26 million postmenopausal Koreans, or 22.5% of all females. Thirteen and fifteen million people will be postmenopausal in 2030, making up almost half of all women. As a result, one of the most crucial concerns in our society will be how these postmenopausal women are treated.

Many health issues arise during the postmenopausal period when there is low estrogen. Unlike vasomotor symptoms, which frequently improve with time, genitourinary symptoms are persistent, rarely go away on their own, and frequently worsen if left untreated. Despite not being life-threatening, these symptoms are progressive and may significantly lower postmenopausal women's quality of life (QOL) by impairing their intimacy with partners and sense of self (Sternfeld et al., 2004).

The Clarifying Vaginal Atrophy's Impact on Sex and Relationships (CLOSER) study, which was just published, discovered that vaginal discomfort directly affected intimacy (women, 58 percent; men, 78 percent) and led to libido loss (64% and 52%, respectively). Overall, vaginal symptoms were found to have a more negative effect on intimate relationships than anticipated by 38% of women and 39% of their male partners. According to women who participated in the REalWomen's Views of Treatment Options for Menopausal Vaginal Changees (REVIVE) survey, vaginal symptoms made it harder for them to enjoy sexual activity (59%), sleep (24%), and life in general (23%).

In addition, gonadotropin-releasing hormone (GnRH) agonist use, surgical menopause, hypothalamic amenorrhea, and cancer treatments such as chemotherapy, pelvic radiation, or endocrine therapy can all result in induced hypoestrogenic states that can cause GSM. The management of menopausal symptoms has become increasingly important for these patients because the genitourinary symptoms associated with abrupt menopause tend to present in relatively younger women and cause greater sexual dysfunction and poorer QOL outcomes (Sturdee and Panay, 2010).

3.3.3. Treatment of GSM

The primary goal of treating GSM is to relieve symptoms. For women with vulvovaginal symptoms unrelated to sexual activity, first-line therapies include long-acting vaginal moisturizers and a short course of low-dose vaginal estrogen. For women with vulvovaginal symptoms related to sexual activity, stepwise treatment is required (Sturdee, 2008). Currently, available treatment options include non-hormonal vaginal lubricants to be used during intercourse, long-acting vaginal moisturizers, systemic hormonal therapies (oral and transdermal), and low-dose vaginal estrogen therapies (e.g., vaginal creams, intravaginal tablets, or intravaginal rings). Although there is still insufficient data on the use of local estrogen in the management of lower urinary tract symptoms, such therapy has been described in some studies. Black cohosh, which has been the most commonly used phytotherapy as a hormone substitute in Western countries, also has been studied widely for the treatment of menopausal symptoms. However, its effect on genitourinary symptoms is still controversial, and a recent Korean study reveals that black cohosh does not exert estrogenic effects on the vaginal atrophy (Hong et al., 2012).

3.3.4. Systemic Treatment

3.3.4.1. Hormone Therapy (HT)

Menopausal symptoms, including vulvovaginal symptoms, can be effectively managed with HT using estrogen alone or in combination with a progestogen. Vaginal symptoms are typically satisfactorily resolved when systemic HT is required to treat other menopausal symptoms. However, 10 to 15% of women experience a lack of resolution of vaginal symptoms with systemic HT; therefore, additional low-dose vaginal estrogen may be required. It is not advised to use HT as the only treatment for sexual function issues, including decreased libido, as there is currently insufficient evidence to support a significant effect of HT on sexual interest, arousal, and orgasmic response. Systemic HT may also exacerbate or cause stress incontinence (Suckling et al., 2006).

3.3.4.2. Selective ER modulators (SERMs)

SERMs have been developed with the goal of having positive effects on targeted tissues with minimal negative effects on other tissues due to concerns about the possible stimulatory effects of systemic estrogen on breast and endometrial tissues, as well as long-term adverse effects (Tan et al., 2012). The use of SERMs to treat menopausal women's vulvovaginal symptoms has been the subject of several studies. Lasofoxifene and ospemifene have a beneficial effect on vaginal tissue in postmenopausal women, but raloxifene and tamoxifene do not have an estrogen agonist effect on the vagina. The clinical development of lasofoxifene has been put on hold, even though multiple studies have demonstrated significant improvements in vaginal pH and vaginal maturation index.

The US Food and Drug Administration (FDA) has approved only one SERM, ospemifene, to treat moderate to severe dyspareunia. An oral non-estrogen medication called espemifene has an estrogen agonistic effect on the tissue lining the vagina. According to published research, taking ospemifene 60 mg orally every day improves dyspareunia, vaginal dryness, pH, and maturation index.

3.3.4.3. Bazedoxifene (BZA) and Conjugated Estrogens (CEs)

The goal of combining CE, a tissue-selective estrogen complex (TSEC), with BZA, a SERM for the prevention and treatment of postmenopausal osteoporosis, is to maximize the therapeutic benefits of each individual component. BZA/CE has been developed to prevent bone loss, relieve vasomotor and vulvovaginal symptoms, and protect the breast and endometrium. According to studies, vulvovaginal symptoms and dyspareunia were significantly improved by BZA (20 mg)/ CE (0.45 or 0.625 mg), while BZA by itself had no beneficial vaginal effects (The North American Menopause Society, 2013).

3.3.5. Local Treatment

3.3.5.1. Non-Hormonal Treatment

Several over-the-counter moisturizers and lubricants (oil, silicone, or water based) are frequently used to treat vulvovaginal symptoms in postmenopausal women. According to the North American Menopause Society, using long-acting vaginal moisturizers on a regular basis and using non-hormonal lubricants during sexual activity are the first-line treatments for women experiencing vulvovaginal symptoms. Lubricants can generally be used during sexual activity to lessen the irritation of atrophic tissue caused by friction.

Long-acting vaginal moisturizing agents also do not improve the vaginal maturation index, but they can lower the pH of the vagina to premenopausal levels. According to two recent studies, topical vaginal estrogen and vaginal hyaluronic acid-based moisturizers are equally effective at relieving vulvovaginal symptoms, and they could be a viable substitute for estrogen-based treatment.

The Society of Obstetricians and Gynecologists of Canada (SOGC) guidelines also state that women who wish to refrain from using estrogen due to health concerns should be offered vaginal moisturizers, which have an efficacy equivalent to topical vaginal estrogen for relieving vulvovaginal symptoms like itching, irritation, and dyspareunia. Recently developed in Korea, Hyallin® is a vaginal hyaluronic acid-based moisturizer that is currently available on prescription. More research is necessary, though, as there have not been many clinical studies done on the long-term safety and effectiveness of these non-hormonal products (The North American Menopause Society, 2012).

3.3.5.2. Hormonal Treatment

Whereas local vaginal estrogen therapy (estrogen tablets, creams, or a vaginal ring) is preferred when genitourinary symptoms are the only complaint, systemic estrogen therapy is preferred if vasomotor symptoms are also present. When non-hormonal treatment fails to alleviate the clinical signs and symptoms of GSM, short-term therapy with local estrogen preparations can help.

Subjective results, such as an improvement in vulvovaginal symptoms and lower urinary tract symptoms like dysuria, frequency, urgency, and nocturia, as well as SUI and UTI, have been reported in studies on the efficacy of vaginal estrogen. Additionally, these studies have shown favorable shifts in vaginal and urethral cytology, an increase in the number of vaginal lactobacilli, a decrease in vaginal pH, an improvement in the gross appearance of the vaginal mucosa, and favorable changes in urine culture results.

However, women have a range of worries about vaginal estrogen treatments, from safety concerns about estrogen-related neoplasms to the inconvenience of vaginal administration. Because low-dose vaginal estrogen produces very low serum levels of estrogen, it is generally thought to have a lower risk of side effects than commonly used doses of systemic estrogen therapy. Low-dose vaginal estrogen use has not been linked to an increased risk of venous thromboembolism, according to a 2006 Cochrane review.

Furthermore, endometrial hyperplasia or adenocarcinoma was extremely rare, and serum estradiol levels stayed within the normal postmenopausal range. Vaginal estrogen therapy is generally safe for the majority of symptomatic GSM women; however, it is controversial in women with estrogen-dependent neoplasia (e.g., vaginal or uterine bleeding) and contraindicated in certain other women either endometrial cancer or breast cancer) (Carberry and Rahn 2014).

3.4. Diagnostic Evaluation

3.4.1. Medical History

A thorough medical history provides valuable insights into a woman's reproductive health, menstrual history, menopausal symptoms, and risk factors, aiding in the accurate diagnosis of menopause and the development of appropriate management strategies (Thurston et al., 2010).

3.4.1.1. Key Components of Medical History

3.4.1.1.1. Menstrual History

A detailed menstrual history is essential for assessing menopausal status. Key aspects to explore include:

- **Age of Menarche:** The age at which menstruation began provides insight into reproductive health and the timing of menopause.
- **Menstrual Regularity:** Changes in menstrual regularity, such as cycle length and flow, are common during perimenopause.
- **Menstrual Symptoms:** Inquire about the presence of symptoms such as heavy bleeding (menorrhagia), irregular bleeding, or skipped periods.
- **Last Menstrual Period (LMP):** Determining the date of the last menstrual period helps establish whether a woman has reached menopause (12 consecutive months without menstruation).
- **Menopausal Symptoms:** Explore the presence and severity of common menopausal symptoms such as hot flashes, night sweats, vaginal dryness, mood changes, and sleep disturbances.

3.4.1.1.2. Reproductive History

Understanding a woman's reproductive history provides context for interpreting menopausal symptoms and hormonal changes:

- **Pregnancy History:** Inquire about the number of pregnancies, deliveries, miscarriages, and abortions.

- **Contraceptive History:** Discuss past and current use of contraception, including oral contraceptives, intrauterine devices (IUDs), and barrier methods.
- **Hormonal Therapy:** Explore any history of hormone replacement therapy (HRT), including estrogen or progesterone use for contraception or menopausal symptom management.

3.4.1.1.3. Gynecological History

A gynecological history helps assess overall reproductive health and the presence of gynecological conditions that may impact menopausal symptoms:

- **Pelvic Pain:** Inquire about the presence of pelvic pain, dyspareunia (pain during intercourse), or other gynecological symptoms.
- **Gynecological Conditions:** Discuss any history of gynecological conditions such as endometriosis, fibroids, polycystic ovary syndrome (PCOS), or pelvic inflammatory disease (PID).

3.4.1.1.4. Medical History

Certain medical conditions and lifestyle factors can influence menopausal symptoms and health outcomes:

- **Chronic Diseases:** Explore the presence of chronic conditions such as diabetes, hypertension, cardiovascular disease, thyroid disorders, or autoimmune conditions.
- **Medication History:** Inquire about current and past medications, including prescription drugs, over-the-counter medications, supplements, and herbal remedies.
- **Smoking and Alcohol Use:** Assess smoking history and alcohol consumption, as these factors can impact menopausal symptoms and bone health.

3.4.1.1.5. Family History

Family history provides insight into genetic predispositions and familial patterns of menopause and related conditions:

- **Menopausal Age:** Inquire about the age at which the patient's mother and sisters reached menopause, as there may be a genetic component to menopausal timing.
- **Osteoporosis and Fractures:** Explore family history of osteoporosis, fractures, and other bone-related conditions.

3.4.2. Physical Examination

Physical examination is an integral component of the clinical evaluation for menopause. While menopause is primarily diagnosed based on a woman's medical history and symptoms, a thorough physical examination provides valuable information about her overall health, identifies signs of hormonal changes, and assesses the impact of menopause on various organ systems (Thurston et al., 2009). A comprehensive physical examination allows healthcare providers to detect any abnormalities, address specific concerns related to menopause, and guide appropriate management strategies.

3.4.2.1. Components of the Physical Examination

3.4.2.1.1. General Examination

1. Vital Signs:
   - **Blood Pressure:** Measurement of blood pressure to assess cardiovascular health and screen for hypertension.
   - **Heart Rate:** Evaluation of heart rate for signs of arrhythmias or autonomic dysfunction.
   - **Temperature:** Assessment of body temperature for signs of fever or hormonal imbalances.
2. **Body Mass Index (BMI):**
   - Calculation of BMI based on weight and height to assess for overweight or obesity, which can impact hormonal balance and cardiovascular health.
3. Skin and Hair:
   - Inspection for signs of estrogen deficiency, such as dry skin, thinning hair, or changes in hair texture.
   - Assessment for striae, acne, or hirsutism, which may indicate underlying endocrine disorders.

3.4.2.1.2. Breast Examination

1. Visual Inspection:
   - Examination of the breasts for symmetry, size, shape, and skin changes.
   - Assessment for dimpling, puckering, or retraction of the skin, which may indicate underlying pathology.
2. Palpation:
   - Manual palpation of the breasts and axillary lymph nodes to detect masses, nodularity, or tenderness.
   - Evaluation of nipple discharge or changes in nipple appearance.

3.4.2.1.3. Pelvic Examination

1. External Genitalia:
   - Visual inspection of the external genitalia for signs of atrophy, inflammation, or lesions.

- Assessment of vaginal introitus for narrowing, dryness, or mucosal changes.

2. Speculum Examination:
   - Insertion of a speculum to visualize the vaginal walls, cervix, and vaginal discharge.
   - Assessment for vaginal atrophy, thinning of vaginal epithelium, and pH changes.
3. Bimanual Examination:
   - Palpation of the uterus, cervix, and adnexa (ovaries and fallopian tubes) to assess size, shape, and mobility.
   - Evaluation for uterine fibroids, ovarian cysts, or pelvic masses.

3.4.2.1.4. Musculoskeletal Examination

1. Posture and Gait:

- Observation of posture and gait for signs of musculoskeletal changes, such as kyphosis or gait abnormalities.
- Assessment for balance and coordination, which may be affected by hormonal changes and bone density loss.

2. Joint Examination:

- Palpation and range of motion testing of major joints, including the spine, hips, knees, and hands.
- Evaluation for signs of arthritis, joint stiffness, or swelling.

3.4.2.1.5. Neurological Examination

1. Cranial Nerves:

- Assessment of cranial nerve function, including visual acuity, extraocular movements, facial sensation, and motor function.
- Evaluation for symptoms of cranial nerve compression or dysfunction.

2. Reflexes:

- Testing of deep tendon reflexes, such as the biceps, triceps, and patellar reflexes, to assess neurological integrity.
- Evaluation for hyperreflexia or hyporeflexia, which may indicate spinal cord pathology.

3.5. Laboratory Tests

3.5.1. Hormone Levels

Menopause marks the end of a woman's reproductive years and is characterized by the cessation of menstrual cycles for 12 consecutive months. This transition is driven by significant hormonal changes, particularly a decline in ovarian function and subsequent decreases in estrogen and progesterone production (Thurston et al., 2005). Diagnosing menopause, especially during the perimenopausal phase, can be complex and often involves evaluating a woman's hormone levels through various tests. These hormone level tests are critical for confirming menopause, understanding the hormonal milieu, and guiding appropriate management strategies.

3.5.1.1. Key Hormones Involved in Menopause

Several hormones play crucial roles during menopause, and their levels can be measured to assess menopausal status:

- Follicle-Stimulating Hormone (FSH): Elevated levels are a hallmark of menopause.

- Luteinizing Hormone (LH): Levels also rise but are less specific than FSH.
- Estrogen (Estradiol): Levels decline significantly during menopause.
- Progesterone: Levels decrease due to the cessation of ovulation.
- Anti-Müllerian Hormone (AMH): Declines as ovarian reserve diminishes.
- Inhibin B: Decreases, reflecting reduced ovarian function.

3.5.1.2. Follicle-Stimulating Hormone (FSH)

- **Role of FSH:** FSH is produced by the pituitary gland and plays a vital role in regulating the menstrual cycle. It stimulates the growth of ovarian follicles and the production of estrogen. During menopause, the decline in ovarian function leads to decreased estrogen production, which results in a lack of negative feedback to the pituitary gland (Thurston et al., 2008). Consequently, FSH levels rise significantly.
- **Testing for FSH:**
  - **Indications:** Testing FSH levels is commonly indicated in women with irregular menstrual cycles, symptoms of menopause, or when the clinical diagnosis of menopause is uncertain.
  - **Procedure:** FSH levels can be measured through a blood test, typically performed on specific days of the menstrual cycle (if the woman is still menstruating) to account for natural fluctuations.
  - **Interpretation:** An FSH level consistently above 30 mIU/mL is suggestive of menopause, although a single measurement may not be definitive due to natural variability.

3.5.1.3. Luteinizing Hormone (LH)

- **Role of LH:** LH, also produced by the pituitary gland, works in conjunction with FSH to regulate the menstrual cycle and ovulation (Thurston et al., 2008). Similar to FSH, LH levels increase as ovarian function declines.
- **Testing for LH:**
  - **Indications:** LH testing is often performed alongside FSH testing to provide a comprehensive picture of pituitary and ovarian function.
  - **Procedure:** Blood samples are taken to measure LH levels, typically along with FSH.
  - **Interpretation:** Elevated LH levels, in conjunction with high FSH levels, support the diagnosis of menopause, although LH is less specific than FSH.

3.5.1.4. Estrogen (Estradiol)

- **Role of Estrogen:** Estrogen, particularly estradiol, is the primary female sex hormone produced by the ovaries. It is crucial for the development and regulation of the female reproductive system and secondary sexual characteristics (Thurston et al., 2006).
- **Testing for Estrogen:**

- **Indications:** Measuring estrogen levels can help confirm menopause and assess the severity of estrogen deficiency.
- **Procedure:** Blood tests are used to measure estradiol levels.
- **Interpretation:** Estradiol levels below 30 pg/mL are typically indicative of menopause. However, estrogen levels can fluctuate, and low levels alone are not definitive without other supporting evidence.

3.5.1.5. Progesterone

- **Role of Progesterone:** Progesterone is produced by the corpus luteum in the ovary after ovulation and is essential for regulating the menstrual cycle and maintaining pregnancy.
- **Testing for Progesterone:**
  - **Indications:** Progesterone levels are less commonly measured in the context of menopause but can be assessed to evaluate ovulatory function.
  - **Procedure:** Blood tests are conducted to measure progesterone, often timed in the luteal phase of the menstrual cycle (if applicable).
  - **Interpretation:** Low progesterone levels, in conjunction with other hormonal changes, can support the diagnosis of menopause.

3.5.1.6. Anti-Müllerian Hormone (AMH)

- **Role of AMH:** AMH is produced by granulosa cells in the ovarian follicles and is a marker of ovarian reserve. It reflects the number of remaining follicles in the ovaries.
- **Testing for AMH:**
  - **Indications:** AMH testing is useful for assessing ovarian reserve and can be an early indicator of declining ovarian function before significant changes in FSH and estrogen levels.
  - **Procedure:** Blood tests are used to measure AMH levels.
  - **Interpretation:** Low AMH levels indicate diminished ovarian reserve and are consistent with the perimenopausal transition. AMH levels decline with age and are typically very low or undetectable in postmenopausal women.

3.5.1.7. Inhibin B

- **Role of Inhibin B:** Inhibin B is produced by ovarian follicles and inhibits FSH production. Levels of inhibin B decline as ovarian function decreases.
- Testing for Inhibin B:
  - **Indications:** Inhibin B testing can provide additional information about ovarian reserve and function.
  - **Procedure:** Blood tests are used to measure inhibin B levels.
  - **Interpretation:** Low or undetectable levels of inhibin B are consistent with decreased ovarian reserve and menopausal transition.

3.5.1.8. Comprehensive Hormonal Assessment

A comprehensive hormonal assessment for menopause typically involves measuring multiple hormones to provide a complete picture of a woman's reproductive status. This approach can help differentiate menopause from other conditions that may present with similar symptoms, such as thyroid disorders or hyperprolactinemia (Thurston et al., 2008).

3.5.1.9. Clinical Implications of Hormone Level Testing

- **Diagnosis of Menopause:** While hormone level testing can support the diagnosis of menopause, it is important to consider the clinical context, including the woman's age, menstrual history, and symptoms (Thurston et al., 2009). Menopause is ultimately a clinical diagnosis based on the cessation of menstruation for 12 consecutive months. Hormone tests are particularly useful in cases of early or premature menopause (before age 40) or when symptoms are atypical.
- **Perimenopause:** Perimenopause, the transition phase leading up to menopause, is characterized by hormonal fluctuations and irregular menstrual cycles. Hormone level testing during perimenopause can be challenging due to the variability in hormone levels. However, elevated FSH and low AMH levels can indicate the onset of perimenopause.
- **Postmenopause:** In postmenopausal women, hormone levels typically stabilize. FSH and LH remain elevated, while estrogen and progesterone levels are low. Monitoring hormone levels in postmenopausal women can be useful for managing symptoms and evaluating the effectiveness of hormone replacement therapy (HRT).

3.5.1.10. Hormone Replacement Therapy (HRT)

Hormone level testing plays a crucial role in the management of menopausal symptoms through HRT. By measuring baseline hormone levels, healthcare providers can tailor HRT to the individual needs of the patient. Follow-up hormone testing can help monitor the effectiveness of HRT and adjust dosages as needed to achieve optimal symptom relief and minimize side effects (Thurston et al., 2008).

3.5.2. Bone Density Test

Bone density tests, or bone densitometry, are crucial in assessing the risk of osteoporosis and guiding appropriate preventive and therapeutic measures for menopausal women.

Bone density tests measure the amount of calcium and other minerals in a segment of bone. The most common and reliable method for assessing bone density is Dual-Energy X-ray Absorptiometry (DEXA or DXA), but other methods such as quantitative ultrasound (QUS) and peripheral quantitative computed tomography (pQCT) are also used (Visvanathan et al., 2005).

3.5.2.1. Importance of Bone Health in Menopause

Estrogen plays a crucial role in maintaining bone density by inhibiting bone resorption (breakdown) and promoting bone formation. During menopause, the decrease in estrogen levels leads to an imbalance between bone resorption and formation, resulting in a net loss of bone mass. This accelerates the decline in bone density, increasing the risk of osteoporosis and fractures, particularly in the spine, hip, and wrist. Early detection of bone density loss is essential for preventing osteoporosis-related complications (Whiteman et al., 2003).

3.5.2.2. Dual-Energy X-ray Absorptiometry (DEXA)

- **Procedure:** DEXA is the gold standard for measuring bone density. It uses low-dose X-rays to assess bone density at various sites, typically the lumbar spine, hip, and sometimes the forearm. The procedure involves the following steps:

1. **Preparation:** Minimal preparation is required. Patients should avoid taking calcium supplements 24 hours before the test. They should wear loose, comfortable clothing without metal zippers, belts, or buttons.
2. **Scanning:** The patient lies on a padded table while a movable arm passes over the body, emitting low-dose X-rays. The scan usually takes 10–30 minutes and is painless.
3. **Analysis:** The machine calculates bone mineral density (BMD) by comparing the amount of X-ray energy absorbed by the bone to the amount absorbed by soft tissue. The results are given as T-scores and Z-scores.

3.5.2.3. Interpretation

- **T-score:** Compares the patient's BMD to the average peak BMD of a young adult of the same sex. It is used to diagnose osteoporosis and assess fracture risk.
  - Normal: T-score -1.0 and above
  - Osteopenia (low bone mass): T-score between -1.0 and -2.5
  - Osteoporosis: T-score -2.5 and below
- **Z-score:** Compares the patient's BMD to the average BMD of people of the same age, sex, and size. It helps identify unusual bone loss for the patient's age.

3.5.2.4. Quantitative Ultrasound (QUS)

- **Procedure:** QUS is a less expensive and more portable method than DEXA. It measures the speed of sound and attenuation of ultrasound waves through bone, typically at the heel (calcaneus), which correlates with bone density and fracture risk (Williams et al., 1995). The procedure involves:
  - **Preparation:** No special preparation is required. The patient removes footwear and places their foot in the ultrasound device.
  - **Scanning:** The device sends ultrasound waves through the heel bone, and the results are obtained within a few minutes.
  - **Analysis:** The device calculates bone density based on the ultrasound wave properties.
- **Interpretation:** QUS results are often reported as T-scores and Z-scores, similar to DEXA, but it is not as precise and is primarily used for screening purposes.

3.5.2.5. Peripheral Quantitative Computed Tomography (pQCT)

- **Procedure:** pQCT provides 3D imaging and measures bone density at peripheral sites such as the forearm or tibia. It is more sensitive than DEXA for detecting changes in bone structure and strength. The procedure involves:
  - **Preparation:** Minimal preparation is required. The patient sits or lies with the limb to be scanned positioned in the device.
  - **Scanning:** The scanner rotates around the limb, taking cross-sectional images.
  - **Analysis:** The images are used to calculate bone density and provide detailed information about bone geometry and strength.
- **Interpretation:** pQCT results provide volumetric BMD (vBMD) and can assess both cortical and trabecular bone density, offering more detailed information than DEXA.

3.5.2.6. Indications for Bone Density Testing in Menopause

Bone density testing is recommended for women at increased risk of osteoporosis, including:

- All women aged 65 and older.
- Postmenopausal women under 65 with risk factors, such as:
  - Family history of osteoporosis or fractures.
  - Personal history of fractures after age 50.
  - Low body weight (BMI < 20 kg/m^2) or significant weight loss.
  - Smoking and excessive alcohol consumption.
  - Long-term use of glucocorticoids or other medications affecting bone health.
  - Medical conditions associated with bone loss, such as rheumatoid arthritis or hyperthyroidism.

3.5.2.7. Clinical Implications of Bone Density Testing

- **Diagnosis of Osteoporosis:** Bone density testing is essential for diagnosing osteoporosis and assessing fracture risk. A T-score of -2.5 or lower confirms the diagnosis of osteoporosis, and further evaluation and management are needed to prevent fractures.
- **Monitoring Bone Health:** Regular bone density testing helps monitor the progression of bone loss and the effectiveness of treatment in menopausal women. The frequency of testing depends on initial results and risk factors, typically every 1–2 years.
- **Guiding Treatment Decisions:** Bone density results guide treatment decisions, including the initiation of pharmacologic therapy such as bisphosphonates, selective estrogen receptor modulators (SERMs), or hormone replacement therapy (HRT). They also inform lifestyle recommendations, including diet, exercise, and fall prevention strategies (Woods et al., 2009).

3.5.2.8. Pharmacologic Therapy

- **Bisphosphonates:** These drugs inhibit bone resorption and are the first-line treatment for osteoporosis. Examples include alendronate, risedronate, and zoledronic acid.
- **Selective Estrogen Receptor Modulators (SERMs):** Raloxifene mimics estrogen's beneficial effects on bone without some of the risks associated with hormone therapy.
- **Hormone Replacement Therapy (HRT):** HRT can prevent bone loss and reduce fracture risk, but it is typically reserved for women with significant menopausal symptoms due to potential risks.
- **Denosumab:** A monoclonal antibody that inhibits bone resorption, used for women at high risk of fracture.
- **Parathyroid Hormone Analogs:** Teriparatide and abaloparatide stimulate bone formation and are used for severe osteoporosis.

A Closer Look

Early Symptoms of Menopause

The early symptoms of menopause often referred to as perimenopause, can begin several years before a woman's final menstrual period. This transitional phase is characterized by fluctuating hormone levels, particularly estrogen and progesterone, which can lead to a variety of physical and emotional changes. One of the hallmark symptoms of early menopause is irregular menstrual cycles. Women may experience changes in the frequency, duration, and flow of their periods. Cycles may become shorter or longer, and the flow can be lighter or heavier than usual.

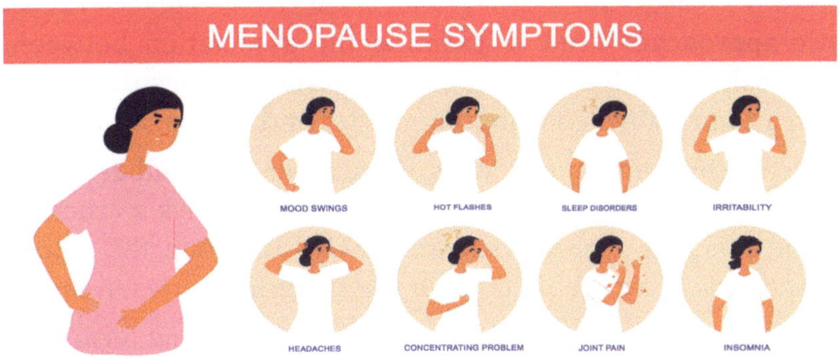

Source:

Hot flashes are another common early symptom of menopause. These sudden feelings of intense heat, often accompanied by sweating and a red, flushed face, can vary in intensity and duration. Night sweats, which are hot flashes that occur during sleep, can disrupt rest and lead to fatigue and irritability. Many women also report sleep disturbances unrelated to night sweats, such as difficulty falling or staying asleep, which can exacerbate feelings of tiredness and mood swings.

Emotional and psychological symptoms are also prevalent during the early stages of menopause. Women may experience mood swings, irritability, anxiety, and depression. These changes can be due to hormonal fluctuations and the stress of adjusting to the physical changes occurring in their bodies. Memory problems and difficulty concentrating, often referred to as "brain fog," are also reported by many women during perimenopause (Woods et al., 2006).

Physical changes such as weight gain, particularly around the abdomen, and changes in skin elasticity and hair texture can also occur. Some women experience joint pain and muscle aches, which can be mistaken for other health issues but are often related to hormonal changes. Additionally, vaginal dryness and changes in libido are common, which can affect sexual health and relationships. Overall, the early symptoms of menopause can be varied and multifaceted, impacting a woman's physical, emotional, and mental well-being. Understanding and recognizing these symptoms can help women seek appropriate medical advice and support to manage this transition more effectively.

Summary

- Menopause, a natural biological process, marks the end of a woman's reproductive years and typically occurs around the age of 45 to 55. It is characterized by the cessation of menstrual periods for 12 consecutive months due to hormonal changes, particularly a decline in estrogen production by the ovaries. The transition through menopause involves various physiological and hormonal fluctuations, leading to a wide range of clinical manifestations that can significantly impact a woman's quality of life.
- Traditionally vasomotor symptoms were reported to begin 5 to 10 years prior to the cessation of the final menstrual cycle, corresponding with the initial decline in circulating gonadal hormones; however, night sweats in particular most often begin in perimenopause.
- VMS, or hot flashes and night sweats, are often considered the cardinal symptoms of menopause. VMS are episodes of profuse heat accompanied by sweating and flushing, experienced predominantly around the head, neck, chest, and upper back.
- The analytic approaches used to examine the association between obesity and VMS primarily use calculated BMI, which encompasses both lean and fat mass, and thereby cannot discern the relative contributions of fat and lean mass as predictors of VMS.
- The urinary tract comprises the kidneys, ureters, bladder, and urethra. Estrogen receptors are present in the bladder and urethra, and estrogen plays a crucial role in maintaining the health and function of these tissues. It helps maintain the mucosal lining, supports blood flow, and influences the function of the smooth muscles in the bladder and urethra.
- The genitourinary syndrome of menopause (GSM) is a new term that describes various menopausal symptoms and signs associated with physical changes of the vulva, vagina, and lower urinary tract. The GSM includes not only genital symptoms (dryness, burning, and irritation) and sexual symptoms (lack of lubrication, discomfort or pain, and impaired function), but also urinary symptoms (urgency, dysuria, and recurrent urinary tract infections [UTI]).
- The female genital tract and lower urinary tract share a common embryonic origin, both arising from the urogenital sinus. As estrogen plays an important role in the function of the lower urinary tract throughout the premenopausal period, estrogen deficiency after menopause causes lower urinary tract symptoms, such as dysuria, urgency, frequency, nocturia, urinary incontinence (UI), and recurrent UTI.
- A thorough medical history provides valuable insights into a woman's reproductive health, menstrual history, menopausal symptoms, and risk factors, aiding in the accurate diagnosis of menopause and the development of appropriate management strategies.
- Physical examination is an integral component of the clinical evaluation for menopause. While menopause is primarily diagnosed based on a woman's medical history and symptoms, a thorough physical examination provides valuable information about her overall health, identifies signs of hormonal changes, and assesses the impact of menopause on various organ systems.

References

1. Adler, N. E., Boyce, W. T., Chesney, M. A., et al. (1993). Socioeconomic inequalities in health: No easy solution. *JAMA, 269*(24), 3140–3145.
2. Alexander, C., Cochran, C. J., Gallicchio, L., et al. (2010). Serum leptin levels, hormone levels, and hot flashes in midlife women. *Fertility and Sterility, 94*(3), 1037–1043.
3. Anderson, G. S. (1999). Human morphology and temperature regulation. *International Journal of Biometeorology, 43*(3), 99–109.
4. Archer, D. F. (2010). Tissue-selective estrogen complexes: A promising option for the comprehensive management of menopausal symptoms. *Drugs & Aging, 27*, 533–544.
5. Avis, N. E., Brockwell, S., Randolph, J. F., Jr., Shen, S., Cain, V. S., Ory, M., et al. (2009). Longitudinal changes in sexual functioning as women transition through menopause: Results from the Study of Women's Health Across the Nation. *Menopause, 16*, 442–452.
6. Barnabei, V. M., Cochrane, B. B., Aragaki, A. K., et al. (2005). Menopausal symptoms and treatment-related effects of estrogen and progestin in the Women's Health Initiative. *Obstetrics & Gynecology, 105*(5 Pt 1), 1063–1073.
7. Barnabei, V. M., Grady, D., Stovall, D. W., et al. (2002). Menopausal symptoms in older women and the effects of treatment with hormone therapy. *Obstetrics & Gynecology, 100*(6), 1209–1218.
8. Beerepoot, M. A., Geerlings, S. E., van Haarst, E. P., van Charante, N. M., & ter Riet, G. (2013). Nonantibiotic prophylaxis for recurrent urinary tract infections: A systematic review and meta-analysis of randomized controlled trials. *Journal of Urology, 190*, 1981–1989.
9. Bolanos, R., Del Castillo, A., & Francia, J. (2010). Soy isoflavones versus placebo in the treatment of climacteric vasomotor symptoms: Systematic review and meta-analysis. *Menopause, 17*(3), 660–666.
10. Brown, J. S., Grady, D., Ouslander, J. G., Herzog, A. R., Varner, R. E., & Posner, S. F. (1999). Prevalence of urinary incontinence and associated risk factors in postmenopausal women. Heart & Estrogen/Progestin Replacement Study (HERS) Research Group. *Obstetrics & Gynecology, 94*, 66–70.
11. Brown, J. S., Vittinghoff, E., Kanaya, A. M., Agarwal, S. K., Hulley, S., & Foxman, B. (2001). Urinary tract infections in postmenopausal women: Effect of hormone therapy and risk factors. *Obstetrics & Gynecology, 98*, 1045–1052.
12. Casper, R. F., & Yen, S. S. (1985). Neuroendocrinology of menopausal flushes: A hypothesis of flush mechanism. *Clinical Endocrinology (Oxf), 22*(3), 293–312.
13. Chae, H. D., Choi, S. Y., Cho, E. J., Cho, Y. M., Lee, S. R., & Lee, E. S., et al. (2014). Awareness and experience of menopausal symptom and hormone therapy in Korean postmenopausal women. *Journal of Menopausal Medicine, 20*, 7–13.
14. Chen, J., Geng, L., Song, X., Li, H., Giordan, N., & Liao, Q. (2013). Evaluation of the efficacy and safety of hyaluronic acid vaginal gel to ease vaginal dryness: A multicenter, randomized, controlled, open-label, parallel-group, clinical trial. *Journal of Sexual Medicine, 10*, 1575–1584.
15. Cody, J. D., Jacobs, M. L., Richardson, K., Moehrer, B., & Hextall, A. (2012). Oestrogen therapy for urinary incontinence in postmenopausal women. *Cochrane Database of Systematic Reviews, 10*, Cd001405.

16. Constantine, G., Graham, S., Portman, D. J., Rosen, R. C., & Kingsberg, S. A. (2015). Female sexual function improved with ospemifene in postmenopausal women with vulvar and vaginal atrophy: Results of a randomized, placebo-controlled trial. *Climacteric, 18*, 226–232.

17. Crandall, C. J., Crawford, S. L., & Gold, E. B. (2006). Vasomotor symptom prevalence is associated with polymorphisms in sex steroid-metabolizing enzymes and receptors. *American Journal of Medicine, 119*(9 Suppl 1), S52–60.

18. Crandall, C. J., Tseng, C. H., Crawford, S. L., et al. (2010). Association of menopausal vasomotor symptoms with increased bone turnover during the menopausal transition. *Journal of Bone and Mineral Research.*

19. Crawford, S. L. (2007). The roles of biologic and nonbiologic factors in cultural differences in vasomotor symptoms measured by surveys. *Menopause, 14*(4), 725–733.

20. den Tonkelaar, I., Seidell, J. C., & van Noord, P. A. (1996). Obesity and fat distribution in relation to hot flashes in Dutch women from the DOM-project. *Maturitas, 23*(3), 301–305.

21. Freedman, R. R., & Blacker, C. M. (2002). Estrogen raises the sweating threshold in postmenopausal women with hot flashes. *Fertility and Sterility, 77*(3), 487–490.

22. Freedman, R. R., & Krell, W. (1999). Reduced thermoregulatory null zone in postmenopausal women with hot flashes. *American Journal of Obstetrics and Gynecology, 181*(1), 66–70.

23. Freedman, R. R., & Woodward, S. (1992). Elevated a2-adrenergic responsiveness in menopausal hot flushes: Pharmacologic and biochemical studies. In P. Lomax & E. Schonbaum (Eds.), *Thermoregulation: The Pathophysiological Basis of Clinical Disorders* (pp. 133–146). Krager.

24. Freeman, E. W., Grisso, J. A., Berlin, J., et al. (2001). Symptom reports from a cohort of African American and white women in the late reproductive years. *Menopause, 8*(1), 33–42.

25. Freeman, E. W., Sammel, M. D., Lin, H., et al. (2005). The role of anxiety and hormonal changes in menopausal hot flashes. *Menopause, 12*(3), 258–266.

26. Gold, E. B., Block, G., Crawford, S., et al. (2004). Lifestyle and demographic factors in relation to vasomotor symptoms: Baseline results from the Study of Women's Health Across the Nation. *American Journal of Epidemiology, 159*(12), 1189–1199.

27. Gold, E. B., Lasley, B., Crawford, S. L., et al. (2007). Relation of daily urinary hormone patterns to vasomotor symptoms in a racially/ethnically diverse sample of midlife women: Study of Women's Health Across the Nation. *Reproductive Sciences, 14*(8), 786–797.

28. Gold, E. B., Sternfeld, B., Kelsey, J. L., et al. (2000). Relation of demographic and lifestyle factors to symptoms in a multi-racial/ethnic population of women aged 40–55 years. *American Journal of Epidemiology, 152*(5), 463–473.

29. Gold, E., Colvin, A., Avis, N., et al. (2006). Longitudinal analysis of vasomotor symptoms and race/ethnicity across the menopausal transition: Study of Women's Health Across the Nation (SWAN). *American Journal of Public Health, 96*(7), 1226–1235.

30. Green, R., Polotsky, A. J., Wildman, R. P., et al. (2010). Menopausal symptoms within a Hispanic cohort: SWAN, the Study of Women's Health Across the Nation. *Climacteric, 13*(4), 376–384.

31. Greendale, G. A., & Gold, E. B. (2005). Lifestyle factors: Are they related to vasomotor symptoms and do they modify the effectiveness or side effects of hormone therapy? *American Journal of Medicine, 118*(Suppl 12B), 148–154.

32. Grimaldi, E. F., Restaino, S., Inglese, S., Foltran, L., Sorz, A., & Di Lorenzo, G., et al. (2012). Role of high molecular weight hyaluronic acid in postmenopausal vaginal discomfort. *Minerva Ginecologica, 64*, 321–329.

33. Hendrix, S. L., Cochrane, B. B., Nygaard, I. E., Handa, V. L., Barnabei, V. M., Iglesia, C., et al. (2005). Effects of estrogen with and without progestin on urinary incontinence. *JAMA, 293*(8), 935–948.

34. Hong, S. N., Kim, J. H., Kim, H. Y., & Kim, A. (2012). Effect of black cohosh on genital atrophy and its adverse effect in postmenopausal women. *Journal of Korean Society of Menopause, 18*, 106–112.

35. Hyde Riley, E., Inui, T. S., Kleinman, K., et al. (2004). Differential association of modifiable health behaviors with hot flashes in perimenopausal and postmenopausal women. *Journal of General Internal Medicine, 19*(7), 740–746.

36. Hyun, H. S., Park, B. R., Kim, Y. S., Mun, S. T., & Bae, D. H. (2010). Urodynamic characterization of postmenopausal women with stress urinary incontinence: Retrospective study in incontinent pre- and post-menopausal women. *Journal of Korean Society of Menopause, 16*, 148–152.

37. Johnston, S. L., Farrell, S. A., Bouchard, C., Farrell, S. A., Beckerson, L. A., Comeau, M., et al. (2004). The detection and management of vaginal atrophy. *Journal of Obstetrics and Gynecology Canada, 26*, 503–515.

38. Kim, M. Y., Im, S. W., & Park, H. M. (2015). The demographic changes of menopausal and geripausal women in Korea. *Journal of Bone Metabolism, 22*, 23–28.

39. Kingsberg, S. A., Wysocki, S., Magnus, L., & Krychman, M. L. (2013). Vulvar and vaginal atrophy in postmenopausal women: Findings from the REVIVE (REal Women's VIews of Treatment Options for Menopausal Vaginal ChangEs) survey. *Journal of Sexual Medicine, 10*, 1790–1799.

40. Lethaby, A. E., Brown, J., Marjoribanks, J., et al. (2007). Phytoestrogens for vasomotor menopausal symptoms. *Cochrane Database of Systematic Reviews, 4*, CD001395.

41. Levine, K. B., Williams, R. E., & Hartmann, K. E. (2008). Vulvovaginal atrophy is strongly associated with female sexual dysfunction among sexually active postmenopausal women. *Menopause, 15*, 661–666.

42. Link, B. G., & Phelan, J. (1995). Social conditions as fundamental causes of disease. *Journal of Health and Social Behavior, Spec No*, 80–94.

43. Lobo, R. A., Pinkerton, J. V., Gass, M. L., Dorin, M. H., Ronkin, S., Pickar, J. H., et al. (2009). Evaluation of bazedoxifene/conjugated estrogens for the treatment of menopausal symptoms and effects on metabolic parameters and overall safety profile. *Fertility and Sterility, 92*, 1025–1038.

44. Lüthje, P., Hirschberg, A. L., & Brauner, A. (2014). Estrogenic action on innate defense mechanisms in the urinary tract. *Maturitas, 77*, 32–36.

45. Malacara, J. M., Perez-Luque, E. L., Martinez-Garza, S., et al. (2004). The relationship of estrogen receptor-alpha polymorphism with symptoms and other characteristics in post-menopausal women. *Maturitas, 49*(2), 163–169.

46. Michnovicz, J. J., Hershcopf, R. J., Naganuma, H., et al. (1986). Increased 2-hydroxylation of estradiol as a possible mechanism for the anti-estrogenic effect of cigarette smoking. *New England Journal of Medicine, 315*(21), 1305–1309.

47. Mirkin, S., & Komm, B. S. (2013). Tissue-selective estrogen complexes for postmenopausal women. *Maturitas, 76*, 213–220.
48. Nappi, R. E., & Kokot-Kierepa, M. (2010). Women's voices in menopause: Results from an international survey on vaginal atrophy. *Maturitas, 67*, 233–238.
49. Nappi, R. E., & Kokot-Kierepa, M. (2012). Vaginal health: Insights, views, and attitudes (VIVA)—Results from an international survey. *Climacteric, 15*, 36–44.
50. Nappi, R. E., & Palacios, S. (2014). Impact of vulvovaginal atrophy on sexual health and quality of life at post menopause. *Climacteric, 17*, 3–9.
51. Nappi, R. E., Kingsberg, S., Maamari, R., & Simon, J. (2013). The CLOSER (CLarifying Vaginal Atrophy's Impact on SEx and Relationships) survey: Implications of vaginal discomfort in postmenopausal women and in male partners. *Journal of Sexual Medicine, 10*, 2232–2241.
52. Nelson, H. D., Vesco, K. K., Haney, E., et al. (2006). Nonhormonal therapies for menopausal hot flashes: Systematic review and meta-analysis. *JAMA, 295*(17), 2057–2071.
53. Pennebaker, J. (1982). *The Psychology of Physical Symptoms*. Springer-Verlag.
54. Pinkerton, J. V., & Stanczyk, F. Z. (2014). Clinical effects of selective estrogen receptor modulators on vulvar and vaginal atrophy. *Menopause, 21*, 309–319.
55. Portman, D. J., & Gass, M. L. (2014). Genitourinary syndrome of menopause: New terminology for vulvovaginal atrophy from the International Society for the Study of Women's Sexual Health and the North American Menopause Society. *Menopause, 21*, 1063–1068.
56. Portman, D. J., Bachmann, G. A., & Simon, J. A. (2013). Ospemifene, a novel selective estrogen receptor modulator for treating dyspareunia associated with postmenopausal vulvar and vaginal atrophy. *Menopause, 20*, 623–630.
57. Rahn, D. D., Carberry, C., Sanses, T. V., Mamik, M. M., Ward, R. M., Meriwether, K. V., et al. (2014). Vaginal estrogen for genitourinary syndrome of menopause: A systematic review. *Obstetrics and Gynecology, 124*, 1147–1156.
58. Randolph, J. F., Jr., Sowers, M., Bondarenko, I., et al. (2005). The relationship of longitudinal change in reproductive hormones and vasomotor symptoms during the menopausal transition. *Journal of Clinical Endocrinology and Metabolism, 90*(11), 6106–6112.
59. Raz, R. (2011). Urinary tract infection in postmenopausal women. *Korean Journal of Urology, 52*, 801–808.
60. Rebbeck, T. R., Su, H. I., Sammel, M. D., et al. (2010). Effect of hormone metabolism genotypes on steroid hormone levels and menopausal symptoms in a prospective population-based cohort of women experiencing the menopausal transition. *Menopause, 17*(5), 1026–1034.
61. Robinson, D., & Cardozo, L. D. (2003). The role of estrogens in female lower urinary tract dysfunction. *Urology, 62*, 45–51.
62. Ryan, K., Berkowitz, R., Barbieri, R., et al. (1999). *Kistner's Gynecology and Women's Health* (7th ed.). Mosby, Inc.
63. Sabia, S., Fournier, A., Mesrine, S., et al. (2008). Risk factors for onset of menopausal symptoms: Results from a large cohort study. *Maturitas, 60*(2), 108–121.
64. Schilling, C., Gallicchio, L., Miller, S. R., et al. (2007). Genetic polymorphisms, hormone levels, and hot flashes in midlife women. *Maturitas, 57*(2), 120–131.

65. Simon, J. A., Lin, V. H., Radovich, C., & Bachmann, G. A. (2013). One-year long-term safety extension study of ospemifene for the treatment of vulvar and vaginal atrophy in postmenopausal women with a uterus. *Menopause, 20*, 418–427.

66. Sinha, A., & Ewies, A. A. (2013). Non-hormonal topical treatment of vulvovaginal atrophy: An up-to-date overview. *Climacteric, 16*, 305–312.

67. Sowers, M. R., Wilson, A. L., Karvonen-Gutierrez, C. A., et al. (2006). Sex steroid hormone pathway genes and health-related measures in women of 4 races/ethnicities: The Study of Women's Health Across the Nation (SWAN). *American Journal of Medicine, 119*(9 Suppl 1), S103–110.

68. Sternfeld, B., Wang, H., Quesenberry, C. P., Jr., et al. (2004). Physical activity and changes in weight and waist circumference in midlife women: Findings from the Study of Women's Health Across the Nation. *American Journal of Epidemiology, 160*(9), 912–922.

69. Sturdee, D. W. (2008). The menopausal hot flush—Anything new? *Maturitas, 60*(1), 42–49.

70. Sturdee, D. W., & Panay, N. (2010). Recommendations for the management of postmenopausal vaginal atrophy. *Climacteric, 13*, 509–522.

71. Suckling, J., Lethaby, A., & Kennedy, R. (2006). Local oestrogen for vaginal atrophy in postmenopausal women. *Cochrane Database of Systematic Reviews*, Cd001500.

72. Tan, O., Bradshaw, K., & Carr, B. R. (2012). Management of vulvovaginal atrophy-related sexual dysfunction in postmenopausal women: An up-to-date review. *Menopause, 19*, 109–117.

73. The North American Menopause Society. (2012). The 2012 hormone therapy position statement of: The North American Menopause Society. *Menopause, 19*, 257–271.

74. The North American Menopause Society. (2013). Management of symptomatic vulvovaginal atrophy: 2013 position statement of The North American Menopause Society. *Menopause, 20*, 888–902. [Quiz 3–quiz 4].

75. Thurston, R. C., Blumenthal, J. A., Babyak, M. A., et al. (2005). Emotional antecedents of hot flashes during daily life. *Psychosomatic Medicine, 67*(1), 137–146.

76. Thurston, R. C., Bromberger, J. T., Joffe, H., et al. (2008). Beyond frequency: Who is most bothered by vasomotor symptoms? *Menopause, 15*(5), 841–847.

77. Thurston, R. C., Bromberger, J., Chang, Y., et al. (2008). Childhood abuse or neglect is associated with increased vasomotor symptom reporting among midlife women. *Menopause, 15*(1), 16–22.

78. Thurston, R. C., Kubzansky, L. D., Kawachi, I., et al. (2006). Do depression and anxiety mediate the link between educational attainment and CHD? *Psychosomatic Medicine, 68*(1), 25–32.

79. Thurston, R. C., Sowers, M. R., Chang, Y., et al. (2008). Adiposity and reporting of vasomotor symptoms among midlife women: The Study of Women's Health Across the Nation. *American Journal of Epidemiology, 167*(1), 78–85.

80. Thurston, R. C., Sowers, M. R., Sternfeld, B., et al. (2009). Gains in body fat and vasomotor symptom reporting over the menopausal transition: The Study of Women's Health Across the Nation. *American Journal of Epidemiology, 170*(6), 766–774.

81. Thurston, R. C., Sowers, M. R., Sutton-Tyrrell, K., et al. (2008). Abdominal adiposity and hot flashes among midlife women. *Menopause, 15*(3), 429–434.

82. Thurston, R., Christie, I., & Matthews, K. (2010). Hot flashes and cardiac vagal control: A link to cardiovascular risk? *Menopause, 17*(3), 456–461.

83. Thurston, R., Matthews, K., Hernandez, J., et al. (2009). Improving the performance of physiologic hot flash measures with support vector machines. *Psychophysiology, 46*(2), 285–292.

84. Visvanathan, K., Gallicchio, L., Schilling, C., et al. (2005). Cytochrome gene polymorphisms, serum estrogens, and hot flushes in midlife women. *Obstetrics & Gynecology, 106*(6), 1372–1381.

85. Whiteman, M. K., Staropoli, C. A., Langenberg, P. W., et al. (2003). Smoking, body mass, and hot flashes in midlife women. *Obstetrics & Gynecology, 101*(2), 264–272.

86. Williams, D. R., & Collins, C. (1995). US socioeconomic and racial differences in health: Patterns and explanations. *Annual Review of Sociology, 21*, 349–386.

87. Woods, N. F., Mitchell, E. S., & Smith-Dijulio, K. (2009). Cortisol levels during the menopausal transition and early post menopause: Observations from the Seattle Midlife Women's Health Study. *Menopause, 16*(4), 708–718.

88. Woods, N. F., Mitchell, E. S., Tao, Y., et al. (2006). Polymorphisms in the estrogen synthesis and metabolism pathways and symptoms during the menopausal transition: Observations from the Seattle Midlife Women's Health Study. *Menopause, 13*(6), 902–910.

Chapter

HORMONE REPLACEMENT THERAPY (HRT)

4

Contents

Introduction

Hormone Replacement Therapy (HRT) is a medical treatment aimed at alleviating symptoms associated with hormonal imbalances, particularly in women undergoing menopause. HRT seeks to restore these hormone levels to mitigate symptoms such as hot flashes, night sweats, mood swings, vaginal dryness, and osteoporosis (Abu et al., 2019).

HRT comes in several forms, including oral tablets, skin patches, gels, creams, and implants. The therapy typically involves either estrogen alone (for women who have had a hysterectomy) or a combination of estrogen and progesterone (for women with an intact uterus) to reduce the risk of endometrial cancer associated with estrogen-only therapy.

The benefits of HRT are well-documented. It is highly effective in reducing menopausal symptoms, improving quality of life, and protecting against bone loss that can lead to osteoporosis and fractures. Additionally, some studies suggest HRT may offer protective benefits for the heart when initiated around the time of menopause (Accreditation Commission for Health Care, 2023).

However, HRT is not without risks. Potential side effects and risks include an increased likelihood of blood clots, stroke, and certain types of cancer, such as breast and endometrial cancer. The decision to use HRT should be based on a thorough discussion between a woman and her healthcare provider, considering personal health history, risk factors, and the severity of menopausal symptoms (Allen et al., 2023).

Current guidelines suggest using the lowest effective dose of HRT for the shortest duration necessary to manage symptoms. Regular follow-ups and reassessments are crucial to ensure the therapy remains appropriate and effective.

HRT is a valuable option for managing menopausal symptoms and improving the quality of life for many women. While it offers significant benefits, it is essential to carefully weigh these against the potential risks and to personalize the treatment approach based on individual health needs and circumstances (Anderson et al., 2004).

Orientation and Directional Terms

Term	Definition	Illustration
Estrogen	Estrogen is a steroid hormone that helps develop and regulate the female reproductive system and secondary sex characteristics.	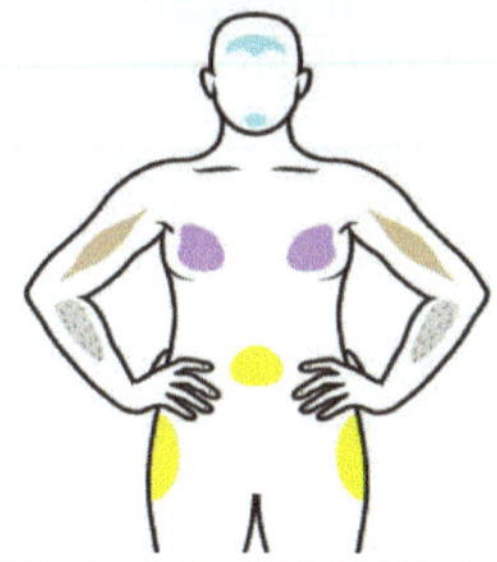
Menopause	Menopause, also known as the climacteric, is the time when a woman's ovaries stop producing hormones and menstrual periods permanently stop.	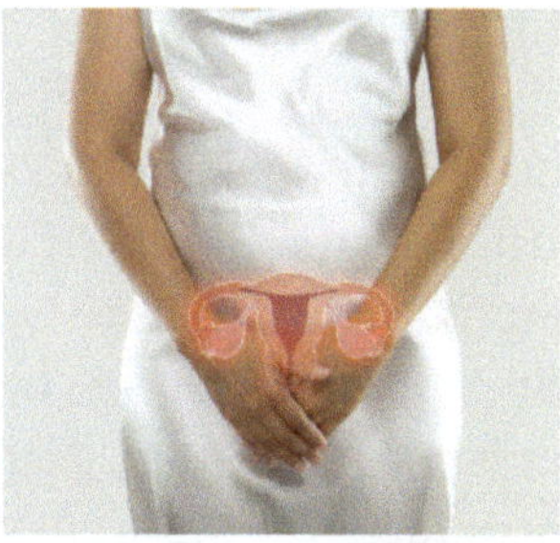
Osteoporosis	Osteoporosis is a bone disease that develops when bone mineral density and bone mass decreases, or when the structure and strength of bone changes.	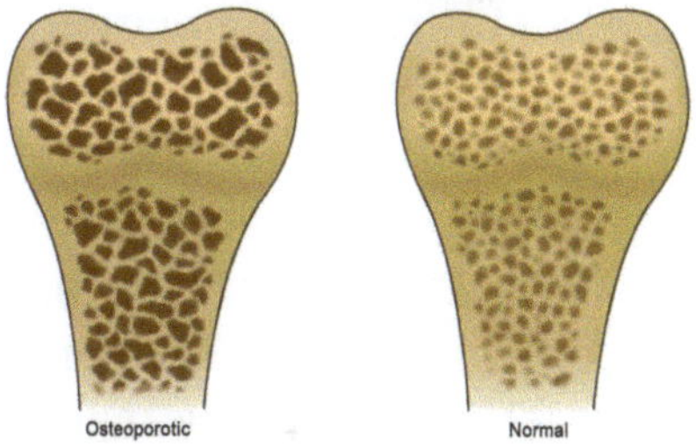
Progestogen	Progestogens are a class of steroid hormones that are either natural or synthetic and bind to progesterone receptors in the body.	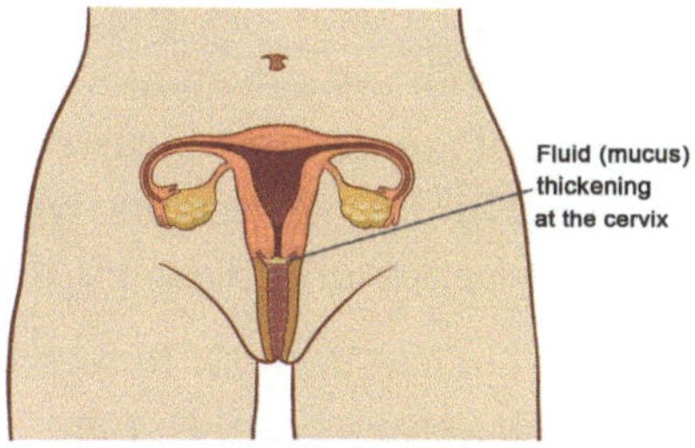
Blood-clotting	Blood clotting, also known as coagulation, is the process by which blood changes from a liquid to a gel to prevent excessive bleeding when a blood vessel is damaged.	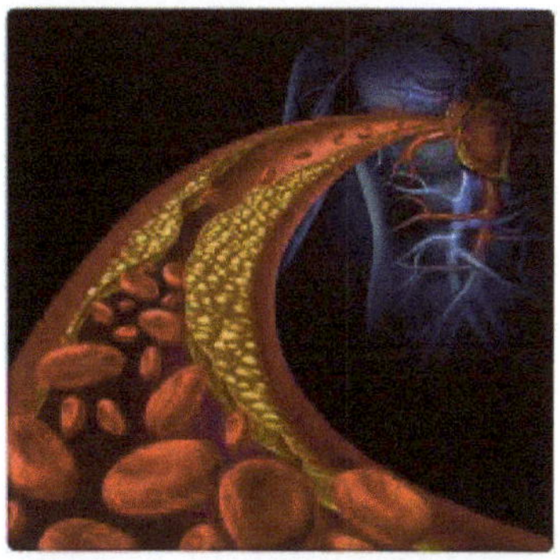

4.1. Overview of Hormone Replacement Therapy

Women who undergo hormone replacement therapy (HRT) are given additional hormones to replace those lost during the menopausal transition. Conventional hormone replacement therapy (HRT) mimics the hormones produced by the human ovary by including an estrogen and progesterone component to relieve menopausal symptoms.

Numerous hormone therapies exist, including those that are naturally occurring in the human ovary, such as estradiol and estriol (Berrodin et al., 2009). Conjugated equine estrogen (CEE), the most often prescribed estrogen in the US, is one of the other estrogenic compounds. Although they have different effects on the human body, they have the same FDA recommendations. This exercise explains when hormone replacement therapy is appropriate and emphasizes the importance of the interprofessional team in treating patients who have postmenopausal symptoms (Barrett-Connor et al., 1991). Hormone Replacement Therapy (HRT) is a treatment that provides women with hormones that are lost during menopause. This therapy aims to alleviate the symptoms of menopause by using a combination of estrogen and progesterone, which are similar to the hormones produced by the ovaries.

The Physicians Desk Reference states that while their effects on the human body are different, they have the same FDA indications. The indications for menopausal issues include:

- Treatment of vasomotor symptoms of menopause
- Treatment of genitourinary syndrome of menopause (previously known as vaginal and vulvar atrophy)
- Prevention of osteoporosis

The term "progestogen" refers to both progesterone produced by the human ovary and progestins, which are substances that resemble progesterone. To prevent endometrial hyperplasia or cancer in her uterus, a woman who wants hormone replacement therapy (HRT) and has an intact uterus needs to take a progestogen with estrogen. The endometrial lining will grow on its own when estrogen is present. Progestogens prevent the lining from growing uncontrollably (Blondon et al., 2021). After a hysterectomy, it is generally believed that a woman no longer requires progestin. Progesterone, on the other hand, is unique since it can alleviate symptoms of mood swings and sleep disturbances, and there is mounting evidence that it protects breast tissue.

FDA-approved indications for progestogens include:

- Amenorrhea, either primary or secondary
- Assisted reproductive technology treatment
- Endometrial hyperplasia
- Dysfunctional uterine bleeding

There are many options for administering estrogen and progestogens, and they can be applied topically or subcutaneously using patches, creams, vaginal inserts, or subdermal pellets. Each administration route has advantages and disadvantages of its own (Bluming, 2022).

- **Oral Estrogen:** Any estrogen administered orally results in increased activated protein-C resistance, increasing the risk of a blood clot. Oral estradiol also induces the hepatic formation of matrix metalloprotease 9, which decreases the formation and rupture of atherosclerotic plaque.

- **Transdermal Estrogen:** Bypasses the hepatic metabolism that produces activated protein-C resistance, and the risk for blood clotting is negated.

The most common way to administer progestin is orally, though some are available in patch form when combined with estrogen. Progesterone can be taken orally and applied vaginally for purposes not authorized by the FDA (Bush et al., 1987).

Sublingual troches, vaginal inserts, and compounded estrogen and progesterone creams are produced by specialty pharmacies.

4.1.1. Adverse Effects

In the US, the Women's Health Initiative (WHI) is the most cited source of information when researching the possible side effects of hormone replacement therapy (Canete et al., 2019).

- **WHI Trial:** This was a complex trial that involved two randomized, double-blind, placebo-controlled studies of postmenopausal hormone therapy. Medroxyprogesterone acetate (MPA) at 2.5 mg per day was combined with CEE at 0.625 mg per day in the first arm. In the second arm, patients who had previous hysterectomies and were solely receiving CEE 0.625 mg were studied.
- **HRT and the Breast:** The CEE/MPA arm was stopped sooner than anticipated because of a 24% (HR=1.24) increase in the incidence of invasive breast cancer. The CEE-only arm was finished in 2004 and has had extended patient follow-up for 11.8 years. It was not terminated early. A statistically significant 23% (HR=0.77) reduction in breast cancer is linked to CEE use for five to nine years. In addition, 63% fewer people in the CEE arm died from breast cancer than in the non-CEE group, and 38% fewer people died from all other causes following a diagnosis of breast cancer (Canonico et al., 2007).

Examining data from European studies—which typically employ non-MPA progesterone or progestins and estradiol derivatives rather than CEE—reveals wildly disparate and inconsistent results. Breast cancer risk was found to be 10% higher when transdermal estradiol was used alone, but 10% lower when combined with progesterone.

- **HRT and the Heart:** Over the course of five years of use, the WHI CEE/MPA arm experienced a 24% increase in the overall incidence of coronary heart disease (CHD). The largest increase in risk occurred in the first year, with an increase of 81% (HR=1.81). This evidence requires cautious interpretation due to the following:
  - The average age of the patient treated in this study was 62 years. In women who started on therapy within ten years of menopause, there was a risk reduction of CAD of 11% (HR=0.89), but this was not statistically significant.
  - In those women who continued CEE/MPA for over six years, the risk of CAD dropped by 30% (HR=0.70).

Treatments based on progesterone and estradiol are not subject to these risks. Numerous mechanisms explain why estradiol, not CEE, provides cardioprotection, according to basic science research (Canonico et al., 2007).

These include lowering coronary artery calcium (CAC) scores, lowering carotid intima-media thickness (CIMT), and stabilizing atherosclerotic plaques. Many later studies conducted in the US and Europe demonstrate that starting hormone replacement therapy (HRT) during the first four years of the menopause transition significantly lowers the risk of cardiovascular disease and death. The "Timing Hypothesis" describes the hypothesis that a cardiovascular benefit is observed when hormone replacement therapy (HRT) is started closer to the menopause transition than when it is started later.

- **HRT and Risk of Stroke:** The WHI trial showed a rise in stroke incidence in both arms: 31% in the CEE/MPA arm and 39% in the CEE arm. There is no change in the incidence of fatal stroke, but there is a similar stroke risk according to inconsistent studies utilizing oral estradiol (Chlebowski et al., 2020).
- **HRT and the Risk of Venous Thromboembolism (VTE):** In the WHI CEE/MPA arm, the risk of VTE, which includes pulmonary embolism and deep vein thrombosis, increased by twofold (HR= 2.06).

Many European studies show that transdermal estradiol does not carry the same thromboembolic risk. A lower overall risk of 0.9 for a blood clot was found in the French ESTHER study. These results are supported by other studies examining various transdermal estradiol dosages and administration methods, with at least no effect on the risk of blood clotting (Cho et al., 2019).

4.1.2. Contraindications

Contraindications for oral or transdermal estrogen-based therapies include:

- Known, suspected, or history of breast cancer
- Known or suspected history of other estrogen-based cancer, i.e., uterine cancer. Women who have had a hysterectomy and have no remaining evidence of disease are still candidates for HRT
- Active deep venous thrombosis (DVT) or a history of DVT or pulmonary embolism (PE)
- History of blood clotting disorder, the most common being Factor V Leiden mutation carriers
- Active or history of arterial thrombotic diseases such as myocardial infarction or stroke
- Chronic liver disease or dysfunction
- Migraine with aura

Transvaginal-based estrogen therapies are exempt from these contraindications because the serum concentration of estrogen obtained through this method is very low. Transvaginal estrogen treatments should not be subject to the same black-box warning as conventional hormone replacement therapy, according to the North American Menopause Society (NAMS).

4.1.3. Monitoring

Progesterone and estradiol levels are not typically monitored by measuring their levels. Rather, the absence of side effects and the alleviation of menopausal symptoms indicate a sufficient medical response.

Adverse side effects may include:

- Abnormal uterine bleeding
- Fluid retention
- Breast tenderness
- Headaches

- Mood changes

There is no scientific proof that HRT causes appreciable weight gain. Serum testing should be used to monitor hormone replacement therapy (HRT), which includes androgen therapies like testosterone but is not the same as conventional HRT (Cold et al., 2022).

4.1.4. Enhancing Healthcare Team Outcomes

Menopausal patients need to be managed by an interdisciplinary team that includes a pharmacist and a nurse. Clinicians shouldn't empirically recommend hormone replacement therapy to improve patient outcomes (Duong et al., 2021). Numerous negative outcomes, such as an elevated risk of breast cancer, stroke, heart disease, and deep vein thrombosis, are associated with these hormones. Close observation is necessary and the course of treatment for these hormones shouldn't exceed a few years. Women who exhibit mild menopausal symptoms should be educated about the advantages and disadvantages of these hormones. In addition to reviewing the patient's medication history, the pharmacist should speak with the prescriber regarding the precise agent and dosage (Gartlehner et al., 2022). Nurses must keep a close eye out for any indications of adverse events, report any concerns to the clinician, and monitor closely on subsequent visits. Using an interprofessional team approach, HRT will yield the best results.

4.2. Medical Uses of Hormone Replacement Therapy

In the US, HRT is approved for the short-term management of menopausal symptoms like vaginal atrophy and hot flashes, as well as the prevention of osteoporosis. The American College of Obstetrics and Gynecology (ACOG) supports the use of hormone replacement therapy (HRT) in suitable situations, approving its use for the symptomatic relief of menopausal symptoms up to the age of 65. The 2016 annual meeting of the North American Menopause Society (NAMS) noted that for women under 60, the benefits of hormone replacement therapy (HRT) may outweigh the risks (Gliemann and Hellsten, 2019).

According to a consensus expert opinion released by The Endocrine Society, HRT carries fewer risks than previously reported and, in most cases, lowers all cause mortality when taken during perimenopause or the early years of menopause. Additionally, position statements endorsing HRT when appropriate have been released by the American Association of Clinical Endocrinologists (AACE). Women who receive this treatment are typically menopausal after surgery, during menopause, or both. Menopause is the term used to describe the period of time that ends permanently twelve months after the last natural menstrual cycle and is caused by ovarian follicular activity loss. Menopause is divided into early and late transition periods known as "perimenopause" and "postmenopause" based on this twelve-month time frame. Surgery to remove the ovaries can cause premature menopause, just as it can be used to treat uterine or ovarian cancer (Gompel et al., 2018).

In terms of demographics, postmenopausal American women with average ages over 60 and concurrent pre-existing conditions make up the great majority of the data that is currently available.

4.2.1. Menopausal Symptoms

HRT is often given as a short-term relief from menopausal symptoms during perimenopause. Potential menopausal symptoms include:

- Hot flashes – vasomotor symptoms
- Vulvovaginal atrophy – atrophic vaginitis and dryness

- Dyspareunia – painful sexual intercourse due to vaginal atrophy and lack of lubrication
- Bone loss – decreased bone mineral density, which can eventually lead to osteopenia, osteoporosis, and associated fractures
- Decreased sexual desire
- Defeminization – diminished feminine fat distribution and accelerated skin aging
- Sleep disturbances and joint pain

The most common of these are loss of sexual drive and vaginal dryness (Sarrel, 2000) (Figure 4.1).

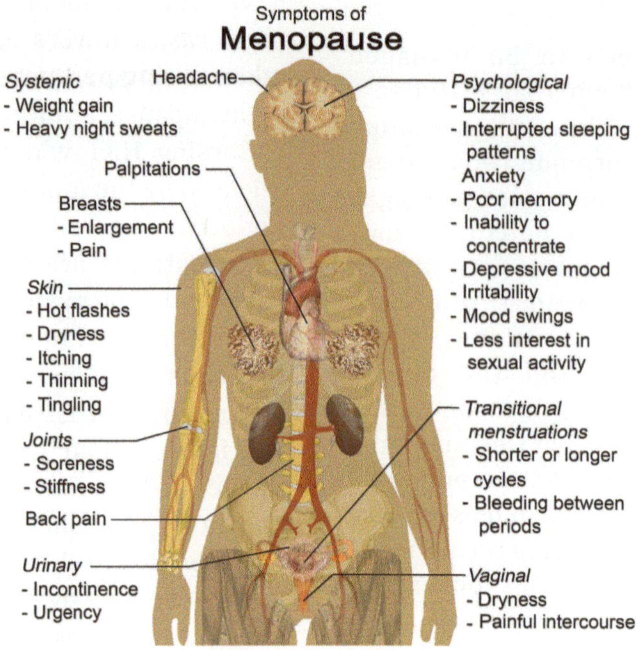

Figure 4.1. *Symptoms of menopause.*

Source: https://upload.wikimedia.org/wikipedia/commons/thumb/9/9f/Symptoms_of_menopause_%28vector%29.svg/450px-Symptoms_of_menopause_%28vector%29.svg.png.

4.2.2. Sexual Function

Menopause-related sexual dysfunction and lack of desire can be managed with HRT. According to epidemiological surveys conducted on women aged 40 to 69, 75% of them continue to engage in sexual activity after menopause. Due to longer life spans, women are now spending at least one-third of their lives in the postmenopausal stage, when maintaining a healthy sexual lifestyle can be crucial to overall well-being (Gordhandas et al., 2019).

Hypoactive sexual desire disorder (HSDD) is a common condition affecting postmenopausal women that can be improved by hormone replacement therapy (HRT). Symptoms of HSDD include decreased libido and sexual dysfunction. During this time, there are several hormonal changes that occur, such as an increase in follicle-stimulating hormone and a decrease in estrogen. Most women experience most of their changes in the late perimenopausal and postmenopausal phases. There are also decreases in inhibitor (A and B) and sex hormone-binding globulin (SHBG). Compared to estrogen and progesterone, women have lower levels of testosterone, which peaks at age 30 and progressively declines with age. There is also less fluctuation in testosterone levels during the menopausal transition (Graham et al., 2022).

Postmenopausal testosterone replacement to premenopausal levels has been recommended as an effective treatment for HSDD in a global consensus position statement. However, after two years of continuous therapy, safety information for testosterone treatment is not available, and dosing above physiologic levels is not recommended. It has been discovered that testosterone patches help postmenopausal women feel more sexually attracted. Since most trials involved women taking progesterone and estrogen concurrently and testosterone therapy itself has a relatively short duration, there is not enough information to assess the effect of testosterone replacement on heart disease or breast cancer. With the available data, testosterone therapy has not been linked to any unfavorable outcomes (Henderson et al., 2016).

Not every woman is receptive, particularly those who have experienced past sexual difficulties. Blood flow, pH levels, and vaginal cells—all of which tend to decline with the onset of menopause—can all be restored with estrogen replacement therapy. The most responsive element to estrogen seems to be pain or discomfort during sexual activity. It has also been demonstrated to benefit the urinary tract. In addition to increasing sexual arousal, frequency, and orgasm, estrogen can also decrease vaginal atrophy (Hodis et al., 2016).

After prolonged use, some women may experience a decrease in the efficacy of hormone replacement therapy. Additionally, libido and arousal can be increased by the combined effects of estrogen and androgen replacement therapy, as opposed to estrogen alone, according to several studies. Europe's supply of tibolone, a synthetic steroid with androgenic, progestogenic, and estrogenic qualities, can help with mood, libido, and physical symptoms. Improvements in vasomotor symptoms, emotional response, sleep disturbances, physical symptoms, and sexual desire have been observed in several placebo-controlled studies; however, the risk profile is comparable to that of conventional hormone replacement therapy (Ziaei et al., 2010) (Figure 4.2).

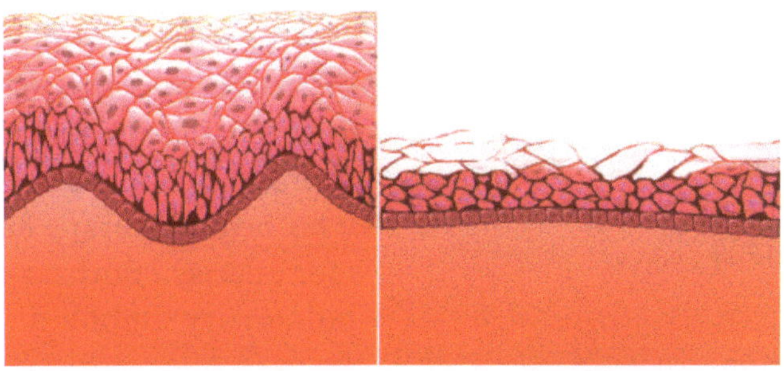

Figure 4.2. *Atrophy of vaginal mucosa that occurs with menopause.*

Source: https://upload.wikimedia.org/wikipedia/commons/thumb/8/85/Vaginal_Mucosa_Normal_vs_Menopause.png/450px-Vaginal_Mucosa_Normal_vs_Menopause.png.

4.2.3. Muscle and Bone

The effects of aging on muscle can be effectively reversed with hormone replacement therapy using androgen and estrogen. In older women, lower free testosterone is linked to a lower incidence of hip fractures, while lower testosterone is linked to lower bone density. In addition to improving reduced sexual function, testosterone therapy can build muscle and bone density.

4.2.4. Side Effects

Side effects in HRT occur with varying frequency and include:

- Common
  - Headache
  - Upset stomach, stomach cramps or bloating
  - Diarrhea
  - Appetite and weight changes
  - Changes in sex drive or performance
  - Nervousness
  - Brown or black patches on the skin
  - Acne
  - Swelling of hands, feet, or lower legs due to fluid retention
  - Changes in menstrual flow
  - Breast tenderness, enlargement, or discharge
  - Sudden difficulty wearing contact lenses
- Uncommon
  - Double vision
  - Severe abdominal pain
  - Yellowing of skin or eyes
  - Severe depression
  - Unusual bleeding
  - Loss of appetite
  - Skin rash
  - Lassitude
  - Fever
  - Dark-colored urine
  - Light colored stool
  - Chorea

4.2.5. Health Effects of HRT

4.2.5.1. Heart Disease

HRT appears to have a divergent effect on menopause, with no effect after ten years and a lower risk of heart disease when started within five years. Hormone replacement therapy (HRT) carries a minimal risk of cardiovascular events for women who are in early menopause and do not have any cardiovascular health concerns. Twenty years after menopause, taking HRT could lead to a rise in heart disease. Because of this variability, some reviews have concluded that there is no discernible impact on morbidity. The fact that long-term mortality from HRT is unchanged with age is significant (Jewett et al., 2014).

Women who began taking hormone replacement therapy (HRT) less than ten years after menopause may have a decreased risk of death and coronary heart disease, but there may not be a significant impact on their risk of stroke or pulmonary embolism. There was little change in mortality and coronary heart disease but a higher risk of stroke in those who began therapy more than ten years after menopause. Both treatments were linked to pulmonary emboli and venous clots.

Progesterone and estrogen replacement therapy (HRT) lowers cholesterol as well. HDL falls and lipoprotein, triglycerides, and LDL rise during menopause; these trends change when estrogen levels rise. In addition, HRT enhances coronary blood flow, sugar metabolism, heart contraction, and reduces plaque development and platelet aggregation. Through the induction of cholesterol ABC transporters, HRT may facilitate reverse cholesterol transport. HRT slows the development of new vascular lesions but does not stop the progression of lesions that already exist, according to atherosclerosis imaging trials. A significant decrease in the pro-thrombotic lipoprotein a is another effect of HRT (Kantarci et al., 2016).

Research on the relationship between testosterone therapy and cardiovascular disease has been inconsistent; while some studies have found no effect or a slight negative effect, others have found improvements in surrogate markers like weight, triglycerides, and cholesterol. Menopause-related low sex hormone-binding globulin has been linked to an elevated body mass index and a higher risk of type 2 diabetes (Shifren et.al., 2017) (Figure 4.3).

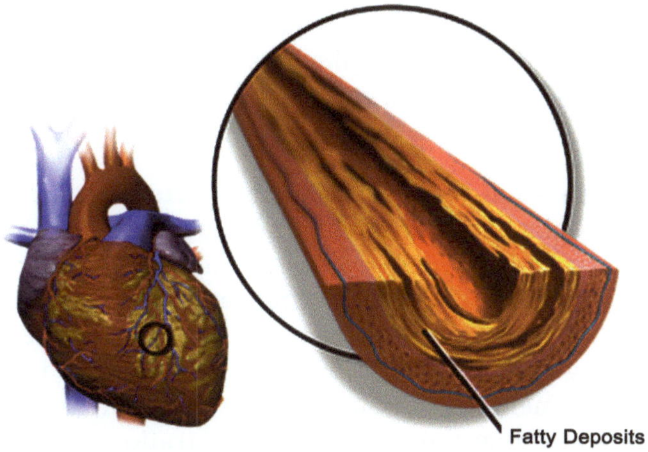

Figure 4.3. *The risks of coronary heart disease with HRT vary depending on age and time since menopause.*

Source: https://upload.wikimedia.org/wikipedia/commons/thumb/d/d1/Blausen_0257_CoronaryArtery_Plaque.png/330px-Blausen_0257_CoronaryArtery_Plaque.png.

4.2.5.2. Blood Clots

Different estrogen and progestogen therapies, as well as different dosages and application techniques, may have different effects on the development of venous blood clots and the risk of pulmonary embolism from hormone replacement therapy. Comparisons between the routes of administration indicate that the risk of blood clots is lower when estrogens are applied topically or vaginally, while the risk of pulmonary embolism and blood clots is higher when estrogens are taken orally (Langer et al., 2017). The anabolic effects that oral therapy has on liver synthesis of vitamin K-dependent clotting factors are absent from skin and vaginal routes of hormone therapy because they are not subject to first pass metabolism. This could account for the possibility that oral therapy may increase the formation of blood clots (Figure 4.4).

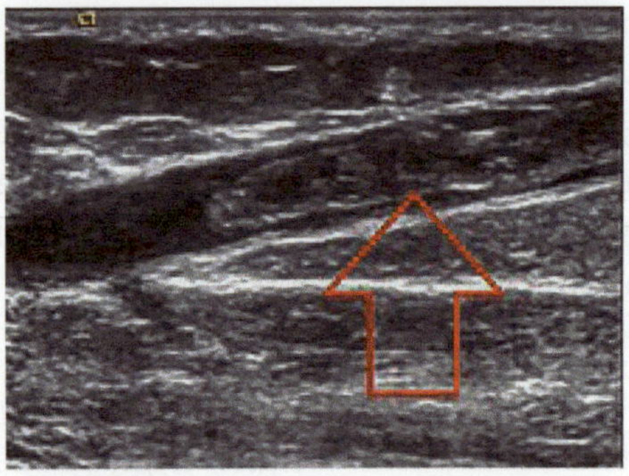

Figure 4.4. *Clot in the greater saphenous vein; oral estrogen is associated with increased risk of venous blood clots due to increased liver formation of vitamin K-dependent clotting factors.*

Source: https://upload.wikimedia.org/wikipedia/commons/thumb/e/e6/Great_saphenous_vein_thrombosis_05091312009.jpg/330px-Great_saphenous_vein_thrombosis_05091312009.jpg.

4.2.5.3. Stroke

According to several research studies, if treatment is started within five years of menopause, there is no chance of an HRT-related stroke. If treatment is administered by non-oral routes, there may even be no correlation at all. The risk of an ischemic stroke increased in the WHI during the intervention period, but this effect did not significantly change after treatment ended or in long-term follow-up mortality. Cohort studies in Swedish women have indicated a possible link between oral synthetic estrogen or combined estrogen-progestogen treatment and hemorrhagic and ischemic stroke when treatment is postponed until five years after menopause. Another sizable group of Danish women revealed that the mode of administration mattered, concluding that while oral estrogen raised the risk of stroke, skin absorption had no effect and vaginal estrogen actually lowered the risk (Manson et al., 2013).

4.2.5.4. Endometrial Cancer

Continuous combined estrogen plus progestin lowers the incidence of endometrial cancer in postmenopausal women. To prevent endometrial disease, progestogen therapy should be administered for a minimum of 14 days each cycle.

Two types of endometrial cancer have been identified in relation to hormone replacement therapy. The most prevalent type, Type 1, is often low-grade and is linked to estrogen therapy. Type 2 is typically higher grade and has a worse prognosis; it is unrelated to estrogen stimulation. Progesterone can be administered concurrently with estrogen therapy to prevent the endometrial hyperplasia that results in endometrial cancer. There is a theory that the widespread use of high-dose estrogens for birth control during the 1970s contributed significantly to the rise in type 1 endometrial cancer cases (Manson et al., 2003).

Contrary to popular belief, progestogens actually accelerate the growth of uterine fibroids. To ensure that there are no underlying endometrial or uterine lesions, a pelvic ultrasound can be done before starting HRT. In postmenopausal women, androgens do not promote endometrial proliferation; rather, they seem to partially block the proliferation that estrogen causes.

There is not enough high-quality evidence to advise women who are thinking about hormone replacement therapy following endometrial cancer treatment (Manson et al., 2003) (Figure 4.5).

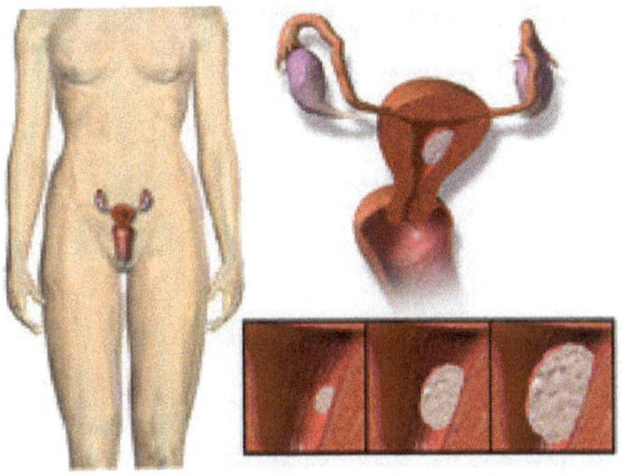

Figure 4.5. *Endometrial cancer can be associated with HRT, particularly in those not taking a progestogen.*

Source: https://upload.wikimedia.org/wikipedia/commons/thumb/9/9b/Blausen_0348_EndometrialCancer.png/330px-Blausen_0348_EndometrialCancer.png.

4.2.5.5. Breast Cancer

The use of hormone replacement therapy to treat menopause is generally not linked to a significant increase in the risk of breast cancer. The kind of HRT, how long the treatment lasts, and the patient's age all affect the degree of risk. Those who had a hysterectomy and took estrogen-only hormone replacement therapy (HRT) had a very low risk of breast cancer. The most widely used kind of combined hormone replacement therapy (HRT) has a slightly increased risk of breast cancer. Older women have a higher risk and women in their 50s have a lower risk. The longer HRT is administered, the higher the risk. There is no higher risk of breast cancer when HRT is used for a year or less (Marjoribanks et al., 2017). There is a higher risk associated with HRT used for longer than five years, but that risk goes down when the therapy is discontinued.

Hormone replacement therapy with synthetic progestogens is associated with a non-statistically significant increased risk of breast cancer. Bioidentical progesterone may lower the risk, but the one prospective study that found evidence of this was underpowered because breast cancer was uncommon in the control group. As of 2018, there were no randomized controlled trials. The length of time between menopause and HRT, as well as the method of synthetic progestin administration, all affect the relative risk of breast cancer (Mendelsohn and Karas, 1999).

The Women's Health Initiative participants who took equine estrogen alone after a hysterectomy had a lower incidence of breast cancer, according to the most recent follow-up study. However, the relative risk rose when estrogen was taken in combination with medroxyprogesterone. Due to the higher risk of vaginal bleeding and uterine cancer associated with unopposed estrogen, estrogen is typically only administered in conjunction with a hysterectomy.

HRT has been more strongly associated with the risk of breast cancer in women with lower body mass indices (BMIs). No breast cancer association has been found with BMIs of over 25. It has been suggested by some that the absence of significant effect in some of these studies could be due to selective prescription to overweight women who have higher baseline estrone, or to the very low progesterone serum levels after oral administration leading to a high tumor inactivation rate (Mikkola et al., 2016).

Women with dense or mixed-dense breast tissue have a higher risk of developing breast cancer than those with low density tissue, so evaluating the response of breast tissue density to HRT using mammography appears to help assess the degree of breast cancer risk associated with therapy.

Micronized progesterone does not appear to be associated with breast cancer risk when used for less than five years with limited data suggesting an increased risk when used for longer duration.

It is advised that women who have experienced breast cancer first explore alternative menopausal treatment options, such as selective estrogen receptor modulators (SERMs) or bisphosphonates for osteoporosis, aspirin and cholesterol-lowering medications for cardiovascular disease, and vaginal estrogen for localized symptoms. Overall, observational studies on systemic hormone replacement therapy following breast cancer are encouraging. If hormone replacement therapy (HRT) is required following breast cancer, combined systemic therapy may not be as safe as estrogen-only or estrogen-progestogen therapy. HRT does not seem to affect the risk of breast cancer in women who carry the BRCA1 or BRCA2 mutation. It has been proposed that one reason for the disparity in breast cancer detection rates between the two groups is the greater proportion of women who use HRT who also get routine screening mammograms than that of women who do not (Miller et al., 2019).

Pre-clinical research on androgen therapy has indicated an inhibitory effect on breast tissue, despite the majority of epidemiological studies indicating a positive association.

4.2.5.6. Ovarian Cancer

Ovarian cancer is linked to hormone replacement therapy (HRT), with approximately one additional case of ovarian cancer for every 1,000 HRT users. Progestogen therapy, as opposed to estrogen alone, lowers this risk when it is administered concurrently. It also gets smaller the longer it has been since stopping HRT. With respect to the particular subtype, there seems to be no correlation with clear cell, endometrioid, or mucous ovarian cancer, but a possible increased risk of serious cancer. Hormonal therapy is generally believed to improve survival rates in patients who have survived ovarian cancer following surgical ovarian excision (Neal-Perry et al., 2023).

4.2.5.7. Other Cancers

- **Colorectal Cancer:** Women who received combined estrogen-progesterone therapy in the WHI were less likely to develop colon cancer. But compared to colorectal cancer in women who do not take hormones, the cancers they did have had a higher chance of spreading to lymph nodes or other remote locations. Usage of HRT is hypothesized to reduce overall mortality and recurrence risk in survivors of colorectal cancer.
- **Cervical Cancer:** In postmenopausal women treated with hormone replacement therapy, there seems to be a marked decrease in the risk of cervical squamous cell cancer and a slight increase in adenocarcinoma. There is no evidence from studies that using HRT with survivors of cervical cancer increases the chance of recurrence.

4.3. Types of Hormone Replacement Therapy

4.3.1. Estrogen

There are three types of estrogen produced by the body that can be supplemented. The primary form of estrogen found in the body after menopause is called estradiol (E1), which is mainly produced in fatty tissue. The strongest form of estrogen, known as estradiol (E2), is present in the body before menopause. The ovaries generate estradiol, but its levels drop significantly after menopause. The body also produces estriol (E3), the weakest form of estrogen, mainly during pregnancy (Nudy et al., 2019).

The most often prescribed oral estrogen replacement is conjugated equine estrogen (CEE). It is made from the urine of pregnant horses and mostly consists of estrone (E1). There are also oral, topical, and vaginal forms of estradiol (E2). Compounding pharmacies can create combinations of different types of estrogen that some clinicians recommend because they may more closely resemble the natural ratios of estrogen found in the body. Though no research has been done, some clinicians think that women with higher levels of estriol (E3), the weakest form of estrogen, may be protected against estrogen-driven cancers such as uterine and breast cancers.

Common starting doses include:

- Conjugated equine estrogen 0.45 to 0.625 mg orally daily
- Micronized 17β-estradiol 0.5 to 1 mg orally daily
- 17β-estradiol 0.0375 to 0.075 mg per day transdermal patch
- Estradiol 10 mcg intravaginally

4.3.2. Progesterone

To prevent endometrial cancer, progesterone must be taken by any woman who has a uterus and is taking oral or transdermal estrogen. Micronized progesterone (MP) is the product of recent developments to increase progesterone absorption and duration of action. Micronized progesterone has a lower risk of invasive breast cancer and is better tolerated than medroxyprogesterone acetate (MPA), with fewer side effects such as irritability and bloating (Ortac et al., 2019).

Common starting doses include:

- medroxyprogesterone acetate 1.5 to 5 mg daily
- norethindrone acetate 0.1 to 0.5 mg daily
- drospirenone 0.25 to 0.5 mg daily
- micronized progesterone 100 to 200 mg daily

4.3.3. Principles of Prescribing Hormone Replacement Therapy

Women who have a history of blood clots, estrogen-sensitive breast and endometrial cancers, elevated triglyceride levels, chronic liver disease, or unexplained vaginal bleeding should not use HRT (Parish et al., 2021). Each woman should make her own decision about hormone replacement therapy (HRT) with the assistance of her clinician, taking into account her medical history, risk factors, attitude toward menopause, time since menopause, and quality of life (Petitti et al., 1987).

- Use the lowest effective dose of HRT to treat symptoms and minimize risks.
- Initiate HRT early and treat for the shortest duration of time, regularly evaluating for ongoing need and effectiveness.

In the words of the Global Consensus Statement on Menopausal Hormone Therapy, "For symptomatic women before the age of 60 or within 10 years after menopause, benefits are more likely to outweigh risks." Due to a slightly increased risk of breast cancer, combined estrogen and progesterone therapy should be reevaluated after three to five years. The length of use can be extended for estrogen-only therapy (Prentice et al., 2005).

- Use the safest preparation of hormones that is associated with the lowest risks.

If vaginal dryness is the only symptom, think about administering HRT vaginally. Think about topical or transdermal estrogen, which avoids the first-pass liver effect and, in comparison to oral preparations, carries a lower risk of venous thromboembolism. To reduce the risk of breast cancer, think about taking oral micronized progesterone instead of synthetic progestins.

- Prescribe a progestin along with estrogen if a uterus is still present to reduce the risk of endometrial cancer.

Progestin should be administered in addition to systemic or transdermal estrogen, advises the North American Menopause Society. If appropriate doses of intravaginal estrogen are prescribed, progestin need not be taken (Pridjian et al., 1987). Despite not having FDA approval for this indication, the levonorgestrel IUD is adequate to guard against this risk.

4.4. Menopausal Hormone Therapy

Estradiol (E2) preserves bone mineral density in postmenopausal women while effectively reducing vasomotor symptoms and those linked to the genitourinary syndrome of menopause, or symptoms of vulvovaginal atrophy (Prior, 2018). Additionally, the data demonstrates that estrogen–E2 is linked to a lower risk of cardiovascular disease and breast cancer.

4.4.1. Why Are Physicians Hesitant to Prescribe Menopausal Hormone Therapy?

The history of menopausal hormone therapy (HT), the Development of scientific knowledge regarding the advantages and disadvantages of hormones, variations in hormone formulations, dosages, and administration methods, and the most recent research substantiating the efficacy and safety of isomolecular (human-identical) forms of progesterone and estradiol are all briefly covered in this Clinical Expert Series.

4.4.2. The History of Menopausal Hormone Therapy

Early in the 20th century, Allen and Doisy's groundbreaking research revealed estrogen to be the hormone associated with women. Soon after, the pharmaceutical industry discovered that pregnant mares' urine was a rich source of estrogen. Premarin, or the urine of pregnant mares, was authorized by the U. S. FDA for the treatment of menopausal symptoms in 1942, and sales continued to rise until a 1975 link between unopposed estrogen use and endometrial hyperplasia or carcinoma was established. By the early 1980s, it was clear that endometrial cancer and overgrowth could be avoided by taking continuous estrogen in combination with a progestin, a synthetic, well-absorbed progesterone derivative. Millions of women were thrilled to have their vaginal symptoms, night sweats, and hot flashes resolved, which caused sales to soar once more (Rott, 2014).

Early in the 1980s, there were studies indicating a decrease in cardiovascular morbidity and mortality, as well as reports of osteoporosis prevention and bone mineral density preservation (Salagame et al., 2018). While the Framingham Heart Study indicated that women taking conjugated equine estrogen and medroxyprogesterone acetate may be at risk for cardiovascular disease (CVD), several later cohort studies—the Nurses' Health Study, the Leisure World Study, and a Kaiser Permanente study—all included long-term follow-up and showed a significant reduction in cardiovascular risk for the cohorts using menopausal hormone therapy (HT). Based on these contradictory results, the claim that cohort studies were skewed by a "healthy user" effect, and the overwhelming impact of CVD in the US and other developed nations, the NIH was given funding for the WHI (Women's Health Initiative), a large-scale, randomized, prospective clinical trial to investigate the effects of menopausal hormone therapy on cardiovascular risk (as well as other health and aging strategies) (Sarrel, 2000).

To lower the incidence of CVD, the WHI was a randomized controlled trial (RCT) to evaluate whether postmenopausal hormone therapy (HT) should be made available to all women. To provide sufficient power for the study, an older cohort was specifically chosen, considering the comparatively low incidence of cardiovascular events among younger women. Enrolling 160, 000 women at a cost of more than $600 million was a huge, costly endeavor. The WHI hormone study's preliminary results were presented at an NIH press conference in July 2002. The study's main focus was on the negative effects of conjugated equine estrogen plus medroxyprogesterone acetate. There was no mention of the substantial advantages of lowering the risk of osteoporosis, osteoporotic fractures, and colon cancer. Prescriptions fell by 79% as a result of the public awareness of the dangers associated with menopausal hormone therapy. Early menopausal patients with symptoms were weaned off hormone therapy due to a generalized sense of uncertainty and anxiety among medical professionals and the general public. For the following decades, the release of the WHI's preliminary data altered the practices of physicians and the education of professionals regarding menopause (Scarabin, 2018).

The advantages and disadvantages of menopausal HT, particularly with E2 and micronized progesterone, for symptom relief and function preservation have been extensively discussed since the 2002 WHI publication. Menopausal hypertensive hormone therapy (HT) should be evaluated primarily for symptoms (lowest dose for the shortest duration) or, alternatively, for the preservation of function (preserving blood vessel elasticity, vulvovaginal epithelium, bone mineral density), which would necessitate long-term, even lifetime therapy? It is important to note that preservation of function is not the same as disease prevention (a distinction that is not discussed here but needs more clarification) (Schierbeck et al., 2012).

Centering the WHI data as the foundation for the majority, if not all, professional society and government agencies (such as the FDA, U.S.current postmenopausal HT guidelines and recommendations from the US Preventive Services Task Force [USPSTF]. The patient group was mostly asymptomatic and nearly ten years older on average than women going through the menopausal transition. Furthermore, even though the hormonal formulations under study were the most often prescribed medications at the time, they were not the most often advised hormones in 2023 (Simon and Kapner, 2020).

4.4.3. Conjugated Equine Estrogen Compared with Estradiol-17

Conjugated equine estrogen and isomolecular estradiol, which has the same chemical structure as human endogenously produced estradiol—than we did twenty years ago. Equine conjugated estrogen has a different structure, receptor binding profile, and cardiovascular impact than estradiol-17β. Conjugated equine estrogen contains many estrogens, at least ten of which structurally resemble human estrogens. Horses also contain other estrogens that are not present in humans (Sizar et al., 2022).

The two distinct estrogen receptors, α and β, were cloned in 1996. Conjugated equine estrogen binds primarily to the β receptor, resulting in more potent overall clinical effects, while estradiol binds equally to the α and β estrogen receptors. Conjugated equine estrogen is far more effective at stimulating matrix metalloproteinase 9, a powerful enzyme that degrades collagen, and other inflammatory markers like C-reactive protein. As a matter of fact, the early increases in cardiovascular events observed during the WHI are now ascribed to the possibility of plaque destabilization and rupture involving these mechanisms. It's interesting to note that cardiovascular events decreased following the first year of the WHI, and by the time the study was stopped, the relative risk for cardiovascular events was less than 1. It is unknown if the sudden decline in events was caused by the attrition of individuals prone to plaque rupture or by the stabilization of pre-existing plaque in elderly patients following their initial exposure to conjugated equine estrogen (Smith et al., 2013).

Numerous studies have shown that estradiol tablets, transdermal patches, and gels improve clinical outcomes, such as vasomotor symptoms, vulvovaginal symptoms, and bone mineral density preservation (gels are not FDA-approved for osteoporosis prevention). The biological activities of conjugated equine estrogen and estradiol-17β differ, as shown by a large number of head-to-head comparative trials that are outside the purview of this commentary (Somers, 2005).

4.4.4. Medroxyprogesterone Acetate Compared with Micronized Progesterone

Additionally, we now know that synthetic progestins exhibit unique receptor binding. This could have led to a higher risk of breast cancer and other potentially harmful metabolic effects for medroxyprogesterone acetate, the progestin used in the WHI (Provera and generic versions). Medroxyprogesterone acetate binds to androgen, glucocorticoid, and progesterone receptors. It raises insulin-like growth factor 1, which leads to an increase in insulin resistance. When combined with estrogen therapy, medroxyprogesterone acetate increases the risk of thrombosis. There is no evidence linking micronized progesterone to a higher risk of thrombogenic events or an increased incidence of breast cancer (Sriprasert et al., 2019).

4.4.5. Risks of Breast Cancer Related to Menopausal Hormone Therapy

4.4.5.1. Conjugated Equine Estrogen Plus Medroxyprogesterone Acetate

In the WHI Estrogen Plus Progestin Trial, 16,608 postmenopausal women with uteruses were randomly assigned to receive either a placebo or a daily oral combination of conjugated equine estrogen (0.6625 mg/d) and medroxyprogesterone acetate (2.05 mg/d). Due to "an increased breast cancer incidence," the CEE+MPA (Conjugated Equine Estrogen + Medroxyprogesterone Acetate) trial was terminated early. It is significant to highlight that the randomization was for baseline cardiovascular risk rather than baseline breast cancer risk, indicating that the trial was not a breast cancer trial (Valdes and Bajaj, 2023).

In a 2018 review, Hodis and Sarrel assessed breast cancer risk critically using the WHI studies as a lens. They discovered that in the typical postmenopausal population (women who have never used menopausal HT), conjugated equine estrogen (0.625 mg) combined with medroxyprogesterone acetate (2.5 mg) had no effect on breast cancer risk. Put another way, for as long as 11 years, conjugated equine estrogen plus medroxyprogesterone acetate had no effect on the incidence of breast cancer when compared to a placebo (Figure 4.6).

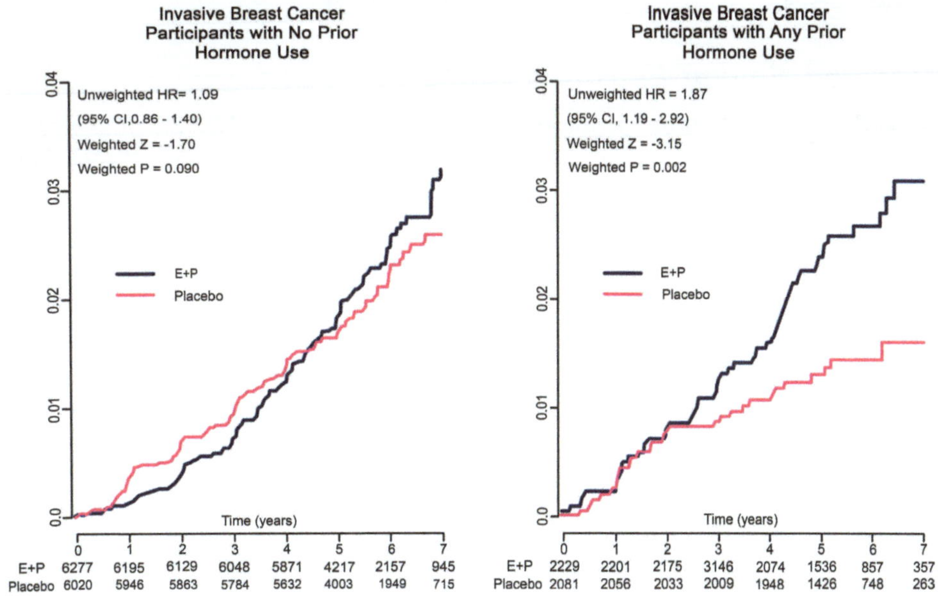

Figure 4.6. *Breast cancer incidence in the Women's Health Initiative trial of conjugated equine estrogen plus medroxyprogesterone acetate (E+P in the figure) compared with placebo, stratified by prior use of hormone therapy, showing similar trends for all the subgroups except for women with prior hormone therapy use randomized to placebo where breast cancer incidence unexpectedly sharply diverges without explanation. It is the divergence in the trend line for women with prior hormone therapy use randomized to placebo that accounts for the elevated hazard ratio for breast cancer, falsely giving the impression that breast cancer incidence was increased in the trial due to conjugated equine estrogen plus medroxyprogesterone acetate, where in fact, the elevated hazard ratio was due to a decreased breast cancer incidence in the placebo-treated group.*

Source: Reprinted with permission from Hodis HN, Sarrel PM. Menopausal hormone therapy and breast cancer: what is the evidence from randomized trials? Climacteric 2018;21:521–8. doi: 10.1080/13697137.2018.1514008.

The contentious breast cancer data were produced by the remarkably low incidence of breast cancer in the placebo group, particularly among those who had previously been on menopausal HT (25% of the study population) and had washed out prior to the start of the WHI study. The WHI authors concentrated on the treatment arm rather than examining why the annualized incidence of breast cancer in the placebo group was so low when compared to all other placebo groups in the WHI studies. The annualized incidence of breast cancer in the treatment group did not differ from that of the cohort of women who were randomized to a placebo and had never used hormones. Breast cancer incidence was remarkably low among participants who had used menopausal hormone therapy prior to being randomly assigned to this placebo group. Stated differently, there was no significant impact of conjugated equine estrogen in combination with medroxyprogesterone acetate on the incidence or mortality of breast cancer. Additionally, Hodis and Sarrel came to the conclusion that the combined risk of breast cancer in this population from conjugated equine estrogen plus medroxyprogesterone acetate was either lower or comparable to the risk of breast cancer from a variety of other factors, such as obesity, low physical activity, and consuming two glasses of wine a day (Van et al., 2023).

4.4.5.2. Conjugated Equine Estrogen Alone

The WHI conjugated equine estrogen–alone trial, which randomized 10,739 postmenopausal women with a history of hysterectomy to either daily conjugated equine estrogen 0.625 mg/d or placebo, received surprisingly little attention. When conjugated equine estrogen alone was compared with a placebo, there was a trend toward a lower risk of breast cancer that has been documented. Chlebowski et al. released the WHI 20-year follow-up data in 2020. The most noteworthy and little-known result of conjugated equine estrogen alone was the statistically significant reduction in breast cancer mortality in the conjugated equine estrogen alone group (45%) compared to the placebo group after 18 years of cumulative follow-up. The findings demonstrate that estrogen (more especially, conjugated equine estrogen alone) dramatically lowers the incidence and mortality of breast cancer. Unfortunately, the previously identified analytical errors in the WHI's CEE+MPA study were not addressed or fixed by Chlebowski et al. It is noteworthy, nevertheless, that the authors did report that, following a lengthy period of follow-up, the group randomized to receive both conjugated equine estrogen and medroxyprogesterone acetate did not experience an increase in breast cancer mortality.

4.4.6. Estradiol-17 and Breast Cancer Risk

In comparison to a group not using hormones or those using combined menopausal HT (isomolecular estradiol plus a progestin), women using isomolecular E2 alone (oral E2, transdermal E2 patches, or transdermal E2 gels) saw a statistically significant reduction in breast cancer mortality, according to the Nationwide Finnish Comparative Study, a large observational trial. When analyzing the data, this Finnish study did not distinguish between E2 delivery methods (oral, transdermal patches, or gels) and doses (1 or 2, 0.025–0.1, and 0.5–1.5 mg, respectively). Delivery mechanism and dosage effect could therefore not be examined.

The authors rationalized that there was no discernible correlation between these factors and the risk of breast cancer in their earlier data analysis. According to this study, E2 was safe for the breast to use for more than ten years. Any history of E2-based menopausal hormone therapy, including when combined with a progestin, was linked to a 50% lower risk of breast cancer death. This held true for all age groups and for over a decade of use.

4.4.7. Estradiol-17 and Cardiovascular Disease

1,006 patients were randomized in the Danish Osteoporosis Prevention Study (DOPS) to receive either no HT or 2 mg of oral E2 plus progestin when necessary. Patients in this study were followed for a maximum of 16 years after they entered menopause. Those randomized to menopausal HT had much lower rates of myocardial infarction, heart failure, or death over the course of the 10-year treatment, compared to placebo, with no increase in thromboembolism, cancer, or stroke. These results differ significantly from the WHI findings. When started in women under 60 years old or within 10 years of the start of menopause, estradiol, as opposed to conjugated equine estrogen, looks to be safe for the cardiovascular system and may be protective against CVD and all-cause mortality. The WHI's published results led to the early termination of DOPS. At 16 years, there was still a significant improvement in the rates of myocardial infarction, heart failure, and mortality 6 years after exposure in the group randomized to menopausal HT, even though the majority of women in DOPS stopped menopausal HT with the 2002 publication of the WHI. Regrettably, the DOPS randomized trial ended prematurely in spite of encouraging results. Extended medical care and monitoring could have addressed open-ended questions, such as whether treatment should be continued indefinitely (Vinogradova et al., 2019) (Figure 4.7).

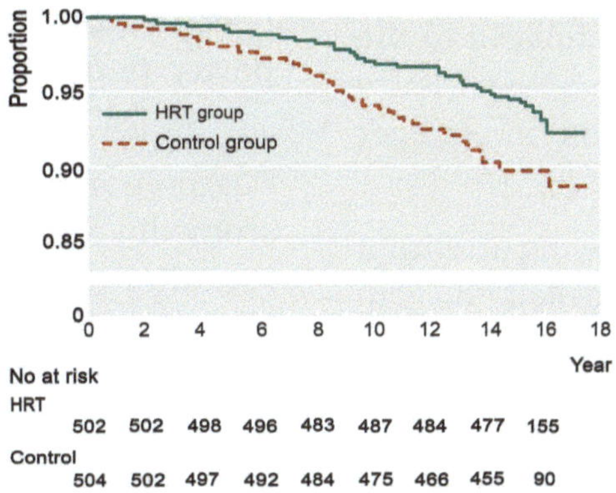

Figure 4.7. *Survival curve from the Danish Osteoporosis Study showing a statistically significant reduction of cardiovascular disease by 52% (HR, 0.48; 95% CI, 0.27–0.89) after 10 years of randomized hormone therapy (estrogen with or without progestogen) relative to no hormone therapy and reduction by 39% (HR, 0.61; 95% CI, 0.39–0.94) after 16 years of total follow-up (10 years of randomized treatment and 6 years of postintervention follow-up). Risk of death or admission to hospital due to heart failure or myocardial infarction (primary end point) over 16 years of follow-up, including 11 years of randomized treatment.*

Source: Reprinted from Schierbeck LL, Rejnmark L, Tofteng CL, Stilgren L, Eiken P, Mosekilde L, et al. Effect of hormone replacement therapy on cardiovascular events in recently postmenopausal women: randomized trial. BMJ 2012; 345:e6409. doi: 10.1136/bmj.e6409.

Endocrine system endogenous 17β is crucial for preserving vascular health. Endogenous E2 has several potential protective mechanisms against CVD. The beneficial impact of estradiol-17β on lipids, its antiplatelet properties, and its anti-inflammatory and antioxidant properties are a few examples of these mechanisms. Research has demonstrated that estrogen enhances endothelium-dependent vasodilatation, that postmenopausal women have more arterial stiffening than premenopausal women do, and that estrogen inhibits monocyte adhesion to vascular endothelium, which is a critical step in the development of atheroma.

The known elevated cardiovascular risk and event rate associated with E2 deprivation, as is observed with primary ovarian insufficiency, whether surgical or natural, strengthens the case for the cardiovascular protective qualities of E2. Treating patients until the age of natural menopause is advised by the American College of Obstetricians and Gynecologists (ACOG) to minimize the harmful health effects of early E2 deprivation in women with primary ovarian insufficiency and in women who are menopausal naturally or through surgery.

The WHI subgroup analysis verified that age and the amount of time since menopause had an impact on CVD risk. The extended 13-year follow-up in the conjugated equine estrogen-alone group showed that the group starting menopausal HT between 50 and 59 years of age had a 40% lower risk of myocardial infarction and lower all-cause mortality compared to the placebo group. Older women did not experience the same significant event reductions as younger women.

As a result, people started paying attention to the timing hypothesis, also called the gap hypothesis. According to the hypothesis, women treated with menopausal hormone therapy (HT) closer to the onset of menopause have greater benefits and lower risks associated with the treatment than women treated with HT later in life, when menopausal hormone therapy (HT) carries fewer benefits and greater risks. This relationship is influenced by age and time since menopause. Consequently, several clinical studies aimed to validate and elucidate the temporal hypothesis (Wilson et al., 1985).

The 4-year Randomized Control Trial (RCT) known as KEEPS (Kronos Early Estrogen Prevention Study) sought to determine how menopausal HT affected the progression of atherosclerosis as indicated by coronary artery calcification and carotid intima-media thickness. In nine U.S. clinical centers, 727 naturally menopausal, healthy women between the ages of 42 and 58 (mean age 52) who had not yet reached menopause were recruited. Three arms were assigned at random, two of which contained 200 mg of cyclical oral micronized progesterone administered every two days. The experimental groups received either a weekly standard-dose Climara (estradiol-17β, 0.05 mg/d) patch, an oral low-dose Premarin (0.45 mg/d), or a placebo. Both Premarin and the Climara (estradiol-17β) patch had no effect on the carotid intima-media thickness progression rate after four years. Premarin was associated with a trend of decreased accumulation of coronary artery calcification. No serious side effects, such as venous thrombosis, were reported. The researchers hypothesized that because of the small sample size or short duration, the study may not have had enough power to detect a difference.

The ELITE (Early Versus Late Postmenopausal Treatment With Estradiol) study did discover a significant benefit for oral estradiol-17β therapy on the accumulation of plaque in the carotid intima-media thickness, in contrast to the KEEPS trial. Carotid intima-media thickness was measured every six months in the randomized, double-blind, placebo-controlled ELITE trial to assess the effects of oral estradiol-17β on subclinical atherosclerosis. At the end of the trial, the coronary artery calcification score was determined by cardiac computed tomography. During a median of five years, 643 postmenopausal women were randomly assigned to receive oral estradiol-17β (1 mg/d) plus sequential micronized vaginal progesterone gel (45 mg/d, days 1–10) or placebo. The women were stratified based on time since menopause (less than six years vs. 10 years or more, early vs. late). In the early-postmenopausal arm, the median age at enrollment was 55.34 years, while in the late-postmenopausal arm, it was 63.06 years. In the early-menopausal treatment arm, the median time since menopause was 30.5 years, while in the late-menopausal treatment arm, it was 14.3 years.

Only women who started estradiol-17β therapy less than 6 years after menopause and only at the 5-year follow-up showed a significant reduction in the progression of carotid intima-media thickness (plaque accumulation) when compared to placebo. It was believed that this result was specific to estradiol-17β and unaffected by progesterone use. The authors proposed that early initiation of estradiol-17β therapy after menopause suppresses the development of atherosclerosis. Adverse events did not differ significantly between the active treatment and placebo groups.

The ELITE research team assessed the relationship between carotid intima-media thickness and serum estradiol-17β levels in a posttrial analysis. They discovered that higher levels of estradiol-17β were linked to an increase in the progression rate of carotid intima-media thickness in the late-postmenopausal group (more than 10 years postmenopausal) and a decrease in the early-postmenopausal group (less than 6 years after menopause). It is unexpected that the ELITE authors, who examined older women (median age 63.6 years) who started HT 10 years or more after menopause (median 14.3 years), a group whose demographics are comparable to those of the WHI study population, did not find any significant adverse cardiovascular events or other adverse events when compared with placebo. This implies that even in women who do not start menopausal HT early, the perceived cardiovascular safety concerns with conjugated equine estrogen found in the WHI may not apply to treatment with estradiol-17β. Possible explanations for this variation are examined elsewhere.

How can we explain the varying positive outcomes of estradiol-17β therapy observed in the KEEPS and ELITE studies? One potential factor to consider is the duration of the studies. KEEPS lasted for only 4 years, while ELITE lasted for 5 years, with the first statistically significant difference in slowing carotid intima-media thickness progression appearing at the 5-year mark. The shorter duration of the KEEPS study may have made it less likely to detect differences in only 4 years, as atherosclerosis is a slow, progressive disease that may require more time to develop and be accurately measured.

4.4.8. Menopausal Hormone Therapy and Venous Thromboembolism

Conjugated equine estrogen greatly raises the risk of pulmonary embolism, stroke, and venous thromboembolism (VTE). In a 2014 population case–control study, patients aged 30–79 from 2003 to 2009 were compared for thrombosis risk, according to a large health maintenance organization in the Pacific Northwest. There was a 68.5% average age. Comparing conjugated equine estrogen to E2, those authors discovered a statistically significant increase in the risk of VTE (odds ratio [OR] 1.78, 95% confidence interval [CI], 1.11–2.84). Additionally, there was a tendency for myocardial infarction to rise. Conjugated equine estrogen users had higher levels of activated protein C in biomarker analyzes of thrombosis, which may account for their increased propensity to clot. Notably, progestin use was taken into account when analyzing these results. Similar to WHI, age was probably a risk factor as well because VTE worsens with age.

A recent analysis of 51,571 veterans from 2003 to 2011, with a mean age of 54 years, found no increase in VTE risk for users of menopausal hormone therapy (HT). There was also no difference in risk between users of conjugated equine estrogen and either oral or transdermal E2. The rate of VTE (1.9 per 1,000 person-years) was similar to the baseline population risk (1–2 per 1,000 person-years). However, VTE rates did rise in individuals with obesity (RR 1.62) or over 75 years of age (RR 2.72) compared to those under 60 years old (Somers, 2006). The goal of the multicenter case-cohort study known as the ESTHER (Estrogen and Thromboembolism Risk) trial was to evaluate the risk of vein-related deaths (VTE) based on the progestogen formulation and the method of administering estradiol, involving women between the ages of 45 and 70 between 1999 and 2005. Using the type of progestogen and the method of estrogen administration, 271 cases of first-time VTE were compared to 670 participants in a control group. The odds ratios (ORs) for oral versus transdermal estrogen were 4.2 (95% confidence interval [CI], 1.5–11.6) and 0.9 (95% confidence interval [CI], 0.4–2.1), respectively, after correcting for potential confounding factors. Pregnane derivatives and micronized progesterone (OR 0.9, 95% CI, 0.4–2.3, and OR 0.7, 95% CI, 0.3–1.9) did not correlate with VTE. On the other hand, medroxyprogesterone acetate and other norpregnane progestogens were linked to a 4-fold higher risk of VTE (OR 3.9, 95% CI, 1.5–10.0).

It is evident that the risk of VTE rises as individuals get older, and there might be a connection between age, the utilization of conjugated equine estrogen with or without medroxyprogesterone acetate, and VTE risk. However, it seems that there is no connection between estradiol-17β when given transdermally or micronized progesterone.

4.4.8.1. Topical and Low-Dose Vaginal Estrogen Therapy

Low-dose topical estrogens (vulvar and vaginal), despite the fears of oncologists and patients alike, seem safe even for those with hormone-sensitive cancers. In a consensus statement on gynecology, ACOG says:

For those with a history of breast cancer, including those taking tamoxifen, low-dose vaginal estrogen may be used if nonhormonal treatments have not been able to effectively address symptoms, following a discussion of the risks and benefits. Low-dose vaginal estrogen may be used in patients using aromatase inhibitors (AIs) following collaborative decision-making involving the patient, gynecologist, and oncologist.

It is important to make it clear to breast cancer survivors that using topical therapies to enhance their quality of life and sexual function will not jeopardize their chances of survival. The safety of systemic HT in breast cancer survivors who have finished their course of treatment with tamoxifen or aromatase inhibitors has been suggested by several recent studies and reviews.

4.4.9. Prevention

A large number of women are experiencing menopausal symptoms without relief as a result of the error of extrapolating trial results from a beautifully designed randomized clinical trial to a population and hormonal formulations not studied in the trial. Additionally, there is a significant lack of understanding among medical professionals regarding the true risks and benefits of different hormone formulations for women during the menopausal transition and beyond. The menopausal transition is currently poorly understood by medical professionals and is not well-trained; fortunately, this has not changed in the last few years (Smith et al., 2014).

Despite data suggesting HT can prevent osteoporosis and maintain cardiovascular health, the USPSTF rated HT as having a D-level effect on disease prevention in 2023. 35 The large majority of studies selected from the WHI trials in older women using conjugated equine estrogen, with its higher risk profile than E2, negated any positive recommendation despite 18 articles showing a marked reduction in osteoporotic fractures. Compared to their 2017 analysis, the USPSTF only included two more RCTs in this 2023 update, both of which examined the structural or cognitive effects of HT on the brain. In an effort to evaluate the timing hypothesis, Henderson et al. examined the impact of 1 mg oral E2 on verbal memory in women who were younger than 6 years old as opposed to those who were older than 10 years after menopause. Neither late treatment with 1 mg oral estradiol compared to placebo nor recent menopause were found to have any appreciable differences in verbal memory as assessed by the tests. Brain magnetic resonance imaging of ninety-five women randomly assigned to receive transdermal E2, conjugated equine estrogen, or a placebo was compared by Kantarci et al. Women taking oral conjugated equine estrogen but not transdermal estradiol showed a marked increase in ventricular volume and a decrease in white matter. There were no discernible changes in any group's cognitive function. The remaining RCTs, which evaluated the effects of conjugated equine estrogen with or without medroxyprogesterone acetate, were all substantially weighted toward different WHI analyzes. Less than 1,000 of the 39,145 patients whose data were included in the USPSTF analysis were from studies that included E2. It is noteworthy that the DOPS study was not included by the authors. Excellent research indicates that estradiol-17β has heart-healthy benefits. A meta-analysis of randomized trials involving young postmenopausal women (mean age 55 years) revealed that HT containing estradiol-17β reduced mortality by 27% (RR 0.73, 95% CI, 0.52–0.96) when compared to no treatment.

Similarly, when started in women under 60 years old or with less than 10 years since menopause, HT may reduce CVD and all-cause mortality by 30–48%, according to meta-analyzes restricted to trial data stratified by age or time since menopause. According to the most recent Cochrane systematic review assessing RCTs of HT for preventing CHD in postmenopausal women, the risk of CHD was reduced by approximately half and the risk of all-cause mortality by 30% among women starting HT before the age of 60 or less than ten years after menopause. The DOPS study's poor quality, which the USPSTF attributed to a lack of blinding of outcomes assessors, led to its exclusion from its revised analysis. Furthermore, the limited number of events and imprecise estimates constrain its findings. Particularly in the setting of a national health care registry, mortality, cancer, and hospitalization for heart failure or myocardial infarction are not outcomes for which a lack of blinding is likely to produce bias. In fact, the timing hypothesis is supported by the low number of events in this earlier-age patient population, which supports WHI's decision to enroll older patients to increase the sample size for a study of CVD outcomes. A statistically significant decrease in the composite outcome of hospital admission or death for cardiovascular disease (heart failure or myocardial infarction) was observed in the DOPS study. The 95% confidence interval for the hazard ratio was 0.28–0.87, or P=. 015), strikingly comparable to the defense against CVD in the population research that served as the catalyst for the WHI. In an editorial published in Menopause, Langer et al. address the public health ramifications of the USPSTF recommendation against using menopausal hormone therapy (HT) for prevention. They skillfully illustrate the risks associated with alternative preventive strategies, such as low-dose aspirin (risk of bleeding and no cardiovascular benefit) or statins for primary cardiovascular prevention (elevated risk of non-insulin-dependent diabetes mellitus), and they contextualize the alleged harms in light of available menopausal hormone therapy options. Ultimately, even taking into account the outcomes of the WHI CEE+MPA trial, the advantages are noteworthy and substantial, with the potential to have a profound impact on public health (Figure 4.8).

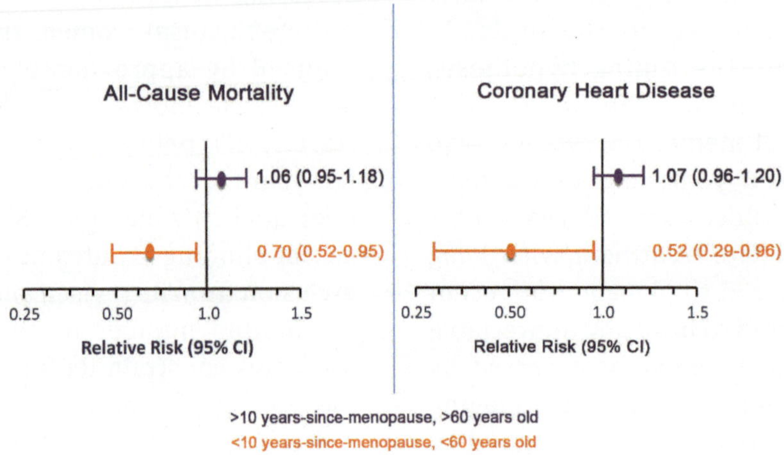

Figure 4.8. *Cochrane meta-analysis validates the Salpeter et al meta-analyzes showing similar reductions in all-cause mortality and coronary heart disease in women initiating hormone therapy <60 year old and/or <10 years-since-menopause relative to placebo. Nineteen randomized controlled trials of 40,410 women comparing hormone therapy of estrogen with or without progestogen with placebo.*

Source: Reprinted with permission from Hodis HN, Mack WJ. Menopausal hormone replacement therapy and reduction of all-cause mortality and cardiovascular disease: it is about time and timing. Cancer J. 2022;28:208–23. doi: 10.1097/PPO.0000000000000591.

4.4.10. Alternative Therapies

The fear of developing breast cancer while using hormone therapy has led many people to look for alternative options. The popularity of "bioidentical" hormone therapy, which is a marketing term often associated with Suzanne Somers, has increased, as well as the exploitation of menopausal women by industries promoting various products and services. However, there is no evidence to support the effectiveness of these interventions.

Leading medical organizations such as ACOG, the Menopause Society, and the National Academies of Sciences, Engineering, and Medicine recommend against using compounded products when FDA-approved formulations are available. FDA-approved oral and transdermal estradiol, as well as oral micronized progesterone, are available options. ACOG also does not recommend routine hormone testing to determine menopausal status. Instead, menstrual history, symptom evaluation, and physical examination are key factors in determining menopausal status. In some cases, hormone level assessment may be helpful for women who have stopped menstruating due to specific medical procedures (Rott, 2014).

The FDA has approved a new neurokinin 3 receptor antagonist for treating vasomotor symptoms related to menopause. Fezolinetant was found to reduce these symptoms in approximately 60%

of patients who received the treatment, which was higher than the 45% response rate seen in those who took a placebo.

4.4.10.1. Testosterone

After treating underlying causes, ACOG recommends transdermal testosterone therapy for postmenopausal women with hypoactive sexual desire disorder. Despite dozens of FDA-approved options for men, there is currently no testosterone product approved for use in women. For women, the recommended initial dosage of testosterone should be approximately one-tenth that of men. The International Society for the Study of Women's Sexual Health has released a detailed "how to do this" guide. Compounding may be required to give patients a convenient way to administer testosterone because it can be challenging to divide the doses meant for men. Clinicians can investigate compounding pharmacies and identify those that have not received state or federal approval and that voluntarily carry out internal quality assurance procedures by consulting with the FDA and the Pharmacy Compounding Accreditation Board. Testing testosterone levels at baseline and 3–6 weeks into therapy is advised by ACOG, not to diagnose hypoactive sexual desire disorder but to make sure that levels do not rise above premenopausal levels while on treatment.

When both formulation and route were variables, we should cease comparing oral conjugated equine estrogen with transdermal E2 and making assumptions about the latter. We are aware that different types of alcohol differ. In the body, methanol behaves differently from ethanol: while the former causes death, the latter has been consumed in social contexts for thousands of years without posing a threat to life. The FDA made a clear distinction between the results of studies on celecoxib (Celebrex), which is still approved, and one cyclooxygenase 2 inhibitor, rofecoxib (Vioxx), which the manufacturer removed from the market in 2004. We do not make recommendations based on the use of all diuretics or β-blockers together.

We know that hormone loss at or near menopause is the beginning of women's increased risk for cardiovascular disease (CVD), bone loss, and dementia. Early hormone loss in women accelerates the development of osteoporosis, heart disease, and cognitive decline (Yasar et al., 2016).

Except for DOPS, more recent studies employing estradiol and progesterone are smaller and have shorter durations, but their conclusions shouldn't be disregarded. It is clear that funding is unlikely for an RCT like the WHI, which is designed to evaluate the advantages and disadvantages of menopausal hormone therapy in a population that is just entering menopause. Therefore, it will be crucial to combine the best data from RCTs with robust and ongoing real-world evidence to support the development of clinical decision support and guidelines related to the effect of menopausal HT on the population of people who are most likely to benefit, those experiencing menopausal symptoms who are typically in their late 40s and early 50s. The tide has shifted too much in favor of not using HT on menopausal women. When taken within ten years of menopause, there is evidence to support the use of estradiol in treating vasomotor symptoms, preventing osteoporosis, and preventing cardiovascular disease and premature death. Micronized progesterone increases bone mineral density without raising the incidence or mortality of breast cancer. It's time we paid attention to what our patients had to say and gave them access to the best therapy out there for holistic care. We should put out our best effort to do this right for our patients.

Age at menopause onset, age at menopausal HT initiation, formulation, and route-specific guidelines should be developed for menopausal hormone therapy. When suitable, real-world evidence data sets should be integrated with RCT evidence to enable fair and significant conclusions to be drawn about important outcomes such as function preservation, symptom resolution, and possibly even long-term morbidity and mortality prevention. Publications' titles and conclusions should be carefully examined to make sure they truthfully and accurately convey the findings of the research presented to protect the public. Lastly, when weighing the advantages and disadvantages of menopausal hormone therapy and developing strong evidence-based guidelines, medical professionals and the general public should be made aware of the significance of each of these factors.

A Closer Look

Estradiol

Estradiol is a potent estrogen steroid hormone and the primary female sex hormone involved in the regulation of the reproductive and menstrual cycle. It is crucial for the development and maintenance of female reproductive tissues, including the breasts, uterus, and vagina. Additionally, estradiol plays a significant role in bone health, cardiovascular function, and the modulation of mood and cognitive function.

Estradiol is predominantly produced by the ovaries, although small amounts are also synthesized by the adrenal glands and, in men, the testes. During the menstrual cycle, estradiol levels fluctuate, peaking just before ovulation to facilitate the release of an egg from the ovary. It also thickens the uterine lining to prepare for potential pregnancy.

In addition to its reproductive functions, estradiol influences several other physiological processes. It helps maintain bone density by inhibiting bone resorption and promoting bone formation, which is why postmenopausal women, who experience a decline in estradiol levels, are at increased risk for osteoporosis. Estradiol also supports skin health, vascular function, and has neuroprotective effects that can impact mood and cognitive abilities.

Medical applications of estradiol include its use in hormone replacement therapy (HRT) for menopausal women to alleviate symptoms such as hot flashes, night sweats, vaginal dryness, and to prevent osteoporosis. Estradiol is also used in contraceptives, often combined with progesterone, to regulate menstrual cycles and prevent pregnancy.

While beneficial, estradiol therapy is not without risks. Potential side effects include an increased risk of blood clots, stroke, and certain cancers, such as breast and endometrial cancer. The decision to use estradiol therapy must consider individual health profiles and be closely monitored by healthcare providers.

Estradiol is a vital hormone with extensive roles in female reproductive health and beyond. Its therapeutic use in HRT and contraception highlights its importance but also necessitates careful consideration of benefits and risks. Regular medical supervision ensures its safe and effective application in managing various health conditions.

Summary

- Hormone Replacement Therapy (HRT) is a medical treatment aimed at alleviating symptoms associated with hormonal imbalances, particularly in women undergoing menopause.
- Hormone replacement therapy (HRT) is supplementing women with hormones that are lost during the menopausal transition.
- Estrogen therapies are numerous and include those indigenous to the human ovary, for example, estradiol and estriol.
- Hormone levels of estradiol and progesterone are not traditionally measured for monitoring purposes.
- HRT is often given as a short-term relief from menopausal symptoms during perimenopause.
- HRT can help with the lack of sexual desire and sexual dysfunction that can occur with menopause.
- The effect of HRT in menopause appears to be divergent, with a lower risk of heart disease when started within five years, but no impact after ten.
- Effects of hormone replacement therapy on venous blood clot formation and potential for pulmonary embolism may vary with different estrogen and progestogen therapies and with different doses or methods of use.
- In postmenopausal women, continuous combined estrogen plus progestin decreases endometrial cancer incidence.
- Androgens do not stimulate endometrial proliferation in post-menopausal women, and appear to inhibit the proliferation induced by estrogen to a certain extent.
- Any woman with a uterus taking oral or transdermal estrogen must also take progesterone to prevent endometrial cancer.
- HRT is contraindicated in women with unexplained vaginal bleeding, estrogen-sensitive breast and endometrial cancers, a history of blood clots, coronary artery disease, and elevated triglyceride levels, or chronic liver disease.

References

1. Abu Zaid, M., Dinh, P. C., Monahan, P. O., Fung, C., El-Charif, O., Feldman, D. R., Hamilton, R. J., et al. (2019). Adverse health outcomes in relationship to hypogonadism after chemotherapy: A multicenter study of testicular cancer survivors. *Journal of the National Comprehensive Cancer Network, 17*(5), 459–468.
2. Accreditation Commission for Health Care. (2024). Compounding pharmacy accreditation. Retrieved from: https://achc.org/compounding-pharmacy (accessed on 10 September 2024).
3. Advisory Panel. (2022). The 2022 hormone therapy position statement of The North American Menopause Society. *Menopause, 29*(7), 767–794. https://doi.org/10.1097/GME.0000000000001985.
4. Allen, J., Laks, S., Zahler-Miller, C., Rungruang, B., Braun, K., & Goldstein, S. R., et al. (2023). Needs assessment of menopause education in United States obstetrics and gynecology

residency training programs. *Menopause, 30*, 1002–1005. https://doi.org/10.1097/GME.0000000000002234.

5. American College of Obstetricians and Gynecologists. (2017). Hormone therapy in primary ovarian insufficiency. *Obstetrics & Gynecology, 129*(5), e134–e141. https://doi.org/10.1097/AOG.0000000000002044.
6. American College of Obstetricians and Gynecologists. (2019). Female sexual dysfunction. *Obstetrics & Gynecology, 134*(1), e1–e18. https://doi.org/10.1097/AOG.0000000000003324.
7. American College of Obstetricians and Gynecologists. (2023). Compounded bioidentical menopausal hormone therapy. *Obstetrics & Gynecology, 142*(6), 1266–1273. https://doi.org/10.1097/AOG.0000000000005395.
8. Anderson, G. L., Limacher, M., Assaf, A. R., Bassford, T., Beresford, S. A. A., Black, H., et al. (2004). Effects of conjugated equine estrogen in postmenopausal women with hysterectomy: The Women's Health Initiative randomized controlled trial. *JAMA, 291*(14), 1701–1712. https://doi.org/10.1001/jama.291.14.1701.
9. Barrett-Connor, E., & Bush, T. L. (1991). Estrogen and coronary heart disease in women. *JAMA, 265*(14), 1861–1867. https://doi.org/10.1001/jama.265.14.1861.
10. Berrodin, T. J., Chang, K. C., Komm, B. S., Freedman, L. P., & Nagpal, S. (2009). Differential biochemical and cellular actions of Premarin estrogens: Distinct pharmacology of bazedoxifene-conjugated estrogens combination. *Molecular Endocrinology, 23*(1), 74–85. https://doi.org/10.1210/me.2008-0366.
11. Blondon, M., Timmons, A., Baraff, A. J., Floyd, J. S., Harrington, L. B., & Korpak, A. M., et al. (2021). Comparative venous thromboembolic safety of oral and transdermal postmenopausal hormone therapies among women veterans. *Menopause, 28*(11), 1125–1130. https://doi.org/10.1097/GME.0000000000001823.
12. Bluming, A. (2022). Hormone replacement therapy after breast cancer: It is time. *Cancer Journal, 28*(2), 183–190. https://doi.org/10.1097/PPO.0000000000000595.
13. Bush, T. L., Barrett-Connor, E., Cowan, L. D., Criqui, M. H., Wallace, R. B., & Suchindran, C. M., et al. (1987). Cardiovascular mortality and noncontraceptive use of estrogen in women: Results from the Lipid Research Clinics Program Follow-Up Study. *Circulation, 75*(6), 1102–1109. https://doi.org/10.1161/01.CIR.75.6.1102.
14. Cañete, M. D., Valle-Martos, R., Martos, R., Cañete, R., Valle, M., & Jiménez-Reina, L. (2019). Effects of growth hormone therapy on metabolic parameters, adipokine, and endothelial dysfunction in prepubertal children. *Acta Paediatrica, 108*(11), 2027–2033. https://doi.org/10.1111/apa.14864.
15. Canonico, M., Oger, E., Plu-Bureau, G., Conard, J., Meyer, G., Lévesque, H., et al. (2007). Hormone therapy and venous thromboembolism among postmenopausal women: Impact of the route of estrogen administration and progestogens: The ESTHER study. *Circulation, 115*(7), 840–845. https://doi.org/10.1161/CIRCULATIONAHA.106.642280.
16. Chlebowski, R. T., Anderson, G. L., Aragaki, A. K., Manson, J. E., Stefanick, M. L., Pan, K., et al. (2020). Association of menopausal hormone therapy with breast cancer incidence and mortality during long-term follow-up of the Women's Health Initiative randomized clinical trials. *JAMA, 324*(4), 369–380. https://doi.org/10.1001/jama.2020.9482.

17. Cho, H. W., Ouh, Y. T., Lee, J. K., & Hong, J. H. (2019). Effects of hormone therapy on recurrence in endometrial cancer survivors: A nationwide study using the Korean Health Insurance Review and Assessment Service database. *Journal of Gynecologic Oncology, 30*(4), e51.

18. Cold, S., Cold, F., Jensen, M. B., Cronin-Fenton, D., Christiansen, P., & Ejlertsen, B. (2022). Systemic or vaginal hormone therapy after early breast cancer: A Danish observational cohort study. *Journal of the National Cancer Institute, 114*(10), 1347–1354. https://doi.org/10.1093/jnci/djac112.

19. Duong, V., Iwamoto, A., Pennycuff, J., Kudish, B., & Iglesia, C. (2021). A systematic review of neurocognitive dysfunction with overactive bladder medications. *International Urogynecology Journal, 32*(11), 2693–2702. https://doi.org/10.1007/s00192-021-04909-5.

20. Endometrial cancer risk was lower in women who used continuous combined HRT than in non-users. (2001). *Evidence-Based Obstetrics & Gynecology, 8*(1–2), 68–69.

21. Gartlehner, G., Patel, S. V., Reddy, S., Rains, C., Schwimmer, M., & Kahwati, L. (2022). Hormone therapy for the primary prevention of chronic conditions in postmenopausal persons: Updated evidence report and systematic review for the US Preventive Services Task Force. *JAMA, 328*(17), 1747–1767. https://doi.org/10.1001/jama.2022.18324.

22. Gliemann, L., & Hellsten, Y. (2019). The exercise timing hypothesis: Can exercise training compensate for the reduction in blood vessel function after menopause if timed right? *Journal of Physiology, 597*(19), 4915–4925. https://doi.org/10.1113/JP277526.

23. Gompel, A., & Plu-Bureau, G. (2018). Progesterone, progestins, and the breast in menopause treatment. *Climacteric, 21*(4), 326–332. https://doi.org/10.1080/13697137.2018.1476483.

24. Gordhandas, S., Norquist, B. M., Pennington, K. P., Yung, R. L., Laya, M. B., & Swisher, E. M. (2019). Hormone replacement therapy after risk-reducing salpingo-oophorectomy in patients with BRCA1 or BRCA2 mutations: A systematic review of risks and benefits. *Gynecologic Oncology, 153*(1), 192–200. https://doi.org/10.1016/j.ygyno.2019.01.022.

25. Graham, S., Archer, D. F., Simon, J. A., Ohleth, K. M., & Bernick, B. (2022). Review of menopausal hormone therapy with estradiol and progesterone versus other estrogens and progestins. *Gynecological Endocrinology, 38*(11), 891–910. https://doi.org/10.1080/09513590.2022.2118254.

26. Henderson, V. W., St John, J. A., Hodis, H. N., McCleary, C. A., Stanczyk, F. Z., & Shoupe, D. (2016). Cognitive effects of estradiol after menopause: A randomized trial of the timing hypothesis. *Neurology, 87*(7), 699–708. https://doi.org/10.1212/WNL.0000000000002980.

27. Hodis, H. N., & Sarrel, P. M. (2018). Menopausal hormone therapy and breast cancer: What is the evidence from randomized trials? *Climacteric, 21*(6), 521–528. https://doi.org/10.1080/13697137.2018.1514008.

28. Hodis, H. N., Mack, W. J., Henderson, V. W., Shoupe, D., Budoff, M. J., Hwang-Levine, J., et al. (2016). Vascular effects of early versus late postmenopausal treatment with estradiol. *New England Journal of Medicine, 374*(13), 1221–1231. https://doi.org/10.1056/NEJMoa1505241.

29. Jewett, P. I., Gangnon, R. E., Trentham-Dietz, A., & Sprague, B. L. (2014). Trends of postmenopausal estrogen plus progestin prevalence in the United States between 1970 and 2010. *Obstetrics & Gynecology, 124*(4), 727–733. https://doi.org/10.1097/AOG.0000000000000469.

30. Kantarci, K., Tosakulwong, N., Lesnick, T. G., Zuk, S. M., Gunter, J. L., Gleason, C. E., et al. (2016).

Effects of hormone therapy on brain structure: A randomized controlled trial. *Neurology, 87*(8), 887–896. https://doi.org/10.1212/WNL.0000000000002970

31. Langer, R. D., Simon, J. A., Pines, A., Lobo, R. A., Hodis, H. N., Pickar, J. H., et al. (2017). Menopausal hormone therapy for primary prevention: Why the USPSTF is wrong. *Menopause, 24*(10), 1101–1112. https://doi.org/10.1097/GME.0000000000000983.
32. Majumdar, S. R., Almasi, E. A., & Stafford, R. S. (2004). Promotion and prescribing of hormone therapy after report of harm by the Women's Health Initiative. *JAMA, 292*(16), 1983–1988. https://doi.org/10.1001/jama.292.16.1983.
33. Manson, J. E., Chlebowski, R. T., Stefanick, M. L., Aragaki, A. K., Rossouw, J. E., Prentice, R. L., et al. (2013). Menopausal hormone therapy and health outcomes during the intervention and extended post-stopping phases of the Women's Health Initiative randomized trials. *JAMA, 310*(13), 1353–1368. https://doi.org/10.1001/jama.2013.278040.
34. Manson, J. E., Hsia, J., Johnson, K. C., Rossouw, J. E., Assaf, A. R., Lasser, N. L., et al. (2003). Estrogen plus progestin and the risk of coronary heart disease. *New England Journal of Medicine, 349*(6), 523–534. https://doi.org/10.1056/NEJMoa030808.
35. Marjoribanks, J., Farquhar, C., Roberts, H., Lethaby, A., & Lee, J. (2017). Long-term hormone therapy for perimenopausal and postmenopausal women. *Cochrane Database of Systematic Reviews, 2017*(1), CD004143. https://doi.org/10.1002/14651858.CD004143.pub5.
36. Mendelsohn, M. E., & Karas, R. H. (1999). The protective effects of estrogen on the cardiovascular system. *New England Journal of Medicine, 340*(23), 1801–1811. https://doi.org/10.1056/NEJM199906103402306.
37. Mikkola, T. S., Savolainen-Peltonen, H., Tuomikoski, P., Hoti, F., Vattulainen, P., Gissler, M., et al. (2016). Reduced risk of breast cancer mortality in women using postmenopausal hormone therapy: A Finnish nationwide comparative study. *Menopause, 23*(11), 1199–1203. https://doi.org/10.1097/GME.0000000000000698.
38. Miller, V. M., Naftolin, F., Asthana, S., Black, D. M., Brinton, E. A., Budoff, M. J., et al. (2019). The Kronos Early Estrogen Prevention Study (KEEPS): What have we learned? *Menopause, 26*(10), 1071–1084. https://doi.org/10.1097/GME.0000000000001326.
39. Neal-Perry, G., Cano, A., Lederman, S., Nappi, R. E., Santoro, N., Wolfman, W., et al. (2023). Safety of fezolinetant for vasomotor symptoms associated with menopause: A randomized controlled trial. *Obstetrics & Gynecology, 141*(6), 737–747. https://doi.org/10.1097/AOG.0000000000005114.
40. NIH Consensus Development Panel on Osteoporosis Prevention, Diagnosis, and Therapy. (2001). Osteoporosis prevention, diagnosis, and therapy. *JAMA, 285*(6), 785–795. https://doi.org/10.1001/jama.285.6.785.
41. Nudy, M., Chinchilli, V. M., & Foy, A. J. (2019). A systematic review and meta-regression analysis to examine the timing hypothesis of hormone replacement therapy on mortality, coronary heart disease, and stroke. *International Journal of Cardiology Heart & Vasculature, 22*, 123–131. https://doi.org/10.1016/j.ijcha.2019.01.001.
42. Ortac, M., Hidir, M., Salabas, E., Boyuk, A., Bese, C., Pazir, Y., & Kadioglu, A. (2019). Evaluation of gonadotropin-replacement therapy in male patients with hypogonadotropic hypogonadism. *Asian Journal of Andrology, 21*(6), 623–627. https://doi.org/10.4103/1008-682X.265345.

43. Parish, S. J., Simon, J. A., Davis, S. R., Giraldi, A., Goldstein, I., Goldstein, S. W., et al. (2021). International Society for the Study of Women's Sexual Health clinical practice guideline for the use of systemic testosterone for hypoactive sexual desire disorder in women. *Journal of Sexual Medicine, 18*(5), 849–867. https://doi.org/10.1016/j.jsxm.2020.10.009.

44. Petitti, D. B., Perlman, J. A., & Sidney, S. (1987). Noncontraceptive estrogens and mortality: Long-term follow-up of women in the Walnut Creek Study. *Obstetrics & Gynecology, 70*(2), 289–293.

45. Prentice, R. L., Langer, R., Stefanick, M. L., Howard, B. V., Pettinger, M., Anderson, G., Barad, D., Curb, J. D., Kotchen, J., Kuller, L., Limacher, M., & Wactawski-Wende, J., & Women's Health Initiative Investigators. (2005). Combined postmenopausal hormone therapy and cardiovascular disease: Toward resolving the discrepancy between observational studies and the Women's Health Initiative clinical trial. *American Journal of Epidemiology, 162*(5), 404–414. https://doi.org/10.1093/aje/kwi237.

46. Pridjian, G., Schmit, V., & Schreiber, J. (1987). Medroxyprogesterone acetate: Receptor binding and correlated effects on steroidogenesis in rat granulosa cells. *Journal of Steroid Biochemistry, 26*(4), 313–319. https://doi.org/10.1016/0022-4731(87)90095-1.

47. Prior, J. C. (2018). Progesterone for the prevention and treatment of osteoporosis in women. *Climacteric, 21*(4), 366–374. https://doi.org/10.1080/13697137.2018.1467400.

48. Rott, H. (2014). Prevention and treatment of venous thromboembolism during HRT: Current perspectives. *International Journal of General Medicine, 7*, 433–440. https://doi.org/10.2147/IJGM.S46310.

49. Salagame, U., Banks, E., O'Connell, D. L., Egger, S., & Canfell, K. (2018). Menopausal hormone therapy use and breast cancer risk by receptor subtypes: Results from the New South Wales Cancer Lifestyle and EvaluAtion of Risk (CLEAR) study. *PLOS ONE, 13*(11), e0205034. https://doi.org/10.1371/journal.pone.0205034.

50. Sarrel, P. M. (2000). Effects of hormone replacement therapy on sexual psychophysiology and behavior in post menopause. *Journal of Women's Health and Gender-Based Medicine, 9*(1), 25–32. https://doi.org/10.1089/jwh.2000.9.25.

51. Scarabin, P. Y. (2018). Progestogens and venous thromboembolism in menopausal women: An updated oral versus transdermal estrogen meta-analysis. *Climacteric, 21*(4), 341–345. https://doi.org/10.1080/13697137.2018.1446931.

52. Schierbeck, L. L., Rejnmark, L., Tofteng, C. L., Stilgren, L., Eiken, P., Mosekilde, L., et al. (2012). Effect of hormone replacement therapy on cardiovascular events in recently postmenopausal women: Randomized trial. *BMJ, 345*, e6409. https://doi.org/10.1136/bmj.e6409.

53. Shifren, J. L., & Davis, S. R. (2017). Androgens in postmenopausal women: A review. *Menopause, 24*(8), 970–979. https://doi.org/10.1097/GME.0000000000000903.

54. Simon, J. A., & Kapner, M. D. (2020). The saga of testosterone for menopausal women at the Food and Drug Administration (FDA). *Journal of Sexual Medicine, 17*(6), 826–829. https://doi.org/10.1016/j.jsxm.2020.01.009.

55. Sizar, O., & Schwartz, J. (2022). Hypogonadism. In *StatPearls*. StatPearls Publishing. Retrieved from: https://www.ncbi.nlm.nih.gov/books/NBK572141/ (accessed on 10 September 2024).

56. Smith, N. L., Blondon, M., Wiggins, K. L., Harrington, L. B., van Hylckama Vlieg, A., Floyd, J. S., et al. (2014). Lower risk of cardiovascular events in postmenopausal women taking oral estradiol compared with oral conjugated equine estrogens. *JAMA Internal Medicine, 174*(1), 25–31. https://doi.org/10.1001/jamainternmed.2013.11074.

57. Somers, S. (2006). *Ageless*. Crown Publishing.

58. Sriprasert, I., Hodis, H. N., Karim, R., Stanczyk, F. Z., Shoupe, D., Henderson, V. W., et al. (2019). Differential effect of plasma estradiol on subclinical atherosclerosis progression in early vs late post menopause. *Journal of Clinical Endocrinology & Metabolism, 104*(1), 293–300. https://doi.org/10.1210/jc.2018-01600.

59. The 2023 nonhormone therapy position statement of the North American Menopause Society. (2023). *Menopause, 30*(5), 573–590. https://doi.org/10.1097/GME.0000000000002200.

60. Treatment of urogenital symptoms in individuals with a history of estrogen-dependent breast cancer. (2021). Clinical Consensus No. 2. *Obstetrics & Gynecology, 138*(5), 950–960.

61. U.S. Food and Drug Administration. (2023). Compounding: Inspections, recalls, and other actions. Retrieved from: https://fda.gov/drugs/human-drug-compounding/compounding-inspections-recalls-and-other-actions (accessed on 10 September 2024).

62. U.S. Food and Drug Administration. (2023). Vioxx (rofecoxib) questions and answers. Retrieved from: https://www.fda.gov/drugs/postmarket-drug-safety-information-patients-and-providers/vioxx-rofecoxib-questions-and-answers (accessed on 10 September 2024).

63. Valdes, A., & Bajaj, T. (2023). Estrogen therapy. In *StatPearls*. StatPearls Publishing. Retrieved from: https://www.ncbi.nlm.nih.gov/books/NBK567793/ (accessed on 10 September 2024).

64. Van Iten, B. (2023). Edgar Allen and Edward A. Doisy's extraction of estrogen from ovarian follicles, (1923). Retrieved from: https://hdl.handle.net/10776/11433 (accessed on 10 September 2024).

65. Vinogradova, Y., Coupland, C., & Hippisley-Cox, J. (2019). Use of hormone replacement therapy and risk of venous thromboembolism: Nested case-control studies using the QResearch and CPRD databases. *BMJ, 364*, k4810. [PMC free article] https://doi.org/10.1136/bmj.k4810.

66. Wilson, P. W., Garrison, R. J., & Castelli, W. P. (1985). Postmenopausal estrogen use, cigarette smoking, and cardiovascular mortality in women over 50: The Framingham study. *New England Journal of Medicine, 313*(17), 1038–1043. https://doi.org/10.1056/NEJM198510243131702.

67. Yaşar, P., Ayaz, G., User, S. D., Güpür, G., & Muyan, M. (2016). Molecular mechanism of estrogen-estrogen receptor signaling. *Reproductive Medicine and Biology, 16*(1), 4–20. https://doi.org/10.1002/rmb2.12006.

Chapter 5

BONE HEALTH AND OSTEOPOROSIS

Contents

Introduction

The most prevalent chronic metabolic bone disease is osteoporosis, which is defined by low bone mass and microarchitectural deterioration of bone tissue. Osteoporosis is a major global health issue that contributes to 8.9 million fractures globally each year, as well as decreased physical and psychological health, a lower quality of life, and a shorter life expectancy. Over 300,000 patients in the UK visit hospitals with osteoporosis-related fractures, which is linked to high health care costs. For instance, osteoporosis was estimated to have cost the UK's health system £1.8 billion in 2000 and is expected to cost the country £2.2 billion by 2025. Osteoporosis is more common as people age, and fractures linked to osteopenia and osteoporosis are more likely to occur in older adults. Known as fragility fractures, they typically result from low energy transfer trauma, such as falling from a standing height, and affect the vertebrae, wrist, hip, and pelvis. The majority of osteoporosis-related fractures, and the ensuing morbidity and mortality, affect octogenarians and nonagenarians. For instance, the death rate in the years after a hip fracture can reach 20%. Disability, chronic pain, decreased function, loss of independence, and the possibility of both short- and long-term institutionalization are examples of specific morbidity.

Understanding the formation, structure, and remodeling process of bone as well as the effects of aging, illness, and drug treatments on bone is necessary to comprehend the mechanism by which osteoporosis develops and the available treatment options. Our goal in this chapter is to examine osteosarcopenia, osteoporosis management, pathology and diagnosis of primary and secondary osteoporosis, and bone physiology and homeostasis as they relate to clinical practice (Arden and Spector, 1997).

Orientation and Directional Terms

Term	Definition	Illustration
Bisphosphonates	Bisphosphonates are a class of drugs that prevent bone density loss and are used to treat osteoporosis and other diseases that cause bone loss. They are the most commonly prescribed drugs for osteoporosis.	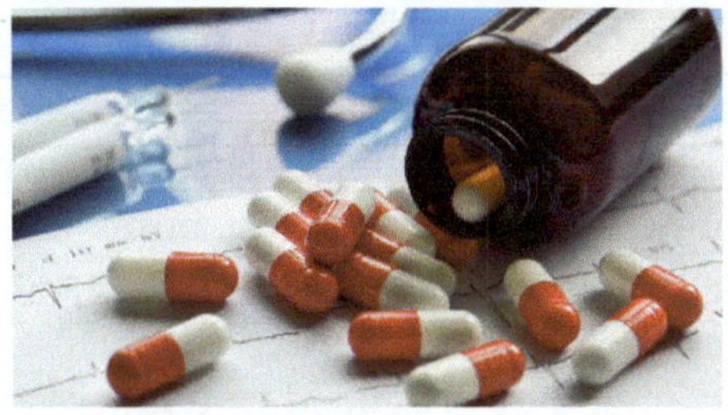
Bone mineral density	Bone mineral density (BMD) is a measurement of the amount of minerals, mainly calcium and phosphorous, in a specific volume of bone. BMD is also known as bone density or bone mass.	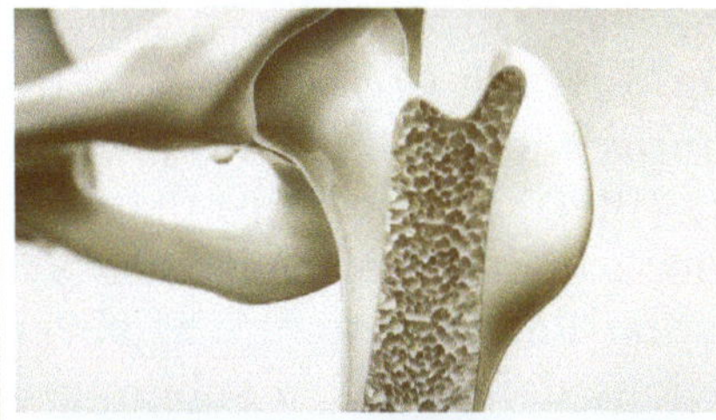
Gaucher Disease	Gaucher disease is a rare metabolic disorder in which lipids, or fats, build up in the body's organs and tissues, including the liver, spleen, and bone marrow.	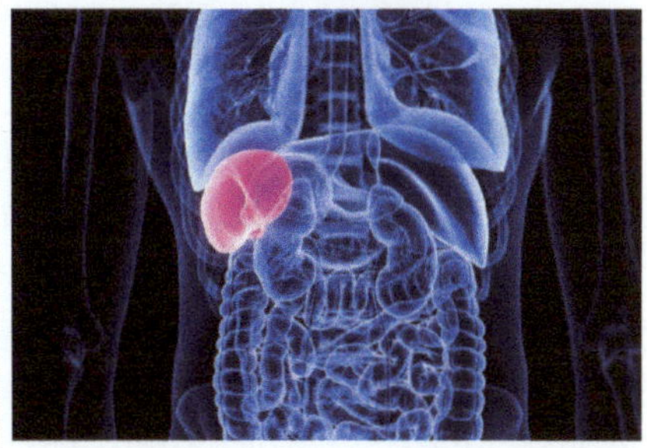
Glucocorticoids	Glucocorticoids are widely used in medical treatment. The prevalence of glucocorticoid use in postmenopausal women was estimated to be between 2.7% and 4.6% in an observational cohort of postmenopausal women.	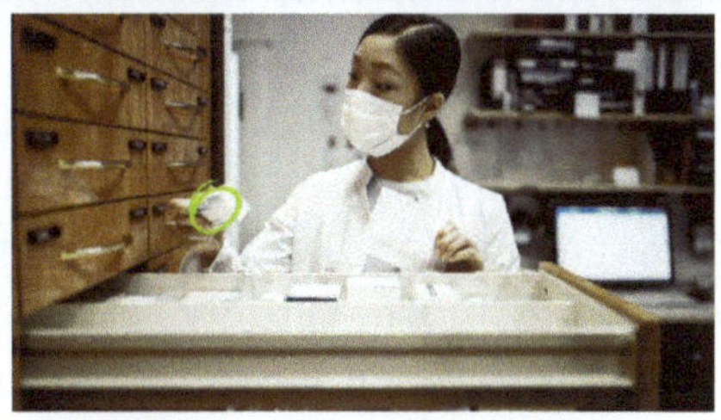
Inflammatory Bowel Disease	Inflammatory bowel disease (IBD) is a chronic autoimmune disorder that causes inflammation in the gastrointestinal (GI) tract. It's made up of two chronic conditions: Crohn's disease and ulcerative colitis.	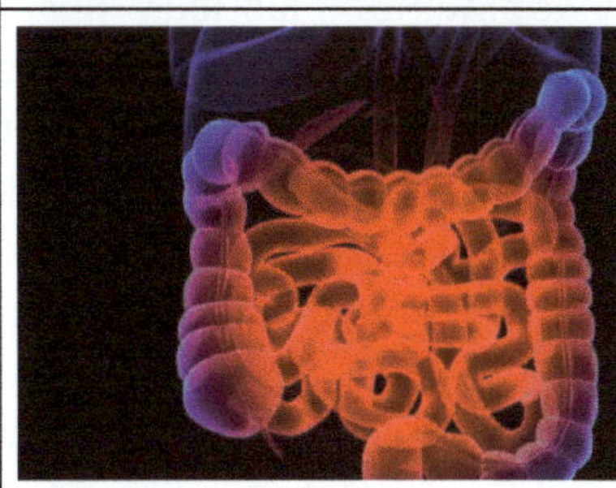

5.1. Epidemiology and Genetics of Postmenopausal Osteoporosis

Osteoporosis is characterized by loss of bone mass and deterioration of the microarchitecture of bone tissue, increasing bone fragility and susceptibility to fractures. Osteoporosis, which is a condition in which bone is normally mineralized but reduced in quantity, is literally translated as "porous bone." A working group of the World Health Organization (WHO) defined osteoporosis in 1994 as having a bone mineral density (BMD) that is more than 2.5 standard deviations below the mean of a young adult population. Because fracture had been included in previous definitions, a subgroup of women with osteoporosis who had also experienced one or more fragility fractures was considered to have severe osteoporosis that was "established."

Osteoporotic fractures have a complicated etiology. There has been a shift toward using the WHO FRAX to assess an individual's 10-year absolute fracture risk based on multiple clinical risk factors, rather than just low bone density. The FRAX tool incorporates family history, specifically pertaining to hip fractures in the parents, which highlights the hereditary aspect of the ailment. The intricate relationship between genetic and environmental factors is becoming more widely acknowledged. The study of gene-environment interactions with developmental plasticity has produced encouraging results, raising the possibility of intervening during fetal development or early life to reduce individual fracture risk and the global burden of osteoporosis. Nevertheless, only a small number of specific genes contributing to osteoporosis risk have been consistently identified. An osteoporotic fracture occurs every three seconds in women, with an estimated 200 million women worldwide suffering from osteoporosis (Johnell and Kanis 2006). This means that one in three women over 50 will experience an osteoporotic fracture. Fragility fractures account for 0.83% of the global non-communicable disease burden. In Europe, fragility fractures cause more disability-adjusted life years (DALYs) than many other chronic diseases, with a rise in this percentage to 1.75%. The current global annual cost of osteoporotic fractures is over $17 billion, and by 2025, it is predicted to reach $25 billion. Osteoporotic fracture treatment is becoming more expensive in the UK and is predicted to reach over £2 billion by 2020. This section will outline the demographic, global, and secular trends in the epidemiology of osteoporosis as well as go over the genetic and early environmental factors linked to the condition.

5.1.1. Genetics

5.1.1.1. Heritability Estimates in Osteoporosis

A significant determinant of BMD in later life is peak bone mass. Twin and family studies have indicated that between 50 and 85% of the variation in BMD is due to heritable factors, which include shared environmental exposures and genetics. These estimates do differ, though, based on the specific skeletal site, with the distal forearm BMD showing a smaller heritable component than the lumbar spine BMD. Age may also affect how much bone outcomes are influenced by heritable factors, according to several studies. Research indicates that the heritable component of bone mineral density (BMD) is lower in postmenopausal women than in premenopausal women. This finding likely reflects the increased influence of lifestyle, nutrition, and disease-related factors in postmenopausal women. Comparably, compared to peak bone mass, which happens much earlier in life, the heritable component of the rate of change in BMD in postmenopausal women is lower.

It is well known that people who have a parent who has had a hip fracture are more susceptible to osteoporotic fractures. Less evidence, on the other hand, points to a substantial hereditary component to this association. Additionally, a heritable component has been identified in the age at menopause, muscle strength, femoral neck geometry, and markers of bone turnover [Arden & Spector, 1997)]. These factors all contribute to a certain degree of susceptibility to osteoporotic fracture. These variables, along with the connections to BMD, imply that the possibility of a role in fracture prediction exists; however, because of the magnitude of the effect, it has proven challenging to prove in epidemiological studies.

5.1.1.2. Genetic Studies in Osteoporosis

Following the discovery that osteoporosis carries a minor but notable genetic component, various genetic studies have been conducted to pinpoint particular genetic loci. The genes causing several uncommon diseases linked to severe osteoporosis, fragility fractures, or high bone mass—all of which are caused by single gene mutations inherited in a classical Mendelian fashion—have been found using linkage studies, which help identify genetic mutations in monogenic disorders. For example, mutations in the COL1A1 and COL1A2 genes, which result in abnormal type 1 collagen formation, are the most common cause of osteogenesis imperfecta. Osteoporosis-pseudoglioma syndrome has been linked to loss of function mutations in the LRP5 gene, which codes for LDL receptor-related protein 5, an essential regulator in osteoblastic bone formation. On the other hand, familial high bone mass syndrome is linked to mutations in the same gene that cause gain of function.

Nonetheless, a multitude of common genetic variants have been linked to postmenopausal osteoporosis, each of which has a negligible impact. Because linkage studies have a low power to detect these common variants, their ability to identify contributory genes has therefore been limited.

Numerous susceptibility loci have been successfully identified by genome-wide association studies (GWAS) and candidate gene association studies (CGAS). Candidate genes for CGAS analysis are selected based on their established involvement in the control of calcium metabolism or bone cell function. Numerous genes responsible for monogenic disorders causing bone fragility have been studied. Common variants, or single nucleotide polymorphisms (SNPs), are found in at least 1% of the population. Either a case-control study for categorical outcomes, like the history of an osteoporotic fracture, or a population study for a quantitative outcome, like BMD, compares the frequency of these SNPs in candidate genes in unrelated subjects. Using this technique, several susceptibility variants have been found. However, because of the studies' limited power and the frequently contradictory results of studies conducted in various populations, false negative results are not uncommon (Burge et al., 2007).

Thanks to the growing acceptance of non-hormone-driven genetic studies, GWAS has identified susceptibility loci for variation in BMD in a clear and repeatable manner. Rather than concentrating on a single candidate gene, a large number (100 000–1 000 000) of common SNPs distributed at close intervals across the genome are analyzed. An important finding in the variant site is taken to mean that functional DNA-sequence variants for the illness or characteristic under study are present in the corresponding region of the genome. These can include variations in gene promoter regions, changes to mRNA degradation, or sequence variants that result in changes to the amino acids in proteins. On the other hand, several putative loci have also been found; their purpose is still unknown. This may also present the chance to discover new pathways and mechanisms related to the growth of bones and the onset of osteoporosis.

Because there are so many tests, GWAS must meet strict statistical thresholds. False negatives are possible, just like with CGAS. The actual effects of genetic polymorphisms are being ascertained through the growing application of meta-analysis. Initially established to conduct a prospective meta-analysis of CGAS, the GENOMOS consortium (Genetic Markers of Osteoporosis) has discovered SNP variants in COL1A1 and LRP5 linked to BMD in the lumbar and femoral spines. Later on, it evolved into the GEFOS (Genetic Factors for Osteoporosis) consortium, which is currently conducting a meta-analysis of ongoing GWAS and has found or verified several loci linked to BMD in the femoral neck or lumbar spine.

5.1.1.3. Genes Involved in Osteoporosis

CGAS and GWAS have revealed several genes that may be involved in the regulation of bone mass and osteoporotic fracture susceptibility. Many of these can be categorized as having an impact on three biological pathways: the RANKL-RANK-OPG pathway, the Wnt-ß-catenin signaling pathway, and the estrogen pathway. These are briefly summarized below.

- **The Estrogen Pathway:** Bone mass, bone geometry, and skeletal growth are all known to be regulated by estrogen. Monogenic disorders linked to osteoporosis include deficiencies in aromatase and estrogen receptors. Age at menopause, BMD, and postmenopausal bone loss are just a few of the osteoporotic traits and risk factors that have been linked to genetic variation at several SNPs in the estrogen receptor type 1 gene (ESR1).
- **Wnt-ß-catenin Signaling Pathway:** A major function of the Wnt signaling pathway is in many developmental processes. When Wnt binds to LRP5 or LRP6 transmembrane receptors in bone, it activates this pathway, which results in osteoblast differentiation and proliferation, bone mineralization, and a decrease in apoptosis. Osteoporosis-pseudoglioma syndrome is caused by loss of function mutations in LRP5, but subtler polymorphisms have been linked to variations in bone mineral density or fracture risk in the general population. Meta-analysis has verified some of these variants. At the significance level of the entire genome, additional genes related to osteoporosis susceptibility that impact the Wnt-ß-catenin signaling pathway have been identified. These include WLS, which encodes a transmembrane protein that promotes Wnt release; CTNNB1, which encodes ß-catenin, a protein involved in the signaling cascade; FOXC2, which activates the signaling pathway; MEF2C, which may regulate SOST expression; and SOST, which encodes sclerostin, an antagonist of Wnt [Ralston SH, Uitterlinden AG (2010)].
- **RANKL-RANK-OPG Pathway:** On osteoclast precursor cells, RANKL (receptor activator of nuclear factor B ligand) binds to RANK. It initiates bone resorption and promotes

osteoclast differentiation. RANKL is antagonistic to osteoprotegerin (OPG). Using CGAS and GWAS, several SNPs in the coding regions and close to the OPG (TNFRSF11B), RANK (TNFRSF11A), and RANKL (TN-FRSF11) genes have been linked to osteoporotic fracture risk and BMD, which has been further validated by meta-analysis. Despite the small amount of variation in BMD that these genes account for, the discovery of these relationships emphasizes how crucial this pathway is to the upkeep of the skeleton (Cooper et al., 2002).

Furthermore, several candidate genes known to play a role in skeletal maintenance have shown inconsistent association with BMD in CGAS and have not yet reached genome-wide significance in meta-analysis, such as COL1A1 and the vitamin D receptor gene (VDR). These genes have been identified from GWAS, but their function in bone metabolism is still unknown. These inconsistent results may be explained by the impact of environmental exposures on the genome.

5.1.1.4. Early Life, gene-Environment Interactions and Epigenetics

Only a small percentage (1–3%) of the observed variance in BMD in the population can be explained by the numerous putative genetic loci that have been identified by CGAS and GWAS studies. Nonetheless, there is growing awareness that environmental variables impact the likelihood of developing osteoporosis by altering gene expression and utilizing epigenetic mechanisms. Because of this, the phenotype that results from a given genotype varies significantly depending on environmental exposures. It is therefore likely that these epigenetic mechanisms play a significant role in explaining why BMD is highly heritable, with genetic variation accounting for a relatively small portion of the variation.

Regarding a person's risk for osteoporosis, several instances of gene–environment interaction during the fetal and early postnatal stages of life are becoming apparent. For instance, no meaningful correlations between birthweight or the VDR genotype and lumbar spine BMD were found in a UK cohort study. Nonetheless, there was a statistically significant interaction between birth weight and VDR genotype as a determinant of lumbar spine BMD, and the relationship between lumbar spine BMD and VDR genotype varied depending on the category of birth weight. This finding implies a potential interaction between genetic influences and the in utero environment, as birth weight is a measure of fetal nutrition. An analogous investigation additionally revealed a noteworthy correlation between polymorphisms in the human growth hormone (GH1) and infant weight, which is indicative of the early life milieu, in determining the pace of osteoporosis. Genetic variation in the interleukin-6 promoter gene was only linked to hip bone mineral density (BMD) in the Framingham Offspring Cohort in a subset of women who were not on estrogen replacement therapy and in those who did not consume enough calcium, indicating gene-environment interactions in later life.

Stable changes in gene expression that occur during cell division and development are referred to as epigenetics. There are no DNA mutations involved in these changes, which are heritable and may last for several generations (Jaenisch & Bird, 2003). Gene repression or enhanced gene activity is caused by chemical changes to DNA and proteins linked to specific DNA loci. DNA methylation is the most researched of these and is currently thought to play a significant role in the expression of genes. This entails methylating cytosine at the carbon-5 position of CpG dinucleotides. Gene repression typically results from methylation that takes place in a gene's promoter region. The patterns of DNA methylation change as a person develops, but crucially, during fetal development, maternal and environmental factors can change the pattern, which in turn can affect adult gene expression.

While the exact epigenetic mechanisms underlying osteoporosis in humans remain unknown, potential targets include the glucocorticoid receptor and vitamin D response elements. Reduced bone mass in the newborn and middle childhood years has been linked to lower maternal 25(OH)-vitamin D concentration during late pregnancy. The concentration of calcium in umbilical veins plays a role in mediating this. The growth of the fetal skeleton is also determined by the expression of the placental calcium transporter (PMCA3). Thus, the mechanism by which the vitamin D status of the mother influences the bone mass of her offspring may be represented by epigenetic regulation of the PMCA3 gene.

5.1.2. Environmental Influences in Childhood

Childhood longitudinal growth gradually increases along a centile curve and starts to track soon after birth. As evidenced by recent longitudinal studies, tracking of bone traits continues throughout early childhood, the pubertal growth spurt, and the early stages of adulthood. Despite this, environmental factors can have a significant impact on bone mineral accrual during childhood and early adulthood. This is crucial because reaching optimal peak bone mass lowers the likelihood of developing osteoporosis later in life. According to a Finnish cohort study, growth rates during childhood are positively correlated with the chance of hip fractures in later life. The study showed that a low growth rate between the ages of 7 and 15 was associated with a significantly higher risk of hip fracture after adjusting for age and sex. Adults who were born small but reached average height by the age of seven were also at higher risk. The increased fracture risk in these children is thought to result from the skeletal envelope being forced ahead of the capacity to mineralize, a phenomenon that is accelerated during pubertal growth. Numerous factors, including diet, lifestyle, medication, and comorbidities, are known to impact the risk of low bone mineral density (BMD) and fracture in adulthood.

5.1.3. Fracture Epidemiology

Fracture incidence is bimodal, peaking in childhood and geriatric populations. Young animals typically suffer from severe trauma-related fractures, which are less common in females and typically affect the long bones. Throughout childhood, bone mass gradually grows and typically peaks by the age of 30, at which time fracture incidence is minimal. After that, there is a gradual decrease in BMD, which leads to an increase in the prevalence of osteoporosis as people age. Osteoporosis rates are especially high in older women, primarily because of the postmenopausal development of hypoestrogenemia. Fracture risk is directly correlated with bone density loss; research indicates that for every standard deviation decrease in BMD, fracture risk nearly doubles. Because of this, people over 65 account for almost three-quarters of all hip, vertebral, and distal forearm fractures. The frequency of hip, vertebral, and wrist fractures in women increases with age, as demonstrated by Figure 5.1, with the specific nature of the relationship varying depending on the type of fracture. An individual's risk of suffering another fracture increases significantly after they have already had one; a meta-analysis revealed an increase in risk of up to 86%. This could help to explain why some people's fractures tend to cluster together (Cummings and Melton, 2002).

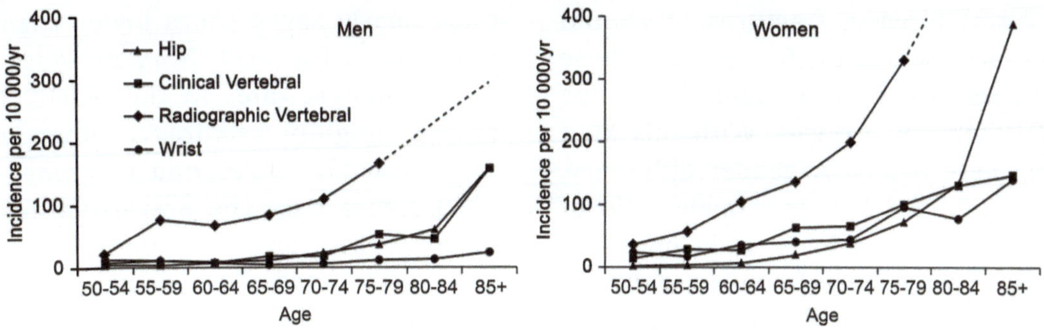

Figure 5.1. *Hip, clinical vertebral, radiographic vertebral and wrist fracture incidence by age in men and women.*

Source: Dale W. Stovall. Osteoporosis Diagnosis and Management. Wiley. ISBN: 9781118316313, 1118316312.

A 2004 US Surgeon General report brought attention to the staggering number of fractures caused by osteoporosis. Approximately 10 million Americans over 50 were estimated to have osteoporosis at that time, and 1.5 million fragility fractures were reported annually. According to a British study on fractures, the proportion of the population at risk is comparable to that of the US. A white woman's lifetime risk of suffering a hip fracture is 1 in 6 (Cummings and Melton 2002). Hip fractures are extremely common in Western populations as people age, accounting for 90% of cases in those over 50. Because women have a roughly twofold higher risk than men in this age group (Melton, 1988), along with the fact that women live longer, women suffer from hip fractures 75% of the time (Jordan and Cooper C 2002).

Hip fractures frequently result in increased dependence, decreased mobility, chronic pain, and disability. After that, a sizable percentage of people need long-term nursing care, and this percentage rises with age. When compared to age and sex-matched individuals without a fracture, survival rates at five years were found to be 80% of those expected. Hip fractures are also associated with an excess risk of mortality in the years immediately following the fracture. Hip fractures are thought to be the cause of about 740,000 deaths worldwide each year. Additionally, they account for more than one-third of the overall financial burden associated with fractures, which is a reflection of the need for hospital inpatient management as well as the high costs of the subsequent residential care. The global direct and indirect costs of hip fractures are predicted to reach $131.5 billion annually by 2050 due to the increasing number of these injuries (Johnell, 1997).

Most vertebral fractures are the result of compressive loading from lifting, shifting positions, or accidental discovery. Postmenopausal women frequently suffer vertebral fractures; a 50-year-old white woman's lifetime risk of experiencing one is 16%. Figure 5.1 illustrates that as people age, there is an almost exponential rise in radiographic vertebral fractures and an approximately linear increase in clinical vertebral fractures. Back pain, height loss, deformity, immobility, and decreased pulmonary function are all symptoms of symptomatic vertebral fractures, even though only about one-third of radiographic vertebral deformities receive clinical attention. Similar to hip fractures, there is an excess mortality associated with them.

Most often, falls on outstretched hands result in distal forearm fractures. It should come as no surprise that the frequency of these fractures peaks in the winter, most likely due to more falls on icy surfaces. With this kind of fracture, there is a clear gender difference, with an age-adjusted female-to-male ratio of 4:1. There is no known increase in mortality rate associated with these fractures, although they can cause significant disability, especially if they affect the dominant limb.

5.1.4. Geography

Globally, fracture incidence varies significantly. Fracture rates are generally higher in areas farther from the equator. Though there are some exceptions to this rule, it is believed that less sun exposure leads to lower levels of vitamin D. Skin exposure to the sun is restricted in nations like Iran where cultural norms mandate covering the majority of the body with clothing. This practice could help to explain why, even though the region is close to the equator, 80% of the population has low vitamin D levels, and fracture rates are high.

All Westernized Caucasian populations, including those in Europe, America, and Oceania, generally have fracture rates that are comparable. However, there is a lot of variation within each of these distinct regions. Ecological variables that have been found to correlate with incidence patterns may be partially to blame for this discrepancy in the US. These include urbanization, socioeconomic status, and the amount of fluoride in the water. Rates are especially high in places where a sizable fraction of the over-65 population lives in poverty.

Parts of southern Europe have hip fracture rates nearly seven times lower than those of Scandinavia, especially Norway, which has some of the highest rates in the world. Increased rates of fragility fractures at other anatomical sites typically correspond to areas with high hip fracture risk. The prevalence of vertebral deformities in European nations was investigated by the EVOS study. They demonstrated a three-fold variation in prevalence, with Scandinavia once more exhibiting the highest frequencies.

Asia exhibits moderate variation, with urbanized nations exhibiting the highest rates. Asia is home to a large proportion of the world's hip fracture cases, estimated to be around 30%, in part because of the region's large population. On the other hand, fracture rates from African populations seem to be low. There isn't much data from this area, though, and its reliability has been questioned. Thus, inaccurate case identification could account for a portion of the low numbers, but population demography might also be important.

5.1.5. Secular Trends

Globally, life expectancy is rising along with the number of elderly people, especially in developing nations. Globally, there are expected to be over 1,500 million individuals 65 years of age or older by the year 2050. Global fracture incidence rose by 25% between 1990 and 2000, and estimates indicate that by 2050, there will be over 6 million hip fractures, up from 1.66 million in 1990. These estimates presuppose a constant incidence of hip fractures according to age; however, the secular trends discovered are significantly location-dependent (Figure 5.2).

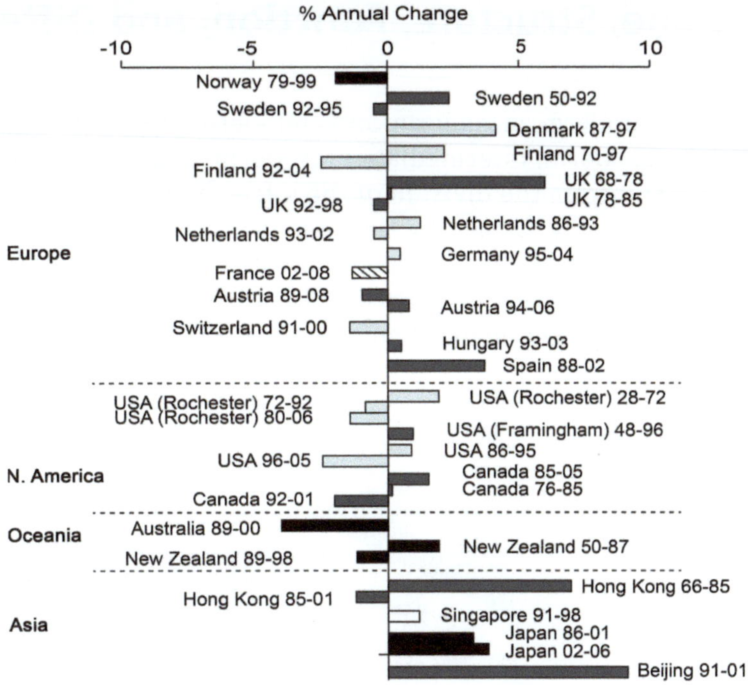

Figure 5.2. *Secular trends in fracture incidence throughout the world.*

Source: Dale W. Stovall. Osteoporosis Diagnosis and Management. Wiley. ISBN: 9781118316313, 1118316312.

It has been demonstrated that age-specific fracture rates increased until about 1980 in most Western populations, including those in Oceania, North America, and the United Kingdom. Reduced physical activity, less time spent outside, and higher rates of vitamin D insufficiency may have contributed to this. Additionally, during this time, a confluence of social and medical factors improved the survival of the elderly who were frail (i.e., those most vulnerable to fracture). Rates have either stayed the same or begun to decrease after this. This trend could be the result of an increase in obesity, the birth cohort effect, or improvements in osteoporosis screening and treatment. Specifically, the introduction of bisphosphonates may have contributed, though this does not explain everything. The rates in the developing world, on the other hand, have not decreased (Dennison et al., 2001).

The fracture burden is predicted to shift toward Asia and the developing world due to a combination of age-specific fracture rates and wildly differing regional changes in population demographics. As a result, it is predicted that by 2050, only about 25% of hip fractures will happen in Europe and North America.

5.2. Origins of Bone, Structure, Function, and Differences in Biological Sex

The blastula divides into the ectoderm, mesoderm, and endoderm, three different cell lineages, during gastrulation. The paraxial mesoderm, intermediate mesoderm, and lateral plate mesoderm are the three paired regions that result from the division of the intraembryonic mesenchymal cells at week four. The limb skeleton is eventually formed by the lateral plate mesoderm. The somites that split off from the paraxial mesoderm are further divided into sclerotomes, myotomes, syndetomes, and dermatomes. Thus, the axial skeleton and muscles develop from the paraxial mesoderm. Given their shared embryonic ancestry, the development of muscle and bone is inextricably linked (Figure 5.3).

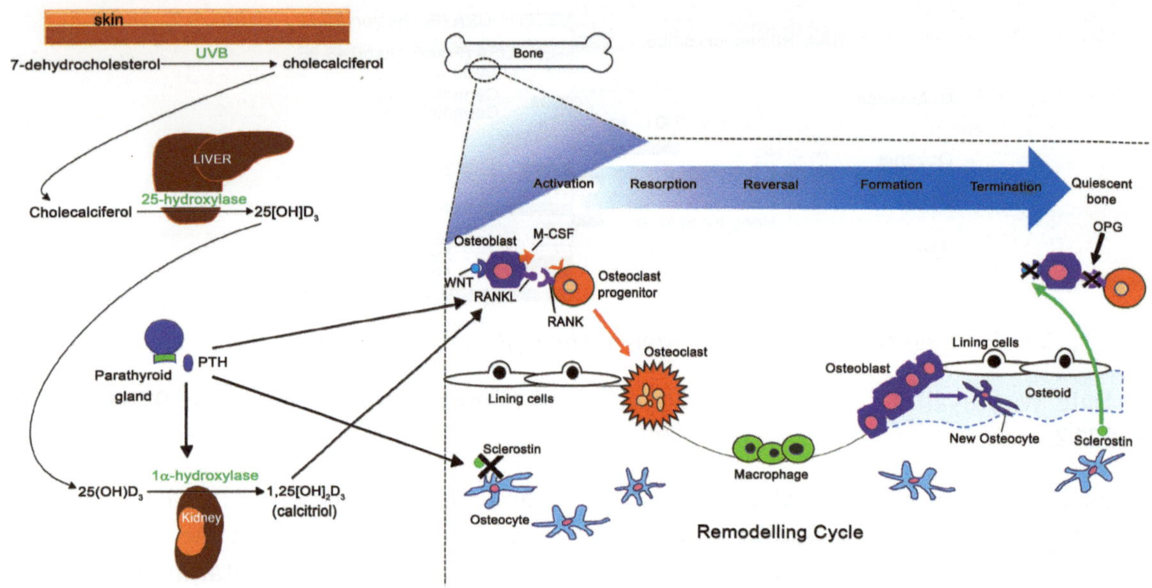

Figure 5.3. *Remodeling cycle and regulators of bone formation. The bone remodeling cycle occurs in 5 stages—activation (during which osteoblastic expression of M-CSF and RANKL stimulate osteoclast progenitor maturation and differentiation into osteoclasts), resorption of bone (by osteoclasts), reversal, formation (new bone laid down by osteoblasts) and termination (bone returns to quiescent phase). Bone remodeling is stimulated by calcitriol and PTH and is inhibited during the quiescent phase by sclerostin, which inhibits WNT-driven bone formation and OPG which inhibits RANK-RANKL interactions.*

Source: J. Barnsley, G. Buckland, P. E. Chan, A. Ong, A. S. Ramos, M. Baxter, F. Laskou, E. M. Dennison, C. Cooper, and Harnish P. Patel. Pathophysiology and treatment of osteoporosis: challenges for clinical practice in older people. Aging Clinical and Experimental Research (2021) 33:759–773. https://doi.org/10.1007/s40520-021-01817-y.

5.2.1. Bone Structure

Bone is an organic and inorganic connective tissue that serves a variety of purposes. Collagenous proteins, of which type I collagen is the most abundant, and a variety of non-collagenous proteins, such as glycosaminoglycans, glycoproteins, and certain serum-derived proteins, make up the organic bone matrix, or osteoid. The many non-collagenous proteins control mineralization, turnover, and deposition in addition to other aspects of bone metabolism. The inorganic component, which makes up between 50 and 70% of the total mass of the bone, is primarily composed of calcium and phosphorus in the form of hydroxyapatite. It gives the bone mechanical rigidity (Ferrari et al,.2004).

About 80% of the adult bone mass in the skeleton is made up of cortical bone, while the remaining 20% is made up of trabecular bone. The mechanical strength and integrity of the bone are preserved by the dense cortical bone, which also has a low turnover rate of about 3% annually. Trabecular bone, on the other hand, is more metabolically active, responsive to hormonal stimuli, and has a lower mineralized content. It is found in long bones and vertebrae, and its turnover rate is about 26% annually. More remodeling occurs in trabecular bone than in cortical bone, which has clinical implications because trabecular bone is more prone to fragility fractures.

Osteocytes, osteoblasts, and osteoclasts make up the majority of the cells that make up bone's cellular component. Osteocytes play a mechano-sensory role in the formation of bone and are located in the matrix's lacunae. Osteoblasts produce osteoid, and osteoclasts break down bone through enzymatic means. For the growth and remodeling of bones throughout the life course, all three subtypes are crucial.

5.2.2. Bone Homeostasis

Bone remodeling involves a careful balance between the action of osteoclasts, tightly coupled with that of osteoblasts, allowing repair of micro-damage and maintaining skeletal structure as well as serum calcium and phosphate homeostasis. Along the surface of the bone, clusters of these cells within multicellular units form active remodeling sites, each of which is covered in a cell canopy. It has been discovered that the mesenchymal stem cells (MSC) that surround the red bone marrow are the source of this cell canopy, which serves as a source of progenitor cells during the remodeling process. Five successive stages of a remodeling cycle—activation, resorption, reversal, formation, and termination—occur on the surface of resting bones (Figure 5.3).

5.2.3. Activation

Osteocytes that express receptor activator of nuclear factor (NF) Kappa-B ligand, or RANKL, interact with the RANK receptor on osteoclast precursors to potently induce differentiation into multinucleated osteoclasts, thereby activating the resting bone surface. The expression of macrophage colony-stimulating factor (M-CSF) by osteoblasts facilitates the survival and differentiation of osteoclast precursors. To attract potential osteoclasts, osteoblasts generate chemokines. Additionally, they secrete matrix metalloproteinases, which break down unmineralized osteoids and reveal adhesion sites where osteoclasts can adhere.

5.2.4. Resorption

Osteoclasts release lysosomal enzymes and hydrogen ions, for example, cathepsin-K into an area below the cell that is "sealed." They remove an old bone tunnel by proteolysis and acidification. By preventing osteoclast differentiation and accelerating their apoptosis, osteoprotegerin (OPG) can inhibit the RANK-RANKL interaction and thereby reduce resorption.

5.2.5. Reversal

Recent years have seen a great deal of research focused on the reversal phase, which starts with osteoclastic signaling that lasts for about 4–5 weeks and is ultimately in charge of the critical coupling of osteoclastic and osteoblastic activity observed at remodeling sites. While "reversal cells" have long been identified, their precise morphology and function are still unknown, despite their obvious distinction from osteoclasts and osteoblasts.

5.2.6. Formation

As the resorbed bone tunnel is entirely replaced by unmineralized osteoid, osteoblasts produce minimal net changes in bone volume during remodeling. As hydroxyapatite is gradually incorporated into the osteoid, bone formation is complete. About 10 to 15% of mature osteoblasts are entombed by the new bone matrix and differentiate into osteocytes by the end of bone formation. Osteocytes at rest express sclerostin, which inhibits osteoblast WNT signaling, which is an inducer of bone formation. Wnt-induced bone formation is made possible by parathyroid hormone (PTH) or mechanical stress, which inhibits sclerostin expression (Hunter et al., 2001).

5.2.7. Termination

A sequence of as-yet-unidentified termination signals marks the end of the remodeling cycle once the tunnel of resorbed bone has been completely replaced. The surface of the resting bone is restored.

5.2.8. Regulation of Bone Remodeling

Signals for remodeling can be mechanical or hormonal in origin. Osteotrophene, growth hormones, and androgens are among the systemic regulators of bone formation. The development, maturation, metabolism, structure, and strength of the musculoskeletal system are all dependent on thyroid hormones, which also influence osteoblast and osteoclast activity to promote bone turnover. Glucocorticoids increase osteoblast apoptosis, which decreases bone formation and prolongs osteoclast survival. Continuous high-dose parathyroid hormone (PTH) release stimulates the expression of RANKL/MCSF and inhibits the expression of OPG, which in turn causes bone resorption indirectly. In the meantime, low intermittent PTH release stimulates osteoblast survival, proliferation, and differentiation, which results in the formation of new bone. Vitamin D3, calcitonin, insulin-like growth factor, prostaglandins, and bone morphogenetic proteins are additional systemic regulators of bone remodeling. Cytokines, growth factors like IGF-1, Sirtuins, protein kinases like mTOR, Forkhead proteins, M-CSF, Wnt, sclerostin, and the RANK/RANKL/OPG system are examples of local regulators of bone remodeling. The remodeling of bones is strictly regulated, and changes in cellular activity, i.e., decreased bone formation and increased bone resorption will result from elevated osteoclastic activity in response to either internal or external stimuli.

All ethnic groups and older people experience a decrease in bone mass and volume. Senescence of MSCs and a change in differentiation potential that favors adipogenesis in the bone marrow cause an imbalance in remodeling within the aged microenvironment. Reduced levels of Sirtuin, for example, can change the intracellular signaling milieu and cause an increase in sclerostin activity, which in turn inhibits WNT and suppresses the formation of new bone. Osteoclastic activity and cathepsin K release are both correlated with increased mTOR activity.

5.2.9. Calcium and Vitamin D Homeostasis

A sufficient supply of calcium is necessary for the mineralization of bone. The synthesis of active vitamin D, renal calcium reabsorption, and bone resorption all occur as a result of PTH's action on these processes. Inactive vitamin D is first hydroxylated by CYP2R1 in the liver and subsequently converted to its active form, calcitriol ($1,25[OH]_2D_3$), in the kidneys by 1a-hydroxylase (CYP27B1). Bone also serves as a calcium reservoir. PTH causes 1α-hydroxylase to increase calcitriol levels. Calcitriol acts on vitamin D receptors (VDRs) to increase intestinal and renal calcium uptake when serum calcium levels are normal or low. But when the amount of calcium in food is not enough to meet the body's need for calcium, i. e. a negative calcium balance develops during periods of undernutrition, which are frequently observed in older individuals (Jaenisch and Bird, 2003). At this point, calcitriol increases the expression of RANKL, which inhibits bone mineralization and promotes bone resorption. At the price of skeletal integrity, these processes mobilize calcium and phosphate from the bone matrix to the serum. When osteocyte VDRs are activated by calcitriol, they produce more fibroblast growth factor 23 (FGF-23), which blocks 1α-hydroxylase and initiates a negative feedback loop.

5.2.10. Peak Bone Mass and Differences in Biological Sex

The greatest quantity of skeletal tissue that a person will have at the end of skeletal maturation is known as peak bone mass. It is believed that peak bone mass is reached between the ages of 25 and 30. After that, it declines at a rate of 0.5 percent annually. Men reach a higher BMD than women, but they do so later. Peak bone mass is attained through a complex process. The strongest evidence for peak bone mass appears to be genetic; genetic factors account for up to 85% of the variation in peak bone mass, which in turn influences bone's physiological metabolism. Increased plasma inorganic phosphate and calcitriol during puberty are thought to be caused by an increase in IGF-1, which in turn causes an increase in bone mass gain during puberty. According to this theory, patients with haploinsufficiency of the IGF-1 receptor have been found to have undesired alterations in bone architecture. Peak bone mass can also be influenced by other factors such as physical activity, intercurrent illness, socioeconomic deprivation, and nutrition (particularly calcium and vitamin D status).

5.3. Secondary Causes of Osteoporosis: Bone Diseases

One inevitable side effect of aging is bone loss. Diseases that make it more difficult for a person to reach their maximum adult bone mass, raise their risk of osteoporosis, and increase their risk of fracture later in life. There are two types of primary osteoporosis: age-related and post-menopausal. Since women's peak bone mineral density is lower than men's, they are more likely to develop primary osteoporosis. The decrease in estrogen that occurs after menopause adds to this risk. It's crucial to remember, though, that about 20% of men who have osteoporosis are hypogonadal.

Because women have higher metabolic rates and are more susceptible to the trophic effects of estrogen, which inhibits osteoclasts and plays a major role in preventing bone resorption, bone loss is most noticeable in the trabecular vertebral bodies in women. For women, a steeper decrease in bone mass starts around age 65–69, and for men, it starts around age 74–79. Compared to men, women over 50 have two times the rate of osteopenia and four times the rate of osteoporosis. For women, the lifetime risk of osteoporotic fractures is about 40%. Smoking, moderate to heavy alcohol consumption, and weight loss in older adults all seem to hasten the thinning of bone in both men and women (Johnell, 1997).

The term "secondary osteoporosis" refers to bone loss, microarchitecural degradation, and fragility fractures brought on by coexisting medical conditions or underlying diseases (Table 5.1). Since it typically affects patient populations (premenopausal women or younger men) who are typically not affected by osteoporosis, secondary osteoporosis presents a diagnostic and treatment challenge. The underlying conditions are varied, and frequently uncommon (Table 5.2), and diagnosis requires specific testing.

Table 5.1. More Common Causes of Secondary Osteoporosis

- Cushing's syndrome or exogenous corticosteroids (e.g. > 5 mg/day for > 3 mths)
- Excessive alcohol use (> 2 units or 18 g/d)
- Primary or secondary hypogonadism
  - e.g. associated with medications (corticosteroids, opioids, androgen deprivation therapy for prostate cancer, aromatase therapy for breast cancer)
- Low calcium intake and vitamin D deficiency or insufficiency (serum 25(OH)D < 60 nmol/L)
- Smoking
- Family history of minimal trauma fracture (possible genetic cause)

Source: Dale W. Stovall. Osteoporosis Diagnosis and Management. Wiley. ISBN: 9781118316313, 1118316312.

Table 5.2. Less Common Causes of Secondary Osteoporosis

- Low BMI (< 20) and associated eating disorders
- Lack of or excessive exercise
- Anti-epileptic drugs (phenytoin, phenobarbitone, primidone, carbamazepine)
- Thyrotoxicosis or thyroxine over-replacement
- Primary hyperparathyroidism
- Chronic liver or kidney disease
- Malabsorption, including coeliac disease
- Hypercalciuria
- Rheumatoid arthritis or ankylosing spondylosis
- Type 1 and type 2 diabetes mellitus
- Multiple myeloma and other monoclonal gammopathies
- HIV or its treatment with protease inhibitors
- Mastocytosis
- Organ transplant or immunosuppressives (cyclo & tacrolimus)
- Osteogenesis imperfecta
- Gaucher and Fabre disease

Source: Dale W. Stovall. Osteoporosis Diagnosis and Management. Wiley. ISBN: 9781118316313, 1118316312.

In addition to the well-known endocrine conditions Cushing's syndrome, hypogonadism (in males or females), hyperthyroidism, and hyperparathyroidism, osteoporosis can also be brought on by diabetes mellitus. Compared to non-diabetic controls, patients with type 1 diabetes mellitus (T1DM) have a 12-fold increased risk of osteoporotic fractures. Type 2 diabetes mellitus (T2DM) patients typically have preserved bone mass, but they also have an increased risk of fractures, which suggests that the material properties and quality of the bone may be compromised. Furthermore, osteoporosis is caused by chronic inflammation, which is a feature of rheumatoid arthritis and inflammatory bowel disease. This is partly due to the proinflammatory cytokine milieu. Another significant factor that has been linked to secondary osteoporosis is bariatric surgery (Johnell and Kanis, 2006).

5.3.1. Pathophysiology

5.3.1.1. Endocrine Diseases

- **Hyperthyroidism:** Overt hyperthyroidism in the past is known to increase the risk of osteoporotic fractures. A 4- and 5-fold increased risk of hip and vertebral fractures, respectively, was linked to a serum TSH level of 0.1 mU/l, according to a large study involving 686 postmenopausal women. Excess thyroid hormone and decreased thyrotropin levels have been linked, based on animal models. Both increased bone resorption and bone loss are brought on by the activation of the thyroid hormone receptor (TR)- on osteoblasts and osteoclasts.
- **Primary Hyperparathyroidism:** Primary hyperparathyroidism, or PHPT, affects women three times more frequently than it does men. Prolonged excess PTH is catabolic to the skeleton and affects cortical bone more often than cancellous bone. As a result, bone loss is more noticeable at skeletal sites that contain cortical bone, such as the femoral neck and middle third of the forearm, but it has less of an impact on the spine, which is primarily made up of cancellous bone. However, PHPT also increases the risk of spinal fractures. Patients with PHPT who are otherwise asymptomatic but have fragility fractures or a T-score <−2.5 should consider parathyroid surgery. A recent observational study conducted over a 15-year period demonstrated that while cortical bone density declined in most subjects without surgery during long-term follow-up, parathyroidectomy restored biochemical indices of bone turnover and preserved BMD. Furthermore, it has been demonstrated that bone density increases after parathyroidectomy at multiple cortical bone sites as well as the spine.
- **Idiopathic Hypercalciuria:** In the context of normocalcemia, idiopathic hypercalciuria arises when the 24-hour urinary calcium excretion surpasses 4 mg/kg/day, irrespective of gender, and when there is no other reason for the elevated urine calcium excretion (e.g., PHPT Cushing's syndrome). Patients with idiopathic hypercalciuria are more likely to develop renal calculi containing calcium, and their bone mineral density (BMD) is frequently decreased despite an increase in bone turnover. It's unclear what causes this condition.

- **Male Hypogonadism:** For men to reach their peak bone mass and maintain their bone strength afterward, androgens are essential. The aromatase enzyme is responsible for converting androgens to estradiol, which is how androgens affect bone in men. Hypogonadism causes increased bone remodeling and rapid bone loss, and it is a major risk factor for low BMD and fragility fractures in men.
- **Pregnancy-Associated Osteoporosis:** Normal pregnancies and lactation both cause bone loss, but it is reversible. Pregnancy-associated osteoporosis exacerbates this bone loss, but the pathophysiological mechanisms are unknown. Preexisting vitamin D deficiency, low calcium and protein intake from diet, low bone mineral density (BMD), elevated levels of parathyroid hormone-related protein (PTHrP), and high rates of bone turnover are all potential contributing factors. Other risk factors include the use of heparins for thromboembolic disorders and multiple pregnancies with extended periods of lactation.
- **Diabetes Mellitus Type 1:** Patients with type 1 diabetes have a twelve-fold increased risk of osteoporotic fractures. Patients with type 1 diabetes may have lower bone mineral density (BMD) and a higher risk of fracture due to a lack of insulin's bone-anabolic effects and those of other beta cell-derived proteins like amylin. Diabetic complications, including retinopathy, polyneuropathy, and nephropathy, are the primary causes of low bone mass and elevated fracture risk in long-term disease. This is partly because of an increased risk of falls. Women with type 2 diabetes had a 20% increased risk of fractures, according to data from the Women's Health Initiative (WHI) Study, even after accounting for increased BMD (4–5 percent higher at the hip) and frequent falls. This might be the result of bone quality deterioration brought on by glycosylation products' effects on bone collagen. The use of thiazolidinedione drugs is a significant additional risk factor for fractures in postmenopausal women with type 2 diabetes. These drugs have been linked to fractures of the hip, proximal humerus, and small hands and feet bones (Jordan and Cooper, 2002).
- **Growth Hormone Deficiency:** Human growth hormone (hGH) stimulates the hepatic receptor, which results in the production of insulin-like growth factor (IGF)-1 and IGF binding proteins (IGFBPs), which are powerful stimulators of osteoblastic functions and bone formation. The degree of osteopenia is correlated with the severity of growth hormone (GH) deficiency, and patients with untreated adult-onset GH deficiency have a 2- to 3-fold increased risk of osteoporotic fractures. Because of their small bone size and short stature, patients with pediatric-onset GH deficiency are difficult to accurately measure areal BMD using DXA; instead, volumetric BMD should be measured using peripheral QCT in these patients.

5.3.1.2. Gastrointestinal Diseases

- **Celiac Disease:** The traditional indicators of celiac disease, chronic diarrhea, and malabsorption from villous atrophy, may not always be present clinically. Osteomalacia and secondary hyperparathyroidism are the results of impaired intestinal absorption of calcium and a common vitamin D deficiency in patients with celiac disease.

Skeletal health may be further hampered by related autoimmune diseases like T1DM, Graves' disease with hyperthyroidism, and type A gastritis with achlorhydria. The recommendation for serologic screening with anti-tissue transglutaminase antibodies in all patients with osteoporosis to rule out celiac disease is supported by a recent study that showed a 17-fold higher prevalence of celiac disease among patients with osteoporosis compared with normal individuals.

- **Inflammatory Bowel Disease:** In patients with Crohn's disease, bone mineral density is lower than in patients with ulcerative colitis, and the pathophysiology of osteoporosis in inflammatory bowel disease is complicated. In patients with inflammatory bowel disease, the main causes of osteoporosis include intermittent or continuous use of systemic glucocorticoid therapy for flare-ups, diarrhea, malabsorption, low body mass index, and chronic inflammation. Low bone mass in patients with short bowel syndrome may also be caused by vitamin D deficiency, functional loss of terminal ileum integrity, recurrent hospital stays, and extended immobility.
- **Gastrectomy and Chronic Proton Pump Inhibitor Therapy:** Up to one-third of patients may develop osteoporosis following a gastrectomy. This condition is brought on by lower calcium absorption as a result of elevated pH levels in the gastrointestinal tract. These results are in line with a report that found postmenopausal women taking the proton pump inhibitor omeprazole had a 3–5-fold increased risk of vertebral fractures. However, bone loss and fractures linked to proton pump inhibitor therapy may not be the result of reduced calcium absorption (Jordan and Cooper, 2002).

5.3.1.3. Bariatric Surgery

Following bariatric surgery, bone loss has emerged as a clinical challenge. Different degrees of reduced fractional calcium absorption and vitamin D malabsorption are linked to the various procedures, such as laparoscopic gastric banding, Roux-en-Y gastric bypass, and biliopancreatic diversion with duodenal switch. Following one of these procedures, bone loss may be moderately severe and appears to be directly correlated with the amount of weight lost. According to an early study, the risk of fractures doubles following bariatric surgery. Furthermore, the resulting calcium and vitamin D deficiency after bariatric surgery may be chronic and challenging to treat.

5.3.2. Hematological and Immunological Diseases

5.3.2.1. Myeloma Bone Disease and Monoclonal Gammopathy of Undetermined Significance

Myeloma cell-secreted cytokines affect bone cells and are primarily responsible for osteoporosis and fractures, affecting the axial skeleton. When myeloma cells express receptor activator of NF-κB ligand (RANKL) and other pro-osteoclastogenic factors (IL-6, Il-11, TGF β), osteoclastogenesis is boosted and bone resorption is accelerated. Furthermore, soluble Wnt signaling inhibitor dickkopf-1, which inhibits osteoblastic differentiation and decreases bone formation, is secreted by myeloma cells. According to a population-based retrospective cohort study that tracked 165 myeloma patients for 537 person-years, there were 16 times more fractures than anticipated in the year before myeloma diagnosis, especially rib or spinal fractures. Monoclonal gammopathy of unknown significance (MGUS) or multiple myeloma may be present in up to 5% of patients with newly diagnosed osteoporosis. In addition to having a 2.7-fold increased risk of axial fractures, patients with MGUS, a condition that can progress to multiple myeloma, also have this risk.

- **Systemic Mastocytosis:** Mastocytosis-related bone loss can occur quickly and severely, affecting the spine as well as the long bones. The overproduction of mast cell products, such as histamine, IL-1, IL-3, and IL-6, which encourage the differentiation of osteoclasts from precursor cells, leads to osteoporosis. Elevated bone resorption is also caused by an activating mutation of tyrosine kinase c-kit (D816V mutation), which is found in more than 90% of adult mastocytosis patients. Patchy osteosclerosis can also happen because histamine and other mediators released by mast cells can promote the formation of new bone.

5.3.2.2. HIV Disease and Highly Active Antiretroviral Therapy (HAART)

Osteoporosis increases the risk of hip, distal radius, spinal, and other fractures in both men and women living with HIV. Compared to non-HIV infected controls, the fracture risk is three to four times higher in older HIV-positive individuals. In a sizable Danish study, it was found that while HIV-positive patients had a higher fracture risk than population controls, this increased risk was only seen in low-energy fractures—not high-energy fractures—and that the increased risk of low-energy fractures was limited to patients receiving highly active antiretroviral therapy (HAART). Vertebral fractures can affect up to 27% of HIV-positive males, compared to 13% of control subjects. Additionally, cases had a higher frequency of multiple vertebral fractures than controls. When compared to controls, HIV-positive individuals have a 3.7-fold higher chance of having osteoporotic bone density. Apart from the use of HAART, low body mass index, hypogonadism, infection, inflammation, vitamin D deficiency, growth hormone deficiency, smoking, and alcohol abuse are associated with an increased risk of osteoporosis. As a result, it's critical to evaluate the bone health of every HIV-positive person, including measuring BMD and vitamin D levels.

While this initial short-term bone loss may not be ongoing, prospective studies, the majority of which have been small and/or nonrandomized, have generally found that starting HAART reduces BMD by 1 percent to 5 percent for 1 to 2 years. More BMD reductions have been linked to tenofovir (TDF) therapy than to stavudine or abacavir (ABC). Patients who were randomized to TDF-emtricitabine (FTC) in a trial involving HAART-naive patients experienced higher increases in markers of bone turnover and greater bone loss over the course of 24 weeks of therapy than patients who were randomized to ABC-lamivudine (3TC). In a TDFemtricitabine (FTC) treatment randomized trial, lower fat mass and baseline bone formation marker levels predicted bone loss later on. The largest prospective study of individuals with HIV (n = 4640) evaluated fractures for five years. The results of this study showed that fracture rates were higher in the first two years after starting HAART (0.53/100 person-years) than in the years that followed (0.30/100 person-years) and that the use of glucocorticoids and current smoking were independently linked to fracture risk, but not with exposure to a particular HAART.

5.3.2.3. Gaucher Disease

Multiple organs are affected by Gaucher disease (GD), an autosomal recessive inherited lysosomal storage disorder. The most prevalent type of GD, known as nonneuronopathic GD (GD1), can manifest as hepatosplenomegaly, anemia, bleeding tendencies, thrombocytopenia, skeletal pathology, growth retardation, and, in extreme situations, pulmonary illness (Jordan and Cooper, 2002). When evaluated by MRI, bone involvement can be found in up to 90% of patients, and it is the main reason for morbidity in GD1 patients. Up to 76% of patients with GD1 have osteoporosis and/or osteopenia, and BMD increases after starting enzyme replacement therapy. These patients also have osteosclerosis, lytic lesions, bone infarcts, avascular necrosis, and, in rare cases, acute osteomyelitis. When no other cause can be found, the diagnosis should be taken into consideration for patients who present with bone infarcts.

5.3.3. Secondary Causes of Osteoporosis Relevant to Older People

Table 5.3 lists several diseases linked to osteoporosis. The following section discusses a handful of those conditions and medication regimens that are relevant to the onset of osteoporosis in the elderly.

Table 5.3. Secondary Causes of Osteoporosis Relevant to older People

Glucocorticoid induced osteoporosis	Monoclonal gammopathy
Proton pump inhibitor use	Multiple myeloma
Antiepileptic drug use	Hyperparathyroidism
Systemic hormonal therapy	Chronic liver disease
Selective serotonin re-uptake inhibitor use	Ankylosing spondylitis
Disorders of the thyroid	Coeliac disease
Loop diuretic use	Rheumatoid arthritis
Chronic kidney disease	Multiple sclerosis
Diabetes	

Source: J. Barnsley, G. Buckland, P. E. Chan, A. Ong, A. S. Ramos, M. Baxter, F. Laskou, E. M. Dennison, C. Cooper, and Harnish P. Patel. Pathophysiology and treatment of osteoporosis: challenges for clinical practice in older people. Aging Clinical and Experimental Research (2021) 33:759–773. https://doi.org/10.1007/s40520-021-01817-y.

5.3.3.1. Glucocorticoids

In many different types of diseases, such as chronic inflammatory, rheumatological, and respiratory conditions, glucocorticoids are a component of the treatment plan. In the United Kingdom, glucocorticoid therapy is thought to be administered for a period of one percent of the population, and the rate of long-term use is progressively rising. However, there are negative effects on bone health in addition to the therapeutic benefits of anti-inflammatory drugs. According to estimates, 30–40% of patients receiving chronic glucocorticoid therapy experience vertebral and non-vertebral fractures; this effect seems to be dose dependent (Kanis et al., 2011). However, after stopping steroids, fracture risk can quickly return to normal. Glucocorticoids cause osteoblasts to function less well, cause osteocytes and osteoblasts to undergo apoptosis, and encourage the formation of osteoclasts, which ultimately suppresses the formation of new bone. Figure 5.4 summarizes the effects of glucocorticoids on hormones and intracellular structures.

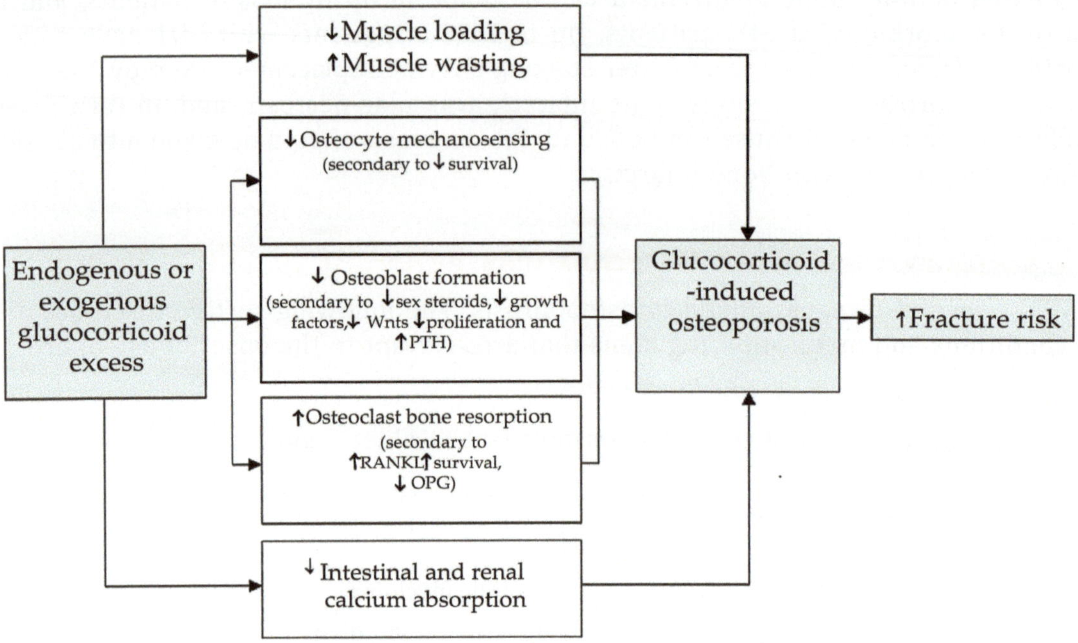

Figure 5.4. *Actions of glucocorticoid excess on bone.*

Source: J. Barnsley, G. Buckland, P. E. Chan, A. Ong, A. S. Ramos, M. Baxter, F. Laskou, E. M. Dennison, C. Cooper, and Harnish P. Patel. Pathophysiology and treatment of osteoporosis: challenges for clinical practice in older people. Aging Clinical and Experimental Research (2021) 33:759–773. https://doi.org/10.1007/s40520-021-01817-y.

5.3.3.2. Proton Pump Inhibitors (PPI)

In the UK, prescriptions for long-term PPIs are becoming more common, and using them has been linked to an increased risk of fracture. There are two primary mechanisms at play. First, osteoclastic precursor stimulation brought on by hypergastrinemia causes a shift in equilibrium that favors higher bone resorption. Second, an increase in osteoclastic activity and hyperparathyroidism result from hypochlorhydria's impact on the absorption of calcium and magnesium. Because of the effects on bone remodeling, reduced mineral absorption, and muscle weakness that impairs physical function and increases the risk of falls, there is an overall increase in the risk of fractures.

5.3.3.3. Antiepileptic Drugs (AED)

The use of AED is linked to an 86% increase in the risk of fractures at any site and a 90% increase in the risk of hip fractures, according to a systematic review and meta-analysis of 22 studies. Compared to those who do not use an enzyme-inducing AED, users of liver-enzyme inducing

AEDs are at a higher risk. Phenobarbiturates, topiramate, and phenytoin are a few examples. AED's impact on bone metabolism is explained by several theories. AED primarily activates the cytochrome P450 enzyme system (CYP2, CYP3) and orphan nuclear and pregnane-X receptors (PXR), which are expressed in the gut, kidneys, and liver. This increases the metabolism of vitamin D to inactive metabolites. Low bone mineral density and bone loss are the subsequent consequences of hypocalcemia and secondary hyperparathyroidism brought on by vitamin D deficiency (Kanis et al., 2011).

5.3.3.4. Systemic Hormonal Therapy

Because they severely deplete estrogen, aromatase inhibitors (AIs), which are used in the treatment of breast cancer, can cause increased bone loss and negative bone balance. When compared to natural postmenopausal bone loss, AI use causes at least twice as much bone loss. Gonadotrophin-releasing hormone (GnRH) agonists inhibit the production of luteinizing hormone and follicle-stimulating hormone by binding to GnRH receptors in the pituitary and downregulating the gonadotropin-producing cells. Following administration, less testosterone and estradiol are produced. Osteocytes, osteoblasts, and osteoclasts are sensitive to both sex hormones and express androgen and estrogen receptors. A decrease in these hormones causes cellular dysfunction and influences the remodeling of bones by favoring resorption rather than formation.

5.3.3.5. Selective Serotonin Reuptake Inhibitor (SSRI)

Serotonin (5-hydroxytryptamine [5-HT]) receptors are found in osteoblasts and osteocytes. 5-HT might play significant regulatory and signaling roles in the remodeling of bone. SSRI use was linked to a higher incidence of non-spine fractures in women with a mean age of 78.5 years. There was a 3.9% reduction in bone mineral density in older men taking SSRIs as opposed to those taking tricyclic antidepressants or no medication at all. It's still unclear exactly which SSRIs increase the risk of fracture, though. On the other hand, it is hypothesized that altering the signaling of bone formation pathways in favor of bone resorption could result in disruption of the serotonin receptors in bone cells.

5.3.3.6. Thyroid Disease

Osteoporosis and increased bone turnover can result from hyperthyroidism. Exogenous (such as primary thyroid disease) and endogenous i.e., levothyroxine over-replacement and long-term therapeutic use are linked to decreased bone mineral density (BMD) and an increased risk of hip and vertebral fractures. Hypothyroidism does not seem to raise the risk of fracture and is linked to a slowing of bone resorption and formation. Subclinical hypothyroidism, however, is linked to a higher risk of fracture and a decreased BMD in postmenopausal women.

5.3.3.7. Loop Diuretics (LD)

Elderly people are frequently prescribed and using LD. Although they also increase calcium excretion and decrease calcium reabsorption, their diuretic action is primarily focused on sodium and chloride reabsorption at the loop of Henle. Reduced BMD and increased bone turnover are possible outcomes of hypocalcemia. The use of LD was linked in clinical studies to a higher fracture risk in postmenopausal women and a lower hip bone mineral density in men. Longer-term studies and practical RCTs are necessary to investigate these effects, though, as renal calcium loss may be compensated for by a PTH-dependent rise in active vitamin D activity, which would keep normocalcemia stable.

5.3.3.8. Chronic Kidney Disease (CKD)

In addition to those with diabetes and hypertension, the incidence of chronic kidney disease (CKD) rises with age. Hypocalcemia, hyperparathyroidism, and disruptions in the kidney's 1α-hydroxylation of vitamin D are the reasons why CKD is linked to osteoporosis and renal osteodystrophy.

5.3.3.9. Diabetes

Diabetes type 1 (T1DM) and type 2 (T2DM) are risk factors for low-energy fractures because they both have low bone strength and quality; however, only T1DM usually lowers bone mineral density (BMD). Throughout life, T1DM is linked to a higher risk of fracture, especially at the hip, even after controlling for co-morbid conditions like chronic kidney disease. It is hypothesized that a partial cause of fracture risk is a deficiency in insulin and IGF-1, which are known to play a significant role in determining peak bone mass. In early adulthood and adolescence, T1DM typically manifests. Now is the moment to put plans into action to raise peak bone mass and increase BMD (Kanis et al., 2011).

T2DM is linked to a higher risk of fractures at the hip, vertebrae, and other susceptible locations but not a lower BMD. Because the gold standard measurement of BMD may understate the true fracture risk for patients with T2DM, this poses a clinical challenge for older adults. In actuality, elevated mechanical loading—which is typically brought on by obesity and hormonal variables like hyperinsulinemia—favors increased bone deposition. Consequently, the elevated risk of fracture is attributed to additional mechanisms. For instance, patients with chronic hyperglycemia produce more advanced glycation end products, which hinder collagen cross-linking in the bone matrix and lower bone strength and quality. Due to peripheral neuropathy, decreased physical function, orthostatic hypotension, poorer vision, and hypoglycemia from medication, patients with diabetes are also more likely to fall.

5.4. Osteoporosis: Diagnosis and Management

Symptoms of common underlying medical conditions and medications that cause bone loss, a thorough physical examination, appropriate laboratory testing, and a detailed history of clinical risk factors for osteoporosis should all be part of the initial evaluation of patients with suspected secondary osteoporosis.

A thorough evaluation of all prescribed drugs is necessary, as is a determination of alcohol and tobacco use in the past and present, as well as any family history of osteoporosis or fractures. Diabetes mellitus, anorexia nervosa, prolonged sex hormone deficiency, and possibly reversible endocrine disorders like acromegaly or Cushing's syndrome should all receive special attention. More laboratory, imaging, and invasive tests might be necessary based on preliminary results and the clinical index of suspicion. For the diagnosis of secondary osteoporosis, bone mineral densitometry with DXA is the preferred technique. Measurements should be taken at the hip and lumbar spine. Hip DXA measurements are more accurate in this population because aortic calcification and osteophytes, which are more prevalent in older men, may artificially raise spinal BMD measurements. An individual who has a Z-score (age- and sex-matched bone mineral density) of <−2 is more likely to have a secondary cause of osteoporosis, and this helps identify those who need further assessment. Fracture risk may rise in the absence of BMD if there is a secondary cause. Patients with Cushing's syndrome or chronic kidney disease (CKD), for instance, may have increased skeletal fragility even in the presence of normal BMD. To find common vertebral fractures, osteolytic lesions, or tumors, spinal X-rays should be taken in patients with localized back pain, recent spinal deformities, or height loss greater than 3 cm. Vertebral fracture assessment (VFA) using digital x-ray angiograms (DXA) offers lateral vertebral morphometry as an alternative to spinal x-rays.

Initial testing should include routine evaluations of the kidneys and liver, a complete blood count, serum calcium and phosphate levels, C-reactive protein, bone-specific alkaline phosphatase, serum 25-hydroxyvitamin D_3, serum levels of thyrotropin, and serum testosterone in men. Other helpful screening tests include serum-free light chains, serum protein electrophoresis, serum parathyroid hormone levels, and 24-hour urinary calcium excretion.

When low levels of 25-hydroxyvitamin D_3 and iron-deficiency anemia are present, it is especially important to measure anti-tissue transglutaminase antibodies. If the results are positive, a duodenal biopsy is necessary to confirm the diagnosis of celiac disease. After taking 1 mg of dexamethasone at midnight the day before, a fasting morning serum cortisol level should be taken to rule out Cushing's syndrome. Measurements of serum tryptase or a 24-hour urine histamine excretion should be made if systemic mastocytosis is suspected. Urinary excretion of Nmethylhistamine or 11-β prostaglandin $F_{2\alpha}$, if accessible, has the potential to be more dependable and sturdy than urinary excretion of histamine. To confirm the osteogenesis imperfecta diagnosis, COL1A genetic testing is necessary.

The use of double tetracycline labeling to measure the rate of bone formation in young people with severe osteoporosis, such as those who have multiple fractures or fractures that occur after antiresorptive treatment, is reserved for iliac crest bone biopsy and bone histomorphometry. In these cases, bone histomorphometry can determine whether systemic mastocytosis or infiltrating malignant diseases like multiple myeloma, lymphoma, leukemia, and disseminated carcinoma are present. It can also distinguish osteomalacia from osteoporosis. When all other possible causes of osteoporosis have been ruled out, premenopausal women or men with idiopathic osteoporosis may also have an osteoblast defect discovered by bone histomorphometry (Kanis et al., 2004).

Despite antiresorptive therapy, biochemical markers of bone turnover may show high rates of bone remodeling, which could be a sign of poor patient adherence to treatment or decreased therapeutic efficacy.

5.4.1. Assessment of Risk

An osteoporosis risk assessment is recommended for all women 65 years of age and older, all men 75 years of age and older, and younger patients with risk factors by the UK National Institute for Health and Care Excellence (NICE). Bone mineral density testing is the gold standard for diagnosing osteoporosis (BMD). The FRAX score can be computed using BMD at the femoral neck, age, sex, smoking, family history, and the use of oral glucocorticoids. The 10-year probability of an osteoporotic-related fracture is estimated by this tool. QFracture and the Trabecular Bone Score are two additional evaluation instruments that have demonstrated strong predictive power. Every risk calculator produces a probability risk instead of a recommendation for a course of action. In both community and secondary care settings, patient-centered management is essential. Treatment decisions should be made in collaboration with the patient, taking into account their preferences, co-occurring conditions, i.e., CKD, the ensuing polypharmacy load, and the social and psychological environment. It should be noted that the dose-dependent effects of smoking, alcohol, and corticosteroids on fracture risk, as well as the elevated risk resulting from multiple prior fractures, are not taken into account by the FRAX score. These elements should be considered when determining the specific fracture risk of an elderly person.

The burden of future fragility fractures may be lessened by screening and intervening for people who are at high risk of fracture. For instance, the UK SCOOP study found that screening with FRAX and pharmacological intervention for post-menopausal women aged 70–85 who were at high risk of fracture was associated with a decrease in hip fracture rate and was cost-effective when compared to usual care. When older patients with hip fractures come to secondary care, they usually have multiple frailty markers, are sarcopenic, and are osteoporotic. Therefore, the process of comprehensive geriatric assessment (CGA) should guide the multidisciplinary assessment and management of these patients, involving orthopedics, older people's specialist teams, pharmacy, therapy, nursing, mental health, dietetics, and speech and language pathologists. While this is the recommended course of action for patients who present with a hip fracture, in cases where the patient is less fragile and more mobile and presents with other fragility fractures, such as i.e., fracture liaison services (FLS), which are usually multidisciplinary coordinated models of care, systematically assess, identify, and provide advice on risk factor management for fractures of the wrist, shoulder, and vertebrae. They are essential in lowering the possibility of more severe fractures down the road. Global programs like the Capture the Fracture initiative (capturethefracture.org) by the International Osteoporosis Foundation facilitate the growth of FLS in secondary care settings. To maintain an individual's independence, general principles include maintaining muscle strength, maintaining bone mineral density, and controlling falls and other risk factors (Kanis et al., 2004).

To identify those who are most likely to suffer a fracture within two years of a sentinel fracture, the notion of imminent fracture was recently developed. Up to 23.2% of patients may experience these events, and risk factors include osteoporosis, comorbidities, older age, recent fracture, and fracture site. e.g., cognitive impairment, polypharmacy in the central nervous system, decreased physical activity, worsening general health, and falls. To lessen the burden of fractures in the future, this supports the idea of early identification, assessment, and treatment of those most at risk using the FLS model.

Sarcopenia is diagnosed by identifying cases using the SARC-F questionnaire, using hand-held dynamometry to detect the presence of decreased grip strength, or by observing poorer performance during repeated chair rises. At this point, a multicomponent intervention involving either nutritional or physical activity interventions is permissible in a probable case of sarcopenia. One can ascertain whether a person has severe sarcopenia by measuring their lean mass using DXA and by taking additional measurements of their physical function, like stroll speed.

5.4.2. Management of Secondary Osteoporosis

The two main goals of managing secondary osteoporosis are to (1) treat the underlying condition; and (2) increase bone mass to ward off fractures in the future. It is necessary to combine a pragmatic strategy with patient-centered, tailored therapy.

5.4.2.1. Treatment of the Underlying Disease

5.4.2.1.1. Endocrine Diseases

In cases when osteoporosis is present, surgical treatment for Cushing's syndrome and primary hyperparathyroidism is recommended. Exogenous hyperthyroidism necessitates adjusting the L-thyroxine dosage with a target serum thyrotropin level between 0.4 and 2.0 mU/l, except cases where TSH-suppressive therapy for differentiated thyroid carcinoma is necessary. Endogenous hyperthyroidism should be treated with antithyroid medications, radioiodine therapy, or surgery.

Men and women with osteoporosis who are premenopausal and lack sex hormones should get replacements. Increases in BMD are observed in hypogonadal men receiving testosterone treatment, even though the treatment's ability to reduce fracture risk has not been investigated. Before beginning treatment, it is important to weigh the advantages and disadvantages of sex hormone therapy, which include the risk of breast cancer and thromboembolic diseases in women and sleep apnea, benign prostatic hypertrophy, and prostate cancer in men.

Growth hormone replacement therapy raises men's bone mineral density (BMD) in cases of adult growth hormone deficiency, but there is no information on how it lowers the risk of fracture and its benefit-risk ratio is still unknown. To reduce the risk of falls, patients with type 1 diabetes (T1DM) who also have low bone mass benefit from aggressively preventing diabetic vascular complications, such as retinopathy, nephropathy, and polyneuropathy. Assessment of the fall risk is necessary for patients with both T1DM and T2DM.

5.4.2.1.2. Gastrointestinal Diseases

Celiac disease patients must follow a gluten-free diet; if they take enough calcium and vitamin D supplements, their bone mineral density (BMD) may rise noticeably. When there is pancreatic insufficiency causing malabsorption, exocrine pancreatic enzymes need to be replenished. As in other inflammatory disorders or after transplantation, efforts should be made to alter the immunosuppressive regimen for patients with inflammatory bowel disease, especially those with Crohn's disease, to control inflammation and lower glucocorticoid doses. When treating Crohn's disease, minimally invasive small bowel surgery is recommended to protect the terminal ileum, and vitamin D deficiency needs to be addressed. Patients undergoing bariatric surgery should have their bone health monitored for the rest of their lives, and any deficiency in calcium or vitamin D should be treated.

5.4.2.2. General Measures

Along with quitting smoking, all patients with secondary osteoporosis should restrict their alcohol intake to no more than two standard drinks per day. A thiazide (12.5–25 mg hydrochlorothiazide per day) may help patients with hypercalciuria by lowering their urine calcium excretion and raising their BMD.

5.4.3. Non-Pharmacological Options for the Treatment of Osteoporosis

Exercise and physical activity have been shown to reduce the risk of osteoporosis-related fractures and falls. Resistance training has been demonstrated to improve bone strength through repeated mechanical loading, which enhances bone mineral density and slows the progression of osteoporosis in addition to maintaining skeletal muscle. For instance, high force exercise, such as progressive resistance strength training of the lower limbs, was found to be the most effective type of exercise for increasing neck of femur bone mineral density in a systematic review of 43 randomized controlled trials. Furthermore, it has been demonstrated that reducing the risk of falls and easing musculoskeletal pain can be achieved by strengthening hip flexion and knee extension and correcting biomechanical imbalance in the abdominal trunk. Moreover, modifiable factors that contribute to the prevention of osteoporosis include quitting smoking, abstaining from excessive alcohol, optimizing calcium intake through diet, and maintaining a balanced diet high in fruits and vegetables with a tendency toward increased protein intake. These guidelines can generally be applied to the treatment of sarcopenia as well. Acute decompensation and the advancement of the frailty syndrome can be lessened by lowering the risk of falls and the resulting fracture through increased bone mineral density (Kanis et al., 2004).

5.4.4. Pharmacological Options for the Treatment of Osteoporosis

There are various pharmacological options for osteoporosis treatment that aim to reduce the risk of fractures. These include:

1. Calcium and vitamin D
2. Antiresorptive therapy—Bisphosphonates, Denosumab.
3. Hormonal treatment—Selective estrogen receptor modulators, Testosterone, PTH analogs.
4. Novel therapies—Romosozumab, Dickkopf-1 (Dkk1) inhibitors.

5.4.4.1. Calcium and Vitamin D

Elderly people frequently lack vitamin D, partly due to physiological changes in the skin's capacity to synthesize the nutrient, but also because they are more likely to be malnourished, have chronic kidney disease, be institutionalized, or be housebound. The recommended daily intake of calcium is 1000 mg and vitamin D is 400 international units (IU) according to national guidelines. It is recommended that elderly individuals who are housebound or residing in a nursing home consume 800 IU of vitamin D daily. Supplementing with calcium and vitamin D lowered the risk of hip fracture by 30% and the risk of fractures overall by 15%, according to a meta-analysis. A study found that patients taking a minimum dose of 1200 mg of calcium and 800 IU of vitamin D had a 12% reduction in all fractures and a lower rate of BMD loss in the hip and spine (Table 5.4).

Table 5.4. Advantages, Adverse Effects and Contraindications of the Main Pharmacological Interventions in Osteoporosis

Treatment	Advantages	Side Effects and Contraindications	Guidance	Posology
Calcium and vitamin D	Reduce the risk of hip fracture and of total fracture Reduce rate of loss of BMD in the hip and spine Reduction in risk of falling Favorable effects on muscle health	Gastrointestinal symptoms Renal stones Some evidence suggests an increased risk of cardiovascular disease (including myocardial infarction) *Contraindicated* in pre-existing hypercalcemia	Housebound older people or those living in a nursing home are advised to take 800 IU of vitamin D per day	1,000 mg of calcium in combination with 400 IU of vitamin D, daily
Bisphosphonates	Reduce the risk of fractures amongst a broad age range of patients Increase BMD (lumbar spine; trochanter; femoral neck; total proximal femur) Reduce the risk of mortality when commenced after a fracture	Gastrointestinal symptoms Bone/muscle/joint pain Hypocalcemia Osteonecrosis of the jaw (rare) Atypical femoral fractures (after 5 years of use) Issues with adherence *Contraindicated* in severe renal impairment; conditions impairing gastric emptying (achalasia, esophageal stricture) and hypocalcemia	For postmenopausal women and men over 50 years of age, who have been confirmed by DXA scan to have osteoporosis Ensure patients have normal serum calcium levels and are replete in vitamin D. Advise good dental hygiene and well-fitting dentures	Alendronate 10 mg PO, once daily or 70 mg once weekly Risedronate 5 mg PO, once daily or 35 mg PO, once weekly Ibandronic acid 150 mg PO, monthly (3 mg every 3 months IV) Zoledronic acid 5 mg IV annually

Denosumab	Reduce the risk of fractures (vertebral, hip, non-vertebral fractures) Increase in BMD without plateau	Hypocalcemia (especially if impaired renal function) Increased risk of bacterial infections Skin rash Increase fracture risk back to pre-treatment level Osteonecrosis of the jaw (rare) Atypical femoral fractures Risk of severe hypocalcemia especially with coexistent Vitamin D deficiency as well as renal impairment	Alongside calcium and vitamin D supplementation Alternative when oral bisphosphonates are not tolerated or are contraindicated Ensure patients have normal serum calcium levels and are replete in vitamin D. Advise good dental hygiene and well-fitting dentures	60 mg SC (6-montly)
Selective estrogen receptor modulators	Reduction in both vertebral and non-vertebral fracture risk Appear to be safe to use in older people	Hot flushes; Lower limb cramps; Joint pain; Can increase risk of venous thromboembolism	Treatment and prevention of osteoporosis in post-menopausal women and are indicated after first line therapies have been considered	Raloxifene 60 mg, daily
Testosterone	Increase in BMD in men who are hypogonadal	Aggression; Prostate cancer; Psychiatric symptoms	For men at high risk for fracture with testosterone levels below 200 ng/dl (6.9 nmol/liter) and have contraindications to other osteoporosis' therapies	
Teriparatide	Appears to increase bone formation within 24 months of use	Nausea; Pain in limbs; Headache; Dizziness; *Contraindicated* in conditions with increased bone turnover (pre-existing hypercalcemia, hyperparathyroidism, Paget's disease); unexplained raised alkaline phosphatase and previous bone radiation therapy; malignancies with bony metastases and severe renal impairment	If intolerant or suffer severe side effects from first line therapies described	20 mcg SC daily (max. 24 months)

Abaloparatide	Lower risks of new vertebral fractures (compared teriparatide) Reduction in risk of non-vertebral Increase in BMD	Appears safe. Further drug safety data pending	Headache, nausea, dizziness, joint pain are key adverse effects	80 mcg SC daily
Romosozumab	Reduces the risk of vertebral and non-vertebral fractures	ARCH study reported an imbalance in serious cardiovascular adverse events. Use may be restricted	Joint pain, hypersensitivity reactions, hypocalcemia are key adverse effects	210 mg (2 × 105 mg injections) SC monthly for 12 months

Source: J. Barnsley, G. Buckland, P. E. Chan, A. Ong, A. S. Ramos, M. Baxter, F. Laskou, E. M. Dennison, C. Cooper, and Harnish P. Patel. Pathophysiology and treatment of osteoporosis: challenges for clinical practice in older people. Aging Clinical and Experimental Research (2021) 33:759–773. https://doi.org/10.1007/s40520-021-01817-y.

Research against calcium supplementation points to a higher risk of heart disease, including myocardial infarction. Other research, however, did not discover a connection between taking supplements of calcium and an increased risk of heart disease (Kanis et al., 2000). Overall, the benefits of supplementation are thought to outweigh the risks, and current recommendations suggest that those receiving treatment for osteoporosis and those at increased risk of insufficiency should take supplements. Supplementing with calcium and vitamin D has also been demonstrated to improve muscle health and lower the risk of falling.

5.4.4.2. Antiresorptive Therapy

5.4.4.2.1. Bisphosphonates (Alendronate, Risedronate, Ibandronate and Zolendronic Acid)

Strong bindings to hydroxyapatite enable bisphosphonates to prevent osteoclast-mediated bone resorption and to promote an increase in bone mineral density. They have been linked to positive outcomes in reducing the risk of fractures in patients of all ages, including those who are frail. Research indicates that taking 10 mg of alendronate every day for ten years improved bone mineral density by 13.7% at the lumbar spine, 10.3% at the trochanter, 5.4% at the femoral neck, and 6.7% at the entire proximal femur. Crucially, it has been demonstrated that starting oral or intravenous bisphosphonate therapy as a secondary preventive measure following a fracture lowers the risk of mortality.

For postmenopausal women and men over 50 with confirmed osteoporosis on DXA, UK NICE guidelines recommend Alendronate 10 mg once daily or 70 mg once weekly; or Risedronate 5 mg once daily or 35 mg once weekly. The typical time frame for BMD evaluation is three to five years. After that, if the patient is still at risk for fracture or has started corticosteroid therapy, treatment is continued. A medication break may be advised if the T-score is >−2.5, pending additional assessment of BMD and fracture risk. On the other hand, compared to those who continue taking bisphosphonates, postmenopausal women who stop taking them at this time may have a 40% increased risk of developing new clinical fractures. It is not advised to use isabronid acid as a first line.

Oral bisphosphonates can cause gastrointestinal distress, pain in the bones and joints, esophageal ulceration, and in rare cases, osteonecrosis of the jaw (with cancer patients having the highest risk). Atypical femur fractures can happen at a rate of 1:1000/year, especially after using bisphosphonates for five years. Oral bisphosphonates should be taken with a glass of water, upright, and on an empty stomach. Because of this complicated dosage schedule, older adults may find it difficult to adhere to bisphosphonates. This problem may be exacerbated by polypharmacy, cognitive decline, and the need for physical care. Moreover, bisphosphonates are unstable and should not be stored in compliance aids. In older people with severe gastro-oesophageal reflux, dysphagia or cognitive impairment, alternative preparations, i.e., yearly intravenous (IV) administration of zoledronic acid or substitutes for bisphosphonates may be employed. Since bisphosphonates are excreted by the kidneys, people with renal impairment should avoid them. Treatment choices can be made based on thresholds provided by estimated glomerular filtration rates (eGFR). For instance, when creatinine clearance is less than 35 mL/min/1.73 m^2 or 30 mL/min/1.73 m^2, respectively, alendronate and risedronate should be avoided. However, in older adults, particularly those with frailty and sarcopenia, eGFR may not be reliable. Therefore, it is appropriate to use Cockcroft and Gault estimation of GFR in these circumstances, particularly when IV Zoledronic is being considered (Table 5.4).

5.4.4.2.2. Denosumab

A humanized monoclonal antibody called denosumab inhibits osteoclastic activity by blocking RANKL. It is administered subcutaneously as an injection (60 mg) every six months to people with a GFR greater than 30 ml/min/1.73 m^2, in conjunction with calcium and vitamin D supplements. In the first three years, postmenopausal women taking denosumab experienced a reduction in fracture incidence of 68% for vertebral fractures, 40% for hip fractures, and 20% for non-vertebral fractures, according to the large multicenter placebo-control trial FREEDOM (Fracture Reduction Evaluation of Denosumab). A 10-year follow-up revealed continued declining fracture incidence and an increase in bone mineral density without plateau. When oral bisphosphonates are not tolerated, are not recommended, or are not possible due to social or psychological issues, denosumab is frequently utilized as a substitute. Usually, treatment lasts five to ten years. Denosumab has anti-resorptive effects that quickly wear off after treatment ends and raise fracture risk to pre-treatment levels within a year of stopping treatment. As a result, patients and doctors must lead 6-monthly reminders (Kanis et al., 2000). In contrast, BMD is preserved with bisphosphonates for a minimum of two years following treatment discontinuation. Side effects include skin rash, increased risk of bacterial infections, osteonecrosis of the jaw, and infrequently, atypical femoral fractures. Hypocalcemia is particularly common in people with impaired renal function (Table 5.4).

Making sure patients have normal serum calcium levels and are fully supplemented with vitamin D reduces the risk of severe hypocalcemia during the treatment when starting denosumab or other anti-resorptive therapy. For people who are vitamin D deficient, there are various loading regimens available. 100,000 IU of cholecalciferol for people who are frail and require rapid loading seems to be well tolerated in the clinical practice of the authors. As an alternative, you could take 20,000 IU three times a week, then 800–1000 IU each day to keep your serum vitamin D level over 50 nmol/L. Excess vitamin D is linked to mineral deposits in soft tissues, hypercalcemia, and hypercalciuria. However, it is thought to be safe to take 800–1000 IU of vitamin D per day to prevent vitamin D deficiency.

5.4.4.3. Hormonal Treatment

5.4.4.3.1. Selective Oestrogen Receptor Modulators (Raloxifene and Lasoxifene)

Raloxifene and Lasoxifene are examples of selective estrogen receptor modulators (SERMs), which work to stop bone resorption brought on by low estrogen levels. They should be used after first-line therapies have been exhausted, mainly for the treatment and prevention of osteoporosis in postmenopausal women. As an illustration of its effectiveness, at three years, women aged 59 to 80 years old who took lasoxifene 0.5 mg had a 42% decrease in the risk of vertebral fractures and a 24% reduction in the hazard rates of non-vertebral fractures. Lower limb cramps and hot flushes are the most frequently reported side effects. The most serious side effect is an increased risk of venous thromboembolism, which is fortunately uncommon (Table 5.4).

5.4.4.3.2. Testosterone

For men with testosterone levels below 200 ng/dl (6.9 nmol/l), who are at high risk of fracture, the Endocrine Society recommends testosterone. Even for patients who do not meet the standard criteria for testosterone therapy but who are not candidates for other osteoporosis treatments, this should be taken into consideration. Increases in prostate-specific antigen as well as effects on the heart and metabolism are possible side effects (Table 5.4).

5.4.4.3.3. PTH Analogs (Teriparatide, Abaloparatide)

Synthetic parathyroid hormone teriparatide is anabolic, not anti-resorptive, in bone. It can be used for both men and women who have severe side effects from the first-line therapies mentioned or who are intolerant. For a maximum of 24 months, teriparatide should be injected subcutaneously at a dose of 20 mcg per day (Kanis et al., 2000). Patients with metabolic bone diseases, such as Paget's disease, skeletal muscle metastases, or a history of bone radiation therapy, should not take teriparatide. Headache, lightheadedness, limb pain, and nausea are some of the side effects. In the ACTIVE trial, 2463 post-menopausal women aged 49–86 years had a significant increase in bone mineral density (BMD). Abaloparatide, a more recent analog of PTH, demonstrated lower risks of new vertebral fractures when compared to both placebo and teriparatide as well as lower risk of non-vertebral fractures when compared to placebo (Table 5.4).

5.4.4.4. Novel Therapies

5.4.4.4.1. Romosozumab

A monoclonal antibody called romozumab binds sclerostin, causing a rise in bone formation and a fall in bone resorption. It is injected subcutaneously once a month at a dosage of 210 mg. In the FRAME study, postmenopausal women with osteoporosis aged 55 to 90 were randomized, double-blind, placebo-controlled, and the treatment was either Romosozumab or a placebo. Monthly denosumab 6 was also administered to both groups. At 24 months, the group receiving romozumab treatment exhibited a 75% reduction in the risk of new vertebral fractures, while adverse event rates remained largely unchanged.

In contrast, a group of postmenopausal women who received alendronate for 24 months was compared to another group that received romosozumab for 12 months, followed by alendronate for an additional 12 months, in the ARCH study. It's interesting to note that patients in the group treated with romosozumab and alendronate had a reduced risk of new vertebral fractures by 48% ($p < 0.001$) and clinical fractures by 27% ($p < 0.001$). There was a 19% reduction in the risk of non-vertebral fractures ($p = 0.04$) and a 38% reduction in the risk of hip fractures ($p = 0.02$). The two groups differed in the number of serious cardiovascular adverse events; 16 patients (0.8%) in the Romosozumab group and 6 (0.3%) in the alendronate group reported cardiac ischemic events (odds ratio 2.65; 95% CI 1.03–6.77); Similarly, 16 patients (0.8%) in the Romosozumab group and 7 (0.3%) in the alendronate group reported cerebrovascular events (odds ratio 2.27; 95% CI 0.93–5.22). But it's important to note this disparity in serious cardiovascular adverse events. To understand this imbalance, more research is required (Table 5.4).

5.4.4.4.2. Dual Inhibition of Dickkopf-1 (Dkk1) and Sclerotin

One of the antagonists in the Wnt signaling pathway, a crucial cascade involved in the formation of bones, is Dkk1. It was discovered that sclerotin inhibition can cause Dkk1 expression to be upregulated. Based on this, a study showed that, in both rodents and primates, the use of an engineered bio-specific antibody against sclerostin and Dkk1 concurrently had a greater effect on bone formation than monotherapies. When dual inhibition was applied, improvements in the ability of fractured bones to heal and repair were also observed. We're currently waiting on clinical trial results.

5.4.4.5. Dementia and Fragility Fracture

Age-related increases in the risk of falls are associated with dementia, which is typified by multimorbidity, behavioral and cognitive issues, and visual and motor impairments. Additionally, the risk of osteoporosis is increased in patients with dementia due to the high prevalence of malnutrition, frailty, and sarcopenia. This coexistence presents a unique therapeutic challenge, and in dementia patients who are at high risk of incident and future fracture, there is a recognized need for pharmaceutical management and bone health assessment. However, due to factors like delirium, worsening cognitive decline, institutionalization, poor adherence, and competing polypharmacy, patients with dementia are less likely to have their fracture risk evaluated or to receive longer-term secondary preventive medications. Furthermore, in this patient group, altered pharmacokinetics work together to increase the risk of adverse drug reactions (ADR). In this sense, it is certain that the risk of fractures rises in direct proportion to the prevalence of dementia. When the risks and benefits of treatment are taken into account in the context of the larger social, physical, and psychological domains, CGA for these patients may only identify short- and medium-term goals that can be achieved.

5.5. The Use of Combination Therapy in the Treatment of Postmenopausal Osteoporosis

Numerous mechanisms underlie pharmacological interventions aimed at preventing fragility fractures. Most frequently used medications are anti-resorptive ones; these include raloxifene, denosumab (a humanized monoclonal antibody to receptor activator of NFB ligand), and the bisphosphonates (alendronate, risedronate, ibandronate, and zoledronic acid). PTH (1–84) and PTH (1–34), or parathyroid hormone (PTH) peptide, are two forms of anabolic skeletal agents that are offered. Lastly, strontium ranelate acts through mechanisms that are not fully understood; its beneficial effects on bone strength and fracture reduction may primarily result from altered properties of the bone material, as its effects on bone remodeling are relatively weak (Melton, 1988).

One may employ combination therapy for several purposes. First, the use of multiple agents may not reduce fractures as much as the synergistic effects of interventions with distinct modes of action or the additive effects of medications with comparable mechanisms of action. Second, other medications might be needed to maintain the positive effects of anabolic agents as their approval is limited to a 24-month treatment period and as BMD decreases after treatment discontinuation. Thirdly, in patients who still have a high risk of fracture, it may be preferable to stop therapy after a maximum of three to five years and continue treatment with other medications. This is especially true for strong anti-resorptive agents. Lastly, it's critical to understand if the initial treatment had an impact on the response in patients who develop treatment-related intolerance and must switch to a different medication.

5.5.1. Combination Anti-Resorptive Therapy

Research has examined the use of combinations of anti-resorptive agents in postmenopausal osteoporosis. These combinations have included raloxifene and alendronate, calcitonin and hormone therapy (HT), estrogen and methyltestosterone, and HT and bisphosphonates. The majority of these studies have shown higher increases in bone mineral density (BMD) when combination therapy is used instead of monotherapy; however, the studies' power to show differences in fracture risk reduction has not been established. It is not usually advised to use two antiresorptive medications at the same time due to the higher cost of combination therapy, the possibility of more side effects, and the lack of evidence of improved anti-fracture efficacy.

5.5.2. Sequential Treatment with Anti-Resorptive Drugs: Alendronate Followed by Denosumab

In clinical practice, changing anti-resorptive medications frequently occurs during treatment. The impact of moving from alendronate to denosumab has been investigated in postmenopausal women who were randomly assigned to continue on alendronate 70 mg once weekly for at least six months or to switch to denosumab 60 mg sc every six months. Compared to women who continued on alendronate, women who switched to denosumab experienced significantly greater increases in bone mineral density (BMD) in the hip and lumbar spine at 6 and 12 months, as well as greater suppression of bone turnover markers. Thus, these data suggest that switching to denosumab increases BMD in patients who need to stop taking bisphosphonates, though it is unclear how this will affect the fracture rate.

5.5.3. Sequential Therapy with Bisphosphonates and Strontium Ranelate

According to a recent study, the BMD response to strontium ranelate is blunted and delayed as a result of prior bisphosphonate therapy. In a prospective study of postmenopausal women with osteoporosis, strontium ranelate (2 g) was given daily along with calcium and vitamin D supplements to 56 women who had never taken a bisphosphonate and 52 women who had been on an oral bisphosphonate for at least a year but had stopped treatment within the previous month. Following a year of treatment, women who had never taken bisphosphonates saw an increase in bone mineral density (BMD) in the lumbar spine of 5.6 percent, while women who had previously taken bisphosphonates saw an increase of 2.1 percent. At both 6 and 12 months, the BMD increase in the former group was significantly lower than in the latter. At one year, the BMD at the total hip did not significantly change in the women who had received bisphosphonate pretreatment, while it increased by 3.4% in the group that had not received treatment. An extension of this research revealed that, after six months, BMD in the spine of pretreated women increased in tandem with treatment-naïve women, while, after two years of treatment, there was still some blunting of the BMD response at the hip (Park et al., 2012). The most plausible explanation for these effects is that bisphosphonates prevent strontium from being absorbed into bone by suppressing bone turnover, which leads to a decrease in newly formed bone.

5.5.4. Combined Anabolic and Anti-Resorptive Therapy

Given that anabolic and anti-resorptive medications have distinct mechanisms of action, combination therapy may be justified because concurrent stimulation of bone formation and inhibition of bone resorption may be more effective than using either medication alone. On the other hand, it's also feasible that anti-resorptives suppress remodeling, which would stop or lessen the rise in the remodeling rate needed for PTH peptides' anabolic skeletal effects.

Deal et al. examined the effects of teriparatide plus raloxifene therapy versus teriparatide alone in osteoporotic postmenopausal women. After six months of treatment, the two groups showed comparable increases in lumbar spine bone mineral density (6.19 percent in the combination group, 5.19 percent in the teriparatide alone group). However, the total hip BMD increased more significantly in the combination therapy group.

PTH (1–84) 100 g/d, alendronate 10 mg/d, or both were randomly assigned to 238 postmenopausal women with low BMD in the Parathyroid Hormone and Alendronate Study (PATH). In all treatment groups, as well as in the combination and PTH alone treatment groups, spine areal BMD had increased after a year of treatment. When comparing the PTH alone group to the other treatment groups, volumetric bone mass (BMD) was almost two times higher as determined by quantitative computed tomography (QCT). Areal bone mineral density (BMD) in the proximal femur increased in the combination group compared to the PTH alone group, but it did not change significantly in the former. Both groups saw an increase in BMD. The PTH group had a significant decrease in volumetric bone mineral density (BMD) throughout the hip, whereas the combination group did not experience a significant change and the alendronate group experienced a slight increase. In contrast, the PTH group showed a significant increase in cortical bone volume at the femoral neck and total hip, while the other two groups did not show any discernible changes. Concurrent use of alendronate was found to mitigate the anabolic effects of PTH, according to the authors, based on changes in hip cortical volume and spine volumetric BMD. Similar findings were reported by two other studies examining the effects of PTH (1–34) in postmenopausal women and men with low BMD, either alone or in combination with alendronate (Ralston and Uitterlinden, 2010).

In a recent study, intravenous zoledronic acid and teriparatide combination therapy were compared to teriparatide treatment alone. Three treatment groups were randomly assigned to postmenopausal women with osteoporosis: a single infusion of 5 mg zoledronic acid combined with 20 µg of teriparatide subcutaneously every day, zoledronic acid alone, or teriparatide alone. At one year, the BMD increases in the lumbar spine were comparable between the teriparatide and combination groups, with the combination group increasing at a faster rate than the other two groups at earlier time points. After a year, the total hip BMD values in the combination and zoledronic acid groups were similar, with the combination group experiencing a higher rate of increase in comparison to the zoledronic acid group at week 13. In the hip, the combination group's increases in BMD were significantly greater than those in the teriparatide alone group at all time points. In the group receiving combination therapy, serum ß-CTX levels decreased quickly, held steady for two months, and then rose to levels above baseline after a year. In the combination therapy group, serum P1NP levels increased from approximately six months to one year. As predicted, in women taking zoledronic acid alone, both markers stayed suppressed for the whole trial.

Comparing this study's findings with those of Black et al. indicates that modifications in the spine's areal BMD following a year of therapy are comparable, however, the research conducted by Cosman et al. made it possible to show that women receiving combination therapy experienced a faster rise in spine BMD at earlier time points. Longer-term studies show that the benefits in spine BMD following PTH monotherapy are higher than those with combination therapy by a two-year margin. In the early phases of treatment, it is evident that combination therapy or treatment with an anti-resorptive agent alone leads to higher increases in BMD in the hip than with PTH monotherapy; however, in longer-term studies, the increase with PTH was greater than that obtained with combination therapy or an anti-resorptive agent. Hip bone mineral density (BMD) is frequently temporarily decreased when PTH is used alone. This is most likely due to increased cortical porosity, and concurrent anti-resorptive therapy prevents this from happening, which is likely caused by decreased cortical remodeling. Patients who are at high risk of hip fracture may benefit most from a combination anti-resorptive and anabolic treatment because early treatment exposure to increased cortical porosity may increase risk. Though hip fracture reduction has been demonstrated for several anti-resorptive agents, this has not been demonstrated with PTH peptides. As a result, the effects of combination therapy on hip fracture risk have not been assessed.

In the PATH study, the combination therapy group and the PTH-treated group experienced higher rates of both hypercalcemia and hypercalciuria than the alendronate group, albeit these effects were usually mild. Significant increases in the mean serum uric acid level were also linked to combination and PTH therapy, and three women—two in the combination group and one in the PTH group—developed gout. When men received combination therapy or PTH therapy alone as opposed to alendronate treatment alone, there was also a higher incidence of hypercalcemia and hypercalciuria. At last, in the research by Cosman et al. The percentages of women in the combination group (13.4%), teriparatide (15%), and zoledronic acid (4%), who had serum calcium levels that were normal at baseline but above the normal range during the study, were reported. In the combination group, one woman experienced significant hypercalcemia (serum calcium >2.89 mmol/l), while two women in the teriparatide group experienced the same condition.

5.5.5. Anabolic and Anti-Resorptive Therapy

5.5.5.1. Sequential Therapy: Anti-resorptive Before Anabolic Therapy

Numerous research studies have demonstrated that the anabolic effects of PTH peptides are diminished by prior bisphosphonate therapy. Ettinger et al. observed higher increases in hip and spine BMD during the first six months of teriparatide therapy in the group of women who had previously received raloxifene as compared to the group of women who had previously received alendronate, in a study of postmenopausal women who were switched from either raloxifene or alendronate to teriparatide. The mean increases in spine BMD at 18 months of teriparatide therapy were 10.2% and 4.1 percent, respectively. Over an 18-month period, BMD in the total hip did not significantly change in women who had previously received alendronate, but it did show a mean increase of 1.8 percent in women who had previously received raloxifene therapy. Teriparatide added to ongoing alendronate therapy significantly increased bone formation markers in postmenopausal women with osteoporosis; after one year of treatment with PTH (1–34) in women previously treated with raloxifene, significant increases in spine and total hip BMD (9.6 percent and 2.7 percent, respectively) were also reported. Both daily and cyclic PTH (1–34) treatment for 15 months was linked to significant increases in hip and spine bone mineral density (BMD), with the increase in spine BMD being significantly greater than that of postmenopausal women with osteoporosis who had been taking alendronate for at least a year. Miller et al. examined the effects of 12-month teriparatide therapy in postmenopausal women with osteoporosis in a prospective, nonrandomized study after the patients had received risedronate or alendronate for at least 24 months. The women who had previously received risedronate treatment showed a noticeably higher increase in the bone formation marker, P1NP, as well as in spine areal and volumetric BMD in comparison to the women who had previously received alendronate treatment. Nevertheless, no comparator group of women receiving PTH peptide therapy who were not yet on treatment was included in any of these studies (Rivadeneira et al., 2009).

In postmenopausal women with established osteoporosis who had or had not received prior anti-resorptive therapy, most commonly alendronate, for a median period of 11 months, the effect of teriparatide therapy on BMD was compared in the European Study of Forsteo (EUROFORS). A secondary subgroup analysis revealed that after 24 months of teriparatide, increases in spine and hip BMD were observed in all four groups (alendronate, etidronate, risedronate, and nonbisphosphonate) of women who had previously received anti-resorptive treatment, with etidronate pretreated women experiencing the largest increase. Previous anti-resorptive treatment was also associated with a modest blunting of the BMD response in the spine and hip. Postmenopausal women receiving HT have also shown that PTH peptide therapy can have anabolic effects even in the face of previous anti-resorptive therapy. Following three years of PTH (1–34) treatment, increases in bone mineral density BMD of 13% and 2.7% in the hip and spine, respectively, were observed. Additionally, women taking both HT and PTH (1–34) were found to have a significantly lower vertebral fracture rate than those receiving HT alone.

When considered collectively, these findings suggest that women who have previously received anti-resorptive therapy—especially more potent agents—may experience some attenuation of the anabolic effect of intermittent PTH therapy. Blunting of the BMD response seems to be generally quite minor; however, it is unknown what effect it may have, if any, on fracture reduction.

5.5.5.2. Sequential Therapy: Anti-Resorptive After Anabolic Therapy

PTH treatment is permitted for a maximum of 24 months. Anti-resorptive therapy should be started after PTH treatment is stopped because loss of bone mineral density (BMD) in the femoral neck, spine, and entire hip has been documented in the year that follows its discontinuation. Further improvements in spine, femoral neck, and total body BMD were observed in the postmenopausal women with osteoporosis who were treated with either PTH (1–84) or placebo for a year, followed by alendronate 10 mg/d for an additional year (Siris et al., 2009). According to Black et al., postmenopausal women who received PTH (1–84) for a year were able to maintain or even enhance their gains in bone mineral density (BMD) in the hip and spine by receiving alendronate therapy for an additional year. Women treated with raloxifene after stopping teriparatide have shown comparable outcomes. Men who took teriparatide for two years saw increases in lumbar spine bone mineral density (BMD) during the next two years when they received bisphosphonate therapy; men who did not receive treatment after stopping teriparatide saw a decrease in BMD.

A Closer Look

The Coexistence of Osteoporosis and Sarcopenia—Osteosarcopenia

Given bone and muscle share similar embryonic origins, both tissues may be influenced by similar metabolic (endocrine and paracrine) and environmental cues to maintain homeostasis. Sarcopenia (muscle failure) is characterized by a decline in skeletal muscle strength, mass and function. Primary sarcopenia occurs with advancing age, whilst secondary sarcopenia is secondary to co-existent illnesses, e.g., diabetes. The prevalence of sarcopenia increases with age and similar to osteoporosis has a multifactorial etiology—undernutrition, decreased physical activity, inflammation, and presence of comorbid diseases. Diagnosis of sarcopenia involves measuring muscle strength (hand grip strength) and function (walking speed or chair rise time), as well as lean mass—Dual-energy X-ray Absorptiometry (DXA) in this situation is a useful method to assess both total and appendicular lean mass as well as a bone mineral density for those suspected to have osteosarcopenia.

The pathophysiology of osteosarcopenia is multifactorial; the common mesenchymal origins of bone and muscle infer a close relationship in their pathogenesis. As such, similar genetic factors can have a pleiotropic influence on both bone and muscle. Polymorphisms of several genes including androgen receptor, estrogen receptor, IGF-1, and vitamin D receptor have been identified that can influence molecular cross-talk and alter cellular mechanisms resulting in an imbalance in muscle and bone turnover. The biomechanical relationship between muscle and bone is evident during aging where lower physical activity and mechanical loading contribute to decreased muscle mass, function and bone mineral density. This supports the 'mechanostat hypothesis,' which postulates that if the mechanical forces of the skeletal musculature acting upon the periosteum reach a given threshold, growth is stimulated as opposed to bone resorbed. In addition, as with caloric intake, dietary vitamin D and protein intake also diminishes with age, contributing to reduced muscle strength, lower bone mineralization and an increase in fall risk. Osteosarcopenia represents an additive burden for older people in terms of their physical and psychological health as well as their quality of life. Understanding the pathophysiology of osteosarcopenia is key to informing combined strategies for treatment and prevention (van Meurs et al., 2008).

Treatments for Osteosarcopenia

There are biochemical and hormonal relationships between bone and muscle through molecular cross-talk between myokines, osteokines and adipokines, secreted from muscle cells, bone cells and marrow adipose tissue, respectively. Abnormal expansion of marrow adipose tissue has been postulated to be a significant factor in the progression of post-menopausal osteoporosis. Similarly, myosteatosis negatively impacts on muscle quality, the force generated per skeletal muscle unit area. Although no single molecule has been implicated in the pathogenesis of either condition, ongoing research may provide new targets for future therapy. Growth hormone, insulin-like growth factor-1, gonadal sex hormones, vitamin D and myostatin have all been associated with a delay in the onset of osteosarcopenia. Though postulated to be novel therapeutic targets for drug development, currently no pharmacological treatments exist for osteosarcopenia.

Summary

- Osteoporosis is a skeletal disease characterized by low bone mass and micro-architectural deterioration of bone tissue with a consequent increase in bone fragility and susceptibility to fracture. The term osteoporosis literally means "porous bone" and refers to a condition in which bone is normally mineralized but reduced in quantity.
- Bone is a specialized and multifunctional connective tissue with both an organic and inorganic component. The organic bone matrix (osteoid) is comprised of collagenous proteins, the predominant being type I collagen as well as a broad range of non-collagenous proteins including glycosaminoglycans, glycoproteins and some serum-derived proteins. The numerous non-collagenous proteins regulate aspects of bone metabolism including deposition, mineralization and turnover.
- Bone remodeling allows repair of micro-damage, maintaining skeletal structure as well as serum calcium and phosphate homeostasis and involves a careful equilibrium between the action of osteoclasts, tightly coupled with that of osteoblasts.
- Peak bone mass is defined as the maximum amount of skeletal tissue an individual will have in their life at the termination of skeletal maturation. Peak bone mass is thought to be attained between 25 and 30 years of age thereafter decreasing at a rate of 0.5% per year. Males attain a higher BMD, albeit later than females. The attainment of peak bone mass is a multifactorial process.
- Bone loss in women is most evident in the trabecular vertebral bodies as they are more metabolically active and are sensitive to the trophic effects of estrogen which has a significant role in preventing bone resorption by inhibiting osteoclasts. A steeper decline in bone mass begins approximately between 65 and 69 years in women and between 74 and 79 years in men. Women aged 50 or over have a four-fold higher rate of osteoporosis and a two-fold higher rate of osteopenia than men. The lifetime risk of osteoporotic fractures in women is approximately 40%. Weight loss in older people, smoking and moderate to high alcohol intake appear to accelerate the loss of bone in both men and women.
- Glucocorticoids form part of the treatment strategy for a wide variety of diseases, including chronic inflammatory, rheumatological and respiratory illnesses. It is estimated that 1% of the population in the United Kingdom are receiving long-term glucocorticoid therapy and the rate of long-term use is gradually increasing.
- Denosumab is a humanized monoclonal antibody that blocks RANKL and hence osteoclastic activity. It is given via subcutaneous injection (60 mg)on a 6-monthly basis alongside calcium and vitamin D supplementation in individuals with a GFR > 30 ml/min/1.73 m^2.
- Teriparatide, a synthetic parathyroid hormone, is anabolic in bone rather than anti-resorptive. It can be used in men and women who are intolerant or who suffer severe side effects from first-line therapies described.
- Romosozumab is a monoclonal antibody that binds sclerostin leading to increased bone formation and a decrease in bone resorption. It is administered as a monthly subcutaneous injection, at a dose of 210 mg.

- Dkk1 is one of the antagonists in the Wnt signaling pathway which is an important cascade involved in bone formation. It was found that inhibition of sclerotin can lead to an upregulation of Dkk1 expression.

References

1. Arden, N. K., & Spector, T. D. (1997). Genetic influences on muscle strength, lean body mass, and bone mineral density: A twin study. *Journal of Bone and Mineral Research, 12*(12), 2076–2081. https://doi.org/10.1359/jbmr.1997.12.12.2076.
2. Burge, R., Dawson-Hughes, B., Solomon, D. H., Wong, J. B., King, A., & Tosteson, A. (2007). Incidence and economic burden of osteoporosis-related fractures in the United States, 2005–2025. *Journal of Bone and Mineral Research, 22*(3), 465–475. https://doi.org/10.1359/jbmr.061113.
3. Cooper, C., Eriksson, J. G., Forsen, T., Osmond, C., Tuomilehto, J., & Barker, D. J. (2001). Maternal height, childhood growth and risk of hip fracture in later life: A longitudinal study. *Osteoporosis International, 12*(8), 623–629. https://doi.org/10.1007/s001980170138.
4. Cummings, S. R., & Melton, L. J. (2002). Epidemiology and outcomes of osteoporotic fractures. *Lancet, 359*(9319), 1761–1767. https://doi.org/10.1016/S0140-6736(02)08657-9.
5. Dennison, E. M., Arden, N. K., Keen, R. W., Syddall, H., Day, I. N., & Spector, T. D., et al. (2001). Birthweight, vitamin D receptor genotype and the programming of osteoporosis. *Paediatric and Perinatal Epidemiology, 15*(3), 211–219. https://doi.org/10.1046/j.1365-3016.2001.00309.x.
6. Ferrari, S. L., Karasik, D., Liu, J., Karamohamed, S., Herbert, A. G., Cupples, L. A., et al. (2004). Interactions of interleukin-6 promoter polymorphisms with dietary and lifestyle factors and their association with bone mass in men and women from the Framingham Osteoporosis Study. *Journal of Bone and Mineral Research, 19*(4), 552–559. https://doi.org/10.1359/JBMR.0301291.
7. Hunter, D. J., De Langhe, S., Snieder, H., MacGregor, A. J., Swaminathan, R., Thakker, R. V., et al. (2001). Genetic contribution to bone metabolism, calcium excretion, and vitamin D and parathyroid hormone regulation. *Journal of Bone and Mineral Research, 16*(2), 371–378. https://doi.org/10.1359/jbmr.2001.16.2.371.
8. Jaenisch, R., & Bird, A. (2003). Epigenetic regulation of gene expression: How the genome integrates intrinsic and environmental signals. *Nature Genetics, 33*(Suppl), 245–254. https://doi.org/10.1038/ng1135.
9. Johnell, O. (1997). The socioeconomic burden of fractures: Today and in the 21st century. *American Journal of Medicine, 103*(2A), 20S–25S. https://doi.org/10.1016/S0002-9343(97)00258-1.
10. Johnell, O., & Kanis, J. A. (2006). An estimate of the worldwide prevalence and disability associated with osteoporotic fractures. *Osteoporosis International, 17*(12), 1726–1733. https://doi.org/10.1007/s00198-006-0176-6.
11. Jordan, K. M., & Cooper, C. (2002). Epidemiology of osteoporosis. *Best Practice & Research: Clinical Rheumatology, 16*(5), 795–806. https://doi.org/10.1053/berh.2002.0197.

12. Kanis, J. A., Hans, D., Cooper, C., Baim, S., Bilezikian, J. P., Binkley, N., et al. (2011). Interpretation and use of FRAX in clinical practice. *Osteoporosis International, 22*(9), 2395–2411. https://doi.org/10.1007/s00198-011-1686-3.

13. Kanis, J. A., Johnell, O., de Laet, C., Johansson, H., Oden, A., Delmas, P., et al. (2004). A meta-analysis of previous fracture and subsequent fracture risk. *Bone, 35*(2), 375–382. https://doi.org/10.1016/j.bone.2004.04.016.

14. Kanis, J. A., Johnell, O., Oden, A., Sembo, I., Redlund-Johnell, I., Dawson, A., et al. (2000). Long-term risk of osteoporotic fracture in Malmo. *Osteoporosis International, 11*(8), 669–674. https://doi.org/10.1007/s001980070058.

15. Melton, L. J., III. (1988). Epidemiology of fractures. In B. L. Riggs & L. J. Melton, III (Eds.), *Osteoporosis: Etiology, Diagnosis, and Management* (pp. 133–154). Raven Press.

16. Park, J. H., Song, Y. M., Sung, J., Lee, K., Kim, Y. S., & Park, Y. S. (2012). Genetic influence on bone mineral density in Korean twins and families: The Healthy Twin Study. *Osteoporosis International, 23*(4), 1343–1349. https://doi.org/10.1007/s00198-011-1777-0.

17. Ralston, S. H., & Uitterlinden, A. G. (2010). Genetics of osteoporosis. *Endocrine Reviews, 31*(5), 629–662. https://doi.org/10.1210/er.2009-0028.

18. Rivadeneira, F., Styrkarsdottir, U., Estrada, K., Halldorsson, B. V., Hsu, Y. H., Richards, J. B., et al. (2009). Twenty bone-mineral-density loci identified by large-scale meta-analysis of genome-wide association studies. *Nature Genetics, 41*(11), 1199–1206. https://doi.org/10.1038/ng.440.

19. Siris, E. S., Selby, P. L., Saag, K. G., Borgstrom, F., Herings, R. M., & Silverman, S. L. (2009). Impact of osteoporosis treatment adherence on fracture rates in North America and Europe. *American Journal of Medicine, 122*(2 Suppl), S3–S13. https://doi.org/10.1016/j.amjmed.2009.01.022.

20. Van Meurs, J. B., Trikalinos, T. A., Ralston, S. H., Balcells, S., Brandi, M. L., Brixen, K., et al. (2008). Large-scale analysis of association between LRP5 and LRP6 variants and osteoporosis. *JAMA, 299*(11), 1277–1290. https://doi.org/10.1001/jama.299.11.1277.

Chapter 6

CARDIOVASCULAR HEALTH

Contents

Introduction

In the US, cardiovascular disease (CVD) kills nearly as many women each year as the next five leading causes of death put together. This is the reason the illness has become a major concern for women's health. It is important to remember that there are gender-specific differences in the pathophysiology and morbidity of ischemic heart disease and that treatment approaches and disease outcomes may not always be the same. Male and female differences in physiology lead to variations in CVD risk, presentation, diagnosis, morbidity, mortality, and therapy (Anagnostis et al., 2019). Studies have revealed differences in women's prognosis, use of medical and interventional therapies, and diagnosis. In relation to ischemic CVD, women are understudied, underdiagnosed, undertreated, and underrepresented when compared to men. Unfortunately, heart failure, atrial fibrillation, peripheral vascular disease, and cerebrovascular disease are among the many CVD conditions that are still not thoroughly investigated for sex-based variations. Several factors uniquely affect women's cardiovascular health. Hormonal influences play a significant role, particularly the protective effects of estrogen before menopause. Estrogen helps maintain healthy blood vessels and favorable cholesterol levels. However, after menopause, the decline in estrogen levels leads to an increased risk of CVD. Women are also at risk from pregnancy-related complications such as preeclampsia, gestational diabetes, and preterm birth, which can have long-term cardiovascular implications. Women with conditions like polycystic ovary syndrome (PCOS) also face a higher risk of developing CVD due to associated metabolic issues.

Lifestyle factors contribute significantly to cardiovascular risk in women. Smoking, physical inactivity, and poor dietary habits are major contributors. Although women generally smoke less than men, they have a higher relative risk of developing CVD from smoking. Furthermore, women are more likely to experience mental health issues like depression and anxiety, which are significant risk factors for cardiovascular diseases. These mental health conditions can exacerbate CVD risk by promoting unhealthy behaviors and increasing physiological stress. Symptom presentation in women often differs from the classic signs of CVD seen in men, which can lead to misdiagnosis or delayed treatment. While men typically experience chest pain as the primary symptom of a heart attack, women are more likely to report atypical symptoms such as fatigue, shortness of breath, nausea, and pain in areas like the back, neck, or jaw. These differences in symptom presentation can result in underdiagnosis and undertreatment of CVD in women. Additionally, women are more prone to microvascular disease, affecting the small arteries of the heart, which is less detectable with standard diagnostic tools used for larger vessel disease common in men. Management of CVD in women requires a comprehensive and tailored approach. Preventive strategies are crucial and include lifestyle modifications such as a heart-healthy diet, regular physical activity, weight management, smoking cessation, and stress reduction. Blood pressure, cholesterol, and blood glucose levels need to be meticulously controlled. Pharmacological treatments must be carefully chosen and monitored, as women may respond differently to medications like statins, antihypertensives, and anticoagulants. Invasive procedures, such as percutaneous coronary intervention (PCI) and coronary artery bypass grafting (CABG), may also have different success rates and complications in women, necessitating gender-specific risk assessments and treatment plans. Increasing awareness among healthcare providers about sex-specific differences in cardiovascular health is essential. More inclusive clinical research is needed to develop evidence-based guidelines that address the specific needs of women.

Orientation and Directional Terms

Term	Definition	Illustration
Cardiovascular Disease (CVD)	General term for conditions affecting the heart or blood vessels. It's usually associated with a build-up of fatty deposits inside the arteries (atherosclerosis) and an increased risk of blood clots.	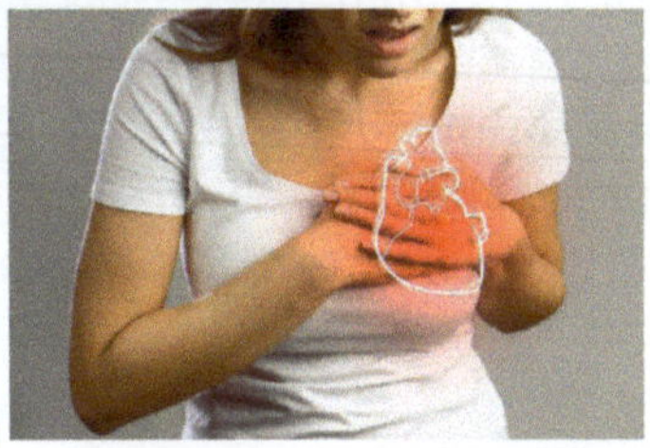
Polycystic Ovary Syndrome (PCOS)	Is a condition in which the ovaries produce an abnormal amount of androgens, male sex hormones that are usually present in women in small amounts. The name polycystic ovary syndrome describes the numerous small cysts (fluid-filled sacs) that form in the ovaries.	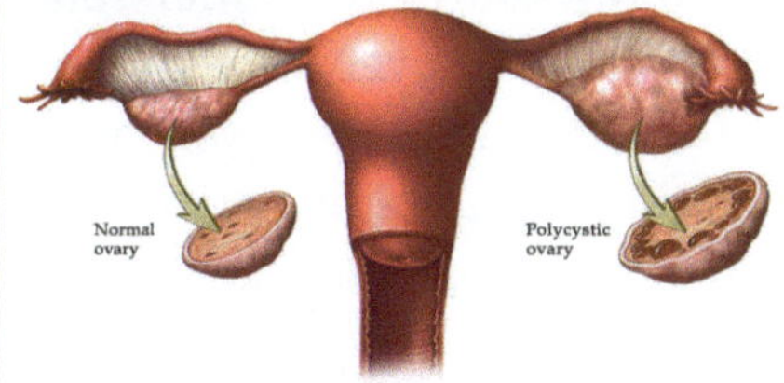
Coronary Artery Bypass Grafting (CABG)	Coronary artery bypass grafting (CABG), also called heart bypass surgery, is a medical procedure to improve blood flow to the heart. It may be needed when the arteries supplying blood to the heart, called coronary arteries, are narrowed or blocked.	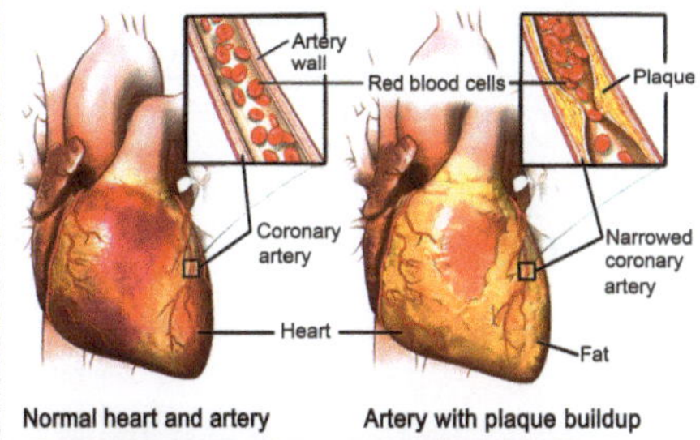
Acute Coronary Syndrome (ACS)	Acute coronary syndrome (ACS) is a syndrome due to decreased blood flow in the coronary arteries such that part of the heart muscle is unable to function properly or dies.	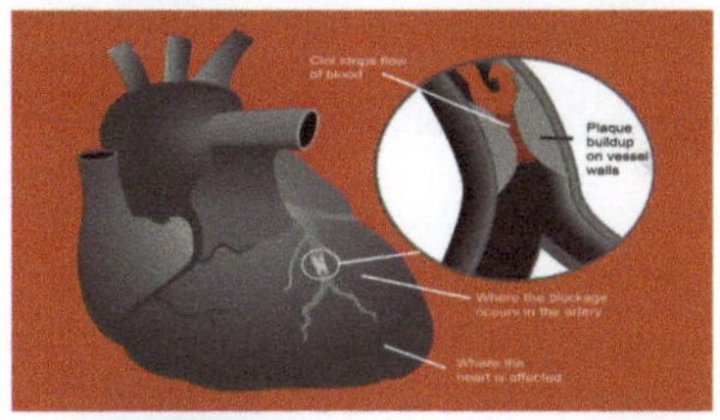
White-Coat Hypertension	White coat syndrome, or white coat hypertension, is the term for when you get a high blood pressure reading in a doctor's office and a normal reading at home.	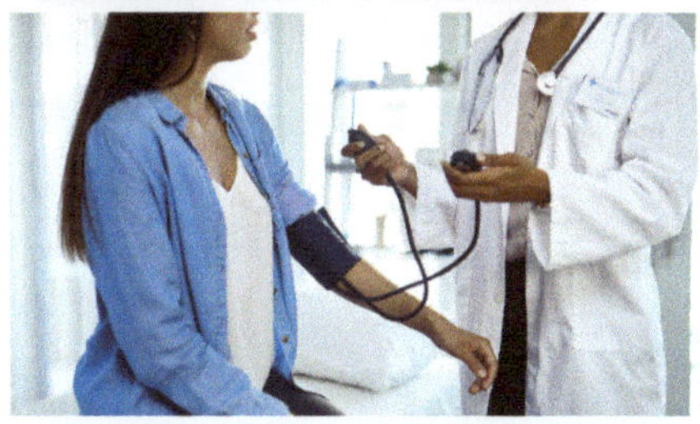
Arterial Hypertension (AH)	Arterial hypertension (AH) is a major cause of cardiovascular diseases (CVD), leading to the dysfunction of many organs, including the heart, blood vessels and kidneys. AH is a multifactorial disease.	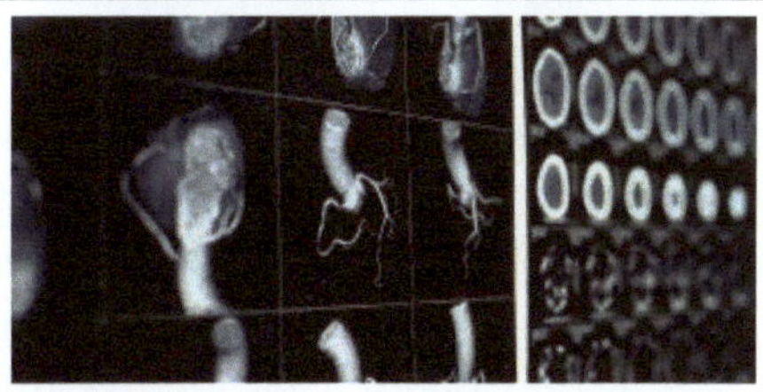

6.1. Sex-Related Differences and Gender Bias

It is estimated that after myocardial infarction (MI) and cardiovascular interventions, 66,000 more women than men pass away annually. In addition to having greater mortality rates than men, women also have worse outcomes (Matthews et al., 2013). The debate revolves around the relative contributions of gender-related biases and real sex-related differences as explanations for the disparate results. True biological differences, such as variations in the structure and function of men's and women's cardiovascular systems, are the cause of sex-related effects. The various anatomical and physiological variations between the cardiovascular systems of men and women are compiled in Table 6.1. On the other hand, psychosocial roles and behaviors that are imposed by society are the source of gender-related bias. Referral bias, for instance, is the phenomenon where bias results in a delayed referral for treatment of acute coronary syndrome (ACS). The combined effect of these factors, as well as their individual effects, is not entirely understood. Research indicates that both are involved in the rise in women's CVD-related morbidity and death. Although education can help reduce gender bias, biological differences between the sexes will always exist.

Table 6.1. Sex-Related Differences in the Cardiovascular System

Parameter	Manifestations
Anatomy	• Dimensions that are smaller in women (adjusted for age and race): left ventricular mass, ventricular wall thickness, left atrial dimension, left ventricular end-diastolic dimension, and vessel size
Hormonal influences	• Estrogen and progesterone are most influential in women; testosterone is predominant in men • Menstruation can affect hematologic and electrocardiographic indices
Cardiovascular function	• Stroke volume in women is 10% less • Pulse rate in women is 3–5 beats/minute faster • Ejection fraction is higher in women
Physiology	• Women have reduced sympathetic and enhanced parasympathetic activity • Women have lower plasma concentrations of norepinephrine
Cardiovascular adaptations	• In response to stress, women experience an increased pulse rate, resulting in increased cardiac output; men increase vascular resistance, resulting in increased blood pressure • Women are more sensitive to altitude or body positioning changes and experience more orthostatic hypotension and syncope
Hematologic indices	• Women have a lower number of circulating red blood cells per unit volume of plasma (resulting in a lower hematocrit) • Because of a lower hemoglobin, women have a lower oxygen-carrying capacity; this is balanced by women having a lower oxygen consumption
Electrocardiographic and electrophysiologic indices	• Women on average have a longer corrected QT interval and a shorter sinus node recovery time • Drug-induced torsades de pointes is more common in women • Sudden cardiac death and atrial fibrillation are less common in women

Source: https://www.accp.com/docs/bookstore/psap/p7b01sample03.pdf.

6.2. Sex-Related Risk of CVD

Pregnancy-related illnesses like preeclampsia, gestational diabetes, and preterm delivery put women at particular risk for cardiovascular disease (CVD) and increase the risk of cardiovascular disease in the future (Manson, 2013). Women with PCOS are also more likely to develop dyslipidemia, hypertension, and metabolic syndrome. Women are also more likely to experience anxiety and depression, two major risk factors for CVD.

6.2.1. Risk Awareness

Women are more likely than men to underestimate the health effects of their risk of CVD. Studies reveal that the majority of women significantly underestimate their vulnerability to heart disease.

The percentage of women who correctly identify heart disease as the leading cause of death for women has increased as a result of educational initiatives aimed at raising awareness. In 2005 surveys, however, minority women and those without a college degree underestimated their own personal risk of illness. Furthermore, a recent study by the American Heart Association (AHA) revealed that while most women acknowledged cardiovascular disease (CVD) as a primary cause of death, few could identify the main risk factors linked to the illness.

6.2.2. Risk Factors

It is important to evaluate women who have both established and new risk factors before starting primary preventive measures like medication, lifestyle changes, or both. Women and men have similar overall risk factors (age, ethnicity, family history) for developing cardiovascular disease (CVD); however, some risk factors—such as diabetes, dyslipidemia, and hypertension—may put them at higher overall risk. Furthermore, women have higher baseline levels of inflammatory markers associated with a higher risk of disease, such as high-sensitivity C-reactive protein (hsCRP), than men do. We don't fully understand the clinical implications of this biomarker in relation to a woman's risk. Strategies for managing risk factors are essentially the same for both sexes at this point. Further studies might yield more prevention techniques tailored to particular sexes.

6.2.2.1. Diabetes

Diabetes increases a woman's risk of developing or dying from coronary heart disease by three to seven times that of a woman without the disease. This is significantly greater than the two- to three-fold elevated risk that men with diabetes encounter. After MI, women with diabetes have a far worse prognosis in the short and long term; they are more likely than men to die, have another MI, or develop heart failure. In the 1990s, women without diabetes saw a 27% decrease in heart disease-related deaths. Contrary to expectations, it rose by 23% in female diabetics. The earlier finding is reinforced by recent data from the National Health and Nutrition Examination Surveys, which indicate that while the mortality rates between women with diabetes and women without the disease have doubled, the mortality rates from all causes and CVD have decreased in men with diabetes. There is a lack of knowledge regarding the causes of these notable discrepancies, and no effective solutions exist (Hodis et al., 2016).

6.2.2.2. Dyslipidemia

Women may be more vulnerable to certain lipid components or lipoproteins than men are, and they may also present a different target for risk reduction. Premenopausal women typically have lower levels of low-density lipoprotein (LDL) cholesterol and higher levels of high-density lipoprotein (HDL) cholesterol than men. Women's LDL and HDL cholesterol levels increase and decrease respectively after menopause. In men, higher total and LDL cholesterol levels are associated with a higher risk of coronary heart disease. On the other hand, women may be more predictive of a low HDL cholesterol and higher triglyceride concentration than men. According to epidemiologic data, women are more protected against CVD than men are by having higher concentrations of HDL cholesterol. Recent studies using a cholesterol ester transfer protein inhibitor to raise HDL cholesterol showed some promise, but torcetrapib patients had a markedly higher risk of cardiovascular events and death, which put an end to further drug development. Nevertheless, genetic research has linked the cholesterol ester transfer protein to an increased risk of MI in the future, indicating the need for more research in this field.

There are two other products in phase II and phase III studies, dalcetrapib and anacetrapib, which are thought to have safer adverse effect profiles. It is currently unknown whether a treatment aimed at increasing HDL cholesterol will have a different impact on cardiovascular events in men and women. Men and maybe even more so women have elevated triglycerides as a risk factor for cardiovascular disease (CVD). A meta-analysis of 17 prospective population-based studies found that women with higher triglyceride concentrations had a 37% increased risk of CVD events, compared to a 14% increased risk in men. Although subgroup analyzes of a prospective study using fenofibrate suggest that lowering triglycerides in this way decreases total cardiovascular events in women but not in men, randomized clinical trials have not consistently demonstrated a reduction in mortality by lowering triglycerides in men and women. At this point, the strength of the outcome data is insufficient to support sex-specific treatment recommendations for hypertriglyceridemia.

6.2.2.4. Hypertension

Women are more vulnerable to hypertension, which is a common modifiable risk factor for both CVD and cerebrovascular disease. By the time they reach their sixth decade of life, women are more likely than men to have hypertension. Compared to other ethnic groups, women of African American descent have a higher prevalence and severity of the disease. Prehypertension, defined as a blood pressure (BP) of 130–139/84–89 mm Hg, is linked to a 2.5 increase in the risk of heart failure, MI, stroke, and cardiovascular death in women but only a 1.6 increase in men. Because women achieve lower rates of blood pressure control than men, these findings highlight the significance of diagnosing and treating hypertension in women. Mexican American, elderly, and postmenopausal women have the lowest rates of blood pressure control. Even though a person's gender significantly influences their blood pressure, antihypertensive medications are equally effective in men and women, despite women having a higher risk than men. Women are more likely to have hypertension due to sex-specific factors such as their shorter stature and arterial tree, which cause lower diastolic blood pressure and faster pulse rates. In comparison to men, women with hypertension are more likely to experience left ventricular hypertrophy and symptomatic heart failure with preserved ejection fraction. Women experience a sharp age-related stiffening of the arterial wall following menopause. The effects of estrogen on the vasculature include lowering sympathetic nervous system activity and preserving endothelial function by producing nitric oxide. Moreover, estrogen lowers the activity of the angiotensin-converting enzyme (ACE) and plasma renin. Moreover, salt sensitivity rises following ovariectomy or menopause-induced estrogen loss. After menopause, dietary factors therefore start to have a greater impact on blood pressure control and could account for some of the variations in blood pressure control rates between the sexes (Hodis et al., 2016).

6.2.2.5. White-Coat Hypertension

The diagnosis of white-coat hypertension is made when an ambulatory blood pressure monitor reads less than 135/85 mm Hg but more than 140/90 mm Hg in the clinic. About

20% of patients with untreated hypertension have white-coat hypertension, which is more common in women than in men. Women's higher resting heart rates could be the cause of this gender-related disparity. Women who experience anxiety-induced tachycardia may see an increase in the brachial arteries' systolic blood pressure while their carotid and aortic pressures remain normal. Future studies should examine the usefulness of ambulatory blood pressure monitoring in the diagnosis and management of hypertensive women.

6.2.2.6. Depression

Psychosocial risks may play a significant role in the pathogenesis of cardiovascular disease (CVD) in both men and women, in addition to traditional cardiovascular risk factors. Women are twice as likely as men to experience depression, the most prevalent psychological disorder. Depression is a major risk factor for women with cardiovascular disease (CVD), as evidenced by its association with an up to 70% increased risk. Moreover, the prognosis for patients with depression and coronary heart disease may be worse than for those without depression (Hodis et al., 2016).

Depression may raise a woman's risk of CVD through increasing inflammatory and atherosclerotic biomarkers, decreasing variability in pulse rate, affecting vascular and hypothalamic-pituitary-adrenal axis function, and increasing platelet activation. Depression raises the risk of drug nonadherence and plays a role in behavioral risk factors for CVD, including poor diet, smoking, and physical inactivity, which is more prevalent in women. A recommendation for primary prevention in women includes screening for depression because depression raises a woman's risk of CVD overall. Until the AHA Depression and Coronary Heart Disease Advisory was published in 2008, women were specifically identified as candidates for depression screening as a primary preventive strategy, as opposed to men. As of right now, depression screening, referral, and treatment are advised for both men and women with heart disease. If antidepressant therapy can partially mitigate the higher mortality rate among women with depressive symptoms, more research is required in this area.

6.2.2.7. Obesity, Physical Inactivity, and Metabolic Syndrome

Obesity, physical inactivity, and metabolic syndrome are important risks contributing to cardiovascular morbidity and mortality. In the United States, the prevalence of obesity and metabolic syndrome is similar between men (33.3% and 34.4%, respectively) and women (35.3% and 34.5%, respectively); however, meta-analyzes of prospective studies have concluded that metabolic syndrome confers a greater overall cardiovascular risk in women, who have a 30% higher relative risk than men. The risk associated with physical inactivity is comparable with that observed for hypertension, dyslipidemia, or cigarette smoking. Yet physical inactivity is reportedly higher in women (12%) than in men (8.4%), and women are less likely than men to engage in vigorous exercise (33.3% vs. 44%). Lifestyle factors contribute significantly to the overall risk of developing coronary events in both sexes, yet women have been observed in epidemiologic studies to be more sensitive to favorable changes in diet, exercise, and alcohol. Future research should focus on lifestyle interventions and their impact on mortality as related to sex (Hodis et al., 2016).

6.2.2.8. Surgical and Pregnancy-Induced Risks

An increasing risk factor for CVD that is particularly important for women is a prior history of pregnancy-related issues. Pregnancy-related hypertension and diabetes may be signs of an increased risk of CVD in older women. Pregnant women who experience preeclampsia or eclampsia have a marked increased risk of hypertension and cerebrovascular disease in later life. Furthermore, women who suffer from placental abruption and infarction, inadequate fetal growth, or intrauterine fetal death are at a higher risk of developing CVD. Although there are numerous causes for these pregnancy-related issues, they all appear to be related to endothelial dysfunction, which may be a sign of early vascular disease in the pregnant woman. These risks associated with pregnancy may be a significant factor in determining a woman's risk of developing CVD, even though they are not taken into account by any CVD risk-scoring systems. Lastly, it has been reported that women who undergo surgical menopause (hysterectomy plus simultaneous bilateral oophorectomy) before going through natural menopause are more likely to experience a cardiovascular event in the future. This is likely due to the premature loss of estrogen's protective effects.

6.2.3. Cardiovascular Risk Equations for Women

6.2.3.1. Framingham Risk Assessment

Because the risk of CVD varies between men and women, researchers have looked for risk equations that can accurately predict the risk of CVD in women. The Framingham risk score (FRS), which was developed in 1976 and is the historical standard, calculates the patient's chance of having a coronary artery disease event within a ten-year period. A woman at high risk can be identified with accuracy if her FRS is more than 20%; however, a lower score may underestimate her actual risk of a CVD event. 98% of asymptomatic women under the age of 59 and 92% of those between the ages of 60 and 69 would be considered low risk, based on data from the Framingham cohort and offspring. A woman under the age of 70 is not likely to receive a score high enough to be eligible for cardiac risk reduction targeted medication. Because of the age-related bias in the FRS, women with subclinical CVD cannot receive intensive preventive therapy earlier in life, which would be more beneficial. Other restrictions on the FRS that are unique to women's risk include its disregard for factors like ethnicity, hysterectomy status, metabolic syndrome or any of its components, and family history. The FRS may poorly predict the risk of CVD in women impacted earlier in life by stroke, angina, and heart failure rather than coronary events (e.g, sudden cardiovascular death, MI), as it was initially intended to predict only CVD events. Only 44% of women and 51% of men had MI as their initial sign of CVD, according to data from the Framingham study. The Women's Health Study (WHS) revealed that women were more likely than men to experience strokes as their first event, highlighting the differences between the sexes. It is important for practitioners to understand the limitations of the FRS when assessing women's cardiovascular risk.

6.2.3.2. Primary Prevention Risk Stratification

It is critical to appropriately assess the wide range of diseases that younger women are at risk for. While the risk of CVD is higher in women over 65 than in men, older women are not the only ones at risk for the disease. The third most common cause of death for women between the ages of 25 and 45 is cardiovascular disease. The presence of one risk factor at age 50 is linked to an increased lifetime risk and a shorter duration of survival from cardiovascular disease (CVD), suggesting that estimating lifetime risk may be more crucial for younger women than for older ones.

According to data from the Framingham Heart Study, healthy women's lifetime risk of CVD is approximately 32% at age 40 and 39% at age 50. This latter percentage is higher than the lifetime risk of colorectal, lung, and breast cancers put together. Moreover, while sudden cardiac death affects more men than women, two-thirds of women who pass away suddenly had no prior coronary disease symptoms, compared to roughly half of men. These data highlight the significance of identifying primary preventive strategies in a woman's early life and determining her risk after a decade. An alternative to the FRS for risk assessment is the AHA's Primary Prevention of CVD in Women Guideline. Some of the FRS's shortcomings, such as addressing a woman's lifetime risk, incorporating a more thorough evaluation of risk factors, and promoting an earlier and more forceful approach to lifestyle modification, may be addressed by the guideline (de Villiers et al., 2016). For instance, the FRS only takes into account smoking as a lifestyle factor. Therefore, the FRS predicted that a middle-aged woman with unhealthy lifestyle choices alone would have a low 10-year risk and might not receive enough information about future cardiovascular health and risk modification. Aggressive risk reduction requires an understanding of the limitations of the FRS among women with unhealthy lifestyle choices. The assessment of lifetime risk in comparison to the FRS's 10-year risk is a second enhancement over the Primary Prevention Risk Assessment. The lifetime risk stratification recommended by the AHA Primary Prevention Guideline for women is shown in Table 6.2. Women using this risk assessment tool are categorized as high risk, at risk, or optimal lifetime risk. This framework takes into account information required to more accurately predict the risk of cardiovascular events during one's lifetime, as well as factors included in the FRS.

Table 6.2. Lifetime Risk Stratification for the Primary Prevention of CVD in Women

Optimal Risk	At Risk	High Risk
• 10-year Framingham global risk score < 10% AND • Healthy lifestyle AND • No risk factors	1 or more of the following: • Smoking • Poor diet • Inactivity • Obesity • Family history of early CVD • Hypertension • Hyperlipidemia • Subclinical vascular disease (i.e., abnormal coronary artery calcium scores and/or carotid intima-media thickness, and high ankle-brachial index) • Poor exercise capacity on a treadmill test • Abnormal pulse rate recovery after exercise	Any one of the following: • Established coronary heart disease • Cerebrovascular disease • Peripheral artery disease • Abdominal aortic aneurysm • Hemodialysis or peritoneal dialysis • Chronic kidney disease • Diabetes • 10-year Framingham global risk score > 20%

Source: https://www.accp.com/docs/bookstore/psap/p7b01sample03.pdf.

Because the AHA guideline takes into account lifestyle factors, family history, premature CVD, and subclinical evidence of vascular disease, it may be able to estimate a woman's risk of cardiovascular events more accurately. The Primary Prevention Risk Assessment includes cardiovascular performance as determined by exercise capacity and pulse rate recovery during stress testing. If any of the aforementioned risks are present, it suggests that the woman may experience a CVD event at some point in her life. According to the Primary Prevention Guideline, treating a woman with multiple marginal cardiometabolic risk factors aggressively would give the clinician greater flexibility, even though the 10-year risk may not increase in the short term. These risk factors become significant over the course of a woman's lifetime. On the other hand, physicians who employ the Third Adult Treatment Panel might postpone starting hyperlipidemia medication until a high-risk FRS status is attained.

6.2.3.3. Other Risk Assessments

Additional women-specific risk assessment scoring evaluations are being investigated and validated. The WHS, which tracked nearly 25,000 women 40 years of age and above for 10.2 years for incident stroke and coronary heart disease events, as well as other outcomes like revascularization, was the source of the Reynolds risk score. Two specific risk factors beyond those in the FRS were found to add greater predictability for CVD events after 35 risk factors were carefully examined. 30% of the women without diabetes and 45% of the women with diabetes were more accurately classified as higher or lower risk when hsCRP and family history were included in the risk algorithm. Like the FRS, the Reynolds model only projects risk for the next ten years. This risk assessment tool's other limitations include the small sample size (95% white).

Therefore, the effectiveness of this tool cannot be generalized to women of various ethnicities. Furthermore, a revised FRS has been proposed to predict the risk of cerebrovascular events, peripheral artery disease, heart failure, and coronary events such as sudden cardiac death and MI over a 10-year period. It is uncertain whether incorporating these additional risk calculations into decision-making will decrease morbidity and mortality in women. These new risk assessments need to be validated in diverse patient populations and directly compared with other tools to determine the most accurate method of assessing a woman's risk. In light of the significant threat of CVD in women, utilizing a lifetime risk assessment seems most appropriate.

6.2.4. Does Transition to Menopause Predispose to Higher CVD Risk?

Menopause is the result of follicle depletion, which causes an estrogen deficit. It is defined as the period of time after the final menstrual period (FMP) or at the time of bilateral oophorectomy. Menopausal transition is linked, compared to premenopausal status, to a higher prevalence of CVD risk factors, including central adiposity, atherogenic dyslipidemia, glucose intolerance, arterial hypertension (AH), and non-alcoholic fatty liver disease (NAFLD). In specifics, body fat is redistributed toward the male pattern of visceral adiposity as a result of the menopause transition. In fact, there are no changes in energy intake associated with the onset of menopause; instead, there is a decrease in energy expenditure and fat oxidation. Postmenopausal women have 36% more thoracic fat and 49% more intra-abdominal fat area than premenopausal women in studies using dual-energy X-ray absorptiometry, CT, or MRI. These variations held true regardless of age or total body fat. Furthermore, compared to premenopausal women, biopsy investigations on postmenopausal women have revealed increased inflammation and fibrosis, as well as hypertrophy of adipocyte cells in both subcutaneous and visceral adipose tissue (Park et al., 2018). The redistribution of body fat following menopause could be attributed to various mechanisms, including the upregulation of lipoprotein lipase activity in adipose tissue and a decrease in lipolysis as a result of lower estrogen concentrations. Another mechanism that controls the distribution of adipose tissue is the loss of 17β-estradiol (17β-E2) activation of estrogen receptor (ER) type α (ERα) in neurons of the ventromedial nucleus of the hypothalamus.

Compared to premenopausal women, postmenopausal women may have up to 50% higher insulin resistance as a result of these alterations in adipose tissue. Animal studies have demonstrated the promotion of β-cell survival and secretion by ERα and ER type β (ERβ). Regardless of age or BMI, postmenopausal women secrete half as much pancreatic insulin as premenopausal women do. Estrogen inhibits gluconeogenesis in the liver by acting through ERα, with the exception of the pancreas. Additionally, it enhances the uptake of glucose in muscles and adipose tissue by primarily translocating glucose transporter 4.

Clinically, women entering menopause may have dysregulated plasma glucose concentrations leading to impaired glucose tolerance (IGT) or no change at all. Independent of BMI, waist-hip ratio, blood pressure, age at menopause, lipid profile, family history of type 2 diabetes (T2DM), and blood pressure, the estimated yearly incidence of IGT after menopause is 6%. A recent meta-analysis, however, revealed that postmenopausal women with a history of EM or POI exhibit a higher risk for T2DM in comparison to women who had a normal age at menopause (>45 years) (odds ratio (OR) 1.12, 95% CI 1.01–1.20 and 1.53, 95% CI 1.03–2.27 and so on, respectively).

Epidemiological evidence points to an increase in blood pressure (BP) following the onset of menopause. Because of decreased vascular elasticity and a higher incidence of atherosclerosis in older age groups, it is unclear whether this is a result of the aging process or menopause in general. Other factors like smoking, obesity, and insufficient physical activity should also be taken into account. In any event, compared to their male counterparts, postmenopausal women have been found to exhibit higher sympathetic activity and a steeper increase in systolic blood pressure. In addition, a recent meta-analysis revealed that women with EM had a marginally but significantly higher risk of AH when compared to women whose menopausal age was over 45 (OR 1.10, 95% CI 1.01–1.19). A lower estrogen-to-androgen ratio during menopause and the production of vasoconstrictive factors like endothelin and angiotensinogen as a result of the drop in estrogen concentrations are two plausible pathogenetic mechanisms.

What is of importance regarding the menopause-associated CVD risk is the changes in lipid profile during the transition to menopause. Concisely, these include an increase in total cholesterol (TC), low-density lipoprotein cholesterol (LDL-C), triglycerides (TG), and a decrease in high-density lipoprotein cholesterol (HDL-C) concentrations. The latter is mainly attributed to the HDL_2-C subfraction. Notably, except for these changes in lipid profile, atherogenic changes in apolipoprotein concentrations and their ratios have also been reported after the onset of menopause. These include an increase in apolipoprotein B (apoB) concentrations and LDL-C/apoB ratio in postmenopausal women, which are evident from the age of 50–55 years, converging with and exceeding the respective values in men. Moreover, despite the rise in apolipoprotein A-I (apoA-I) and apolipoprotein A-II (apoA-II) concentrations in postmenopausal compared with premenopausal women, the HDL-C/apoA-I and HDL-C/apoA-II ratios decrease to the lowest degree seen in men, suggesting a lower cholesterol content of HDL particles. Regarding lipoprotein (a) (Lp(a)), an independent risk factor for atherosclerotic CVD, inconclusive data exist as to whether this increases after menopause (Guthrie et al., 1999).

Moreover, dyslipidemia and insulin resistance promote the development of NAFLD by facilitating an increased influx of free fatty acids into the liver. Other than the lack of estrogen, the relative excess of androgens and the reduction in sex hormone-binding globulin also lead to increased adipose mass in the abdomen and consequent non-alcoholic fatty liver disease. When comparing postmenopausal women to premenopausal women, there is a two-fold increase in the risk of NAFLD. The proportionately high incidence of NAFLD in females. <45 years, 45–55 and > It is 5.3, 18.8, and 27.8% for people 55 years of age. When someone is obese, that number jumps to 48.4%. Among postmenopausal women with T2DM, NAFLD affects over 50% of them. In addition, women over the age of fifty-five have a high prevalence of non-alcoholic steatohepatitis (13.2%), which rises to 14.9% in those who are obese and have non-alcoholic fatty liver disease (NAFLD).

6.2.5. Is There an Independent Association Between Menopause and Increased Risk of CVD Events?

According to the previously mentioned data, women may develop an atherogenic profile during and after menopause, which increases their risk of cardiovascular disease. It's interesting to note that endothelial dysfunction begins early in the postmenopausal era, prior to the onset of subclinical atherosclerosis. This could help explain "undetermined" chest pain and dyspnea, which are frequently linked to stress or menopausal symptomatology. These women also have a two-fold higher risk of IHD. Around menopause, inflammatory co-morbidities like thyroid dysfunction and autoimmune rheumatic diseases (such as rheumatoid arthritis and systemic lupus erythematosus) increase a woman's risk of cardiovascular disease (CVD).

Whether this increased risk is translated into an equivalent risk of CVD events in postmenopausal women, irrespective of the effect of chronological aging, has not been established, as the relevant studies show inconsistent data. On the other hand, both EM and POI have been associated with increased CVD morbidity and mortality, mainly due to IHD. According to a meta-analysis, published in 2016 (32 studies; n = 310,329 postmenopausal women), the history of EM is associated with a 1.5-fold increased risk for IHD (relative risk (RR) for overall IHD 1.50, 95% CI 1.28–1.76) compared with normal age at menopause (>45 years). This was also the case for fatal IHD (RR 1.11, 95% CI 1.03–1.20), CVD mortality (RR 1.19, 95% CI 1.08–1.31) and all-cause mortality (RR 1.12, 95% CI 1.03–1.21). However, no association between overall stroke risk and stroke mortality was observed (Tchernof et al., 2004).

With respect to POI, two meta-analyzes published in 2016, confirmed these results. In particular, the history of POI augments the risk of all-cause and IHD mortality by 39% (pooled RR 1.39, 95% CI 1.10–1.77) and 48% (pooled RR 1.48, 95% CI 1.02–2.16), respectively, compared with normal age at menopause (>45 years). This was also the case with another meta-analysis (10 studies; n =190,588 postmenopausal women), showing an increased risk of IHD (hazard ratio (HR) 1.69, 95% CI 1.29–2.21) and total CVD morbidity or mortality (HR 1.61, 95% CI 1.22–2.12). As with EM, the history of POI was not associated with an increased risk of stroke. A recent cohort study from the UK (n = 144,260 postmenopausal women, aged 40–69 years) showed an increased risk for CVD for natural and surgical premature menopause (<40 years) compared with menopause at age >40 years (HR 1.36, 95% CI 1.19–1.56 and 1.87, 95% CI 1.36–2.58, respectively, after adjustment for conventional CVD risk factors and the use of MHT). This was again mainly attributed to IHD.

6.2.6. Does Menopausal Hormone Therapy Reduce CVD Risk?

6.2.6.1. Menopausal Hormone Therapy and CVD Risk Factors

It naturally arises to ask whether MHT could lower the risk of CVD since menopause increases it, at least in women with EM and POI. A growing body of research backs up the idea that, depending on the formulation (type, dosage, route of administration, and progestogen type), MHT may, to varying degrees, reduce the majority of CVD risk factors, including visceral adiposity, dyslipidemia, and glucose homeostasis. In a dose-dependent manner, estrogen may raise the concentrations of HDL-C and decrease TC, LDL-C, and Lp(a). Comparing conjugated equine estrogen (CEE) to 17β-E_2, which is higher when taken orally as opposed to topically, reveals that the former exhibits more marked changes. On the other hand, TG concentrations may rise in response to oral estrogen while they may fall or stay the same when administered transdermally. However, unlike the oral regimen, the latter does not impact the coagulation system and is not linked to an elevated risk of venous thromboembolism (VTE).

MHT may lower visceral adiposity, waist circumference, blood pressure and BMI, or it may have no effect at all. MHT enhances glucose homeostasis in terms of glucose metabolism by raising insulin sensitivity, secretion, and muscle uptake. Additionally, it may 30% lower the risk of T2DM. Oral and transdermal estrogen have a positive impact on glucose metabolism; however, at similar dosages, oral CEE has a stronger effect. Current research yields conflicting results regarding MHT's impact on NAFLD. Progestogens appear to alter the impact of estrogen on the previously listed risk factors for CVD. Low-dose norethisterone acetate and dydrogesterone are neutral, while medroxyprogesterone acetate (MPA) and levonorgestrel may lessen this effect. Due to their indifferent impact on lipid profile, progestogens that are micronized or dydrogestered are generally the favored option.

6.2.6.2. MHT and CVD Events

Several observational studies have demonstrated the protective effect of MHT on CHD risk in relation to CVD events, particularly between 1980 and 2000. However, a randomized controlled trial (RCT) setting was required to test the idea of CVD primary prevention by MHT. The Women's Health Initiative (WHI) Study served as the model RCT, aimed at examining the impact of MHT on breast cancer risk and CVD (with CHD as the primary outcome). This study was divided into two arms. The first, called WHI-1, examined the effects of CEE 0.625 mg/day plus MPA 2.5 mg/day (n = 8506) and a placebo (n = 8022) on postmenopausal women (aged 50–79) who had an intact uterus. Evidence of an elevated risk of invasive breast cancer (HR 1.26, 95% CI 1.00–1.59) led to the early termination of this study at 5.2 years. The estimated HR for IHD, total CVD, stroke, and VTE was 1.29 (95% CI 1.02–1.63), 1.22 (95% CI 1.09–1.36), 1.41 (95% CI 1.07–1.85), and 2.11 (95% CI 1.58–2.82), according to the study's preliminary findings. MHT did, however, show a lower risk of hip (HR 0.66, 95% CI 0.45–0.98), colorectal cancer (HR 0.63, 95% CI 0.43–0.92), and total fractures (HR 0.76, 95% CI 0.69–0.85). Notably, the risk of coronary heart disease (CHD) was not significant (HR 1.24, 95% confidence interval 0.97–1.60) when the WHI-1 final results were released.

The second arm (WHI-2) recruited 10,739 postmenopausal women, aged 50–79 years, with a history of hysterectomy, who were randomized to CEE 0.625 mg/day (n = 5310) or placebo (n =5329). MHT increased the risk of stroke (HR 1.39, 95% CI 1.10–1.77) and VTE (1.33, 95% CI 0.99–1.7), without any effect on the risk of CHD and colorectal cancer. Interestingly, it decreased the risk of breast cancer (HR 0.77,

95% CI 0.59–1.01), hip (HR 0.61, 95% CI 0.41–0.91) and total fractures (HR 0.70, 95% CI 0.63–0.79).

However, a thorough examination of the WHI trials can dispel their initial unfavorable impression. It is important to remember that the average age of the participants was 63 years old, and two-thirds of them were over 60. Age-stratified women showed a marginally non-significant reduction in CHD risk in the 50–59 year age group (HR 0.56, 95% CI 0.3–1.03) when CEE was used alone, while there was no effect in the 60–69 and 70–79 year age groups. For women aged 50–59 and 60–69, the corresponding absolute risk stratified by age was five and ten fewer cases of fatal and non-fatal CHD per 10,000 women/year, respectively, while there were more than four cases for those aged 70–79. On the other hand, in the estrogen-alone arm, a composite CHD outcome was significantly lower in patients starting treatment before the age of 60, and in the long-term follow-up after the intervention, there was a significant decrease in CHD events when compared to the placebo (Hong et al., 2007).

Moreover, a prospective Danish cohort (n = 698,098 postmenopausal women, aged 51–69 years), published 5 years after the WHI, showed no increased risk of myocardial infarction (MI) (RR 1.03, 95% CI 0.95–1.11) for current MHT users compared with never users. In subgroup analyzes, this risk increased with a longer duration (>4 years) (RR 1.81, 95% CI 1.19–2.77). Interestingly, the risk for MI decreased (RR 0.62, 95% CI 0.42–0.93) with transdermal unopposed estrogen (compared with women who never used MHT) and it was also lower than that of oral regimen.

A Cochrane meta-analysis, published in 2015, showed a decreased risk of CHD (RR 0.52, 95% CI 0.29–0.96) and all-cause mortality (RR 0.70, 95% CI 0.52–0.95) if MHT was commenced within 10 years since menopause, raising the issue of 'window of opportunity.' No effect on the risk of stroke was observed, although the risk of VTE remained high (RR 1.74, 95% CI 1.11–2.73).

More recent RCTs, like the Early vs. Late Intervention Trial with Estradiol study, which randomized 643 seemingly healthy postmenopausal women to either 17β-E_2 (1 mg/day plus vaginal gel of progesterone for non-hysterectomized women) or placebo, supported the timing hypothesis. Only in early postmenopausal women (less than 6 years from their first menopausal period) did 17β-E_2 reduce the rate of carotid intima-media thickness progression after a median of 5 years when compared to placebo. There was nothing different found in late postmenopausal women in this area. Including 502 women between the ages of 45 and 58, the Danish Osteoporosis Prevention Study confirmed the cardioprotective effect of MHT in early postmenopausal women. Its results showed that 2 mg/day of 17β-E_2 was linked to a 52% decrease in the risk of the composite CVD outcome (HR 0.48, 95% CI 0.26–0.87). The risk of breast cancer, stroke, or VTE was the same for all groups.

On the other hand, the coronary artery calcium score, another surrogate marker of atherosclerotic CVD, did not show any benefit of estrogen (either CEE 0.45 mg/day or transdermal 17β-E_2 50 μg/day) over placebo in the Kronos Early Oestrogen Prevention Study, an RCT that included 728 women (aged 42 to 58). The trial lasted only 48 months, which is a very short time. Moreover, the Heart and Estrogen/Progestin Replacement Study (HERS) indicates that MHT has no effect on CVD risk in the context of secondary prevention.

The evidence mentioned above suggests that most international societies agree on the indications for MHT. Since the advantages of MHT outweigh the risks, these include cases of EM or POI, as well as postmenopausal women under 60 years old or within ten years of menopause and at low-to-moderate risk for CVD, for the relief of menopausal symptoms. At this time, MHT should not be used in women who are at high risk for CVD or for the exclusive goal of primary or secondary CHD prevention. Because micronized progesterone and dydrogesterone have no effect on coagulation parameters or CVD risk factors, transdermal estradiol is the first-choice treatment for patients with moderate risk of CVD. This can be applied either alone for women without uteruses or in combination with these hormones. For women who have a high risk of VTE, this is also true.

Clinicians should also consider that CVD mortality increases after MHT discontinuation, concerning either IHD (standardized mortality ratio (SMR) 1.26, 95% CI 1.16–1.37) or stroke (SMR 1.63, 95% CI 1.47–1.79), during the first post-treatment year. However, this risk is dissipated thereafter (SMR 0.75, 95% CI 0.72–0.78 and 0.89, 95% CI 0.85–0.94). This risk is also higher in women <60 years, but not in older women who discontinue MHT (SMR 1.94, 95% CI 1.51–2.48).

Progestogen is primarily responsible for the breast cancer risk associated with MHT. It appears to vanish when MHT is stopped and is comparatively lower with more recent regimens like micronized progesterone and dydrogesterone. For up to five years of treatment, MHT containing micronized progesterone does not raise the risk of breast cancer, per a recent systematic review. There is only a slight indication of an elevated risk if MHT is used for more than five years.

6.3. CVD Among Women

More women die from CVDeach year than from all cancers combined, accounting for 35% of deaths in this category. It has an impact on women of all ages. Yet, there is still a severe lack of research, recognition, diagnosis, and treatment for CVD in women.

6.3.1. Disease Presentation

When it comes to CVD, women typically present with more comorbid conditions and at an older age than men. Poorer outcomes in women may be explained by diagnostic confusion and misdiagnosis brought on by the complex and multifactorial presentations. Women are more likely to present with non-ST-segment elevation ACS without an increase in troponin concentrations than men are with ST-segment elevation MI (STEMI). Women are more likely than men to experience MI that goes undiagnosed or goes unspoken. There is evidence that the sexes perceive pain differently, which could account for some of the variation in symptoms that present differently. Men and women with ACS often develop chest pain; however, women are more likely than men to present with so-called atypical symptoms, such as nausea and vomiting, unexplained weakness and fatigue, indigestion, shortness of breath, middle or upper back pain, dyspnea, and paroxysmal nocturnal dyspnea. Prodromal symptoms, such as unusual tiredness, anxiety, or sleep disturbances reported hours to days before the development of ACS symptoms, have been documented in retrospective data for women (Moreau et al., 2012).

Women may experience referral bias, which is the delay of aggressive medical treatment if both the patient and the doctor fail to identify the presenting symptoms of cardiovascular disease. Timely treatment becomes more complicated because women tend to attribute their symptoms to non-cardiac causes. Women have generally waited longer than men to seek treatment for their acute symptoms in ACS studies. Only 27% of men and 34% of women in a sizable cohort arrived at the hospital after more than 4 hours from the start of ACS symptoms. Men were seen seven minutes on average sooner in the hospital than women after arriving.

Other disparities at ACS presentation are evident. For women, these include a lower likelihood of hospitalization compared with men (2 times less likely if older than 55 and 7 times less likely if younger than 55), less likely to have electrocardiography (ECG), and less likely to have care by a cardiologist (53% vs. 63%) during hospitalization for ACS. Because treatment delays can increase mortality, educating women at risk of disease is essential. Time delays and presenting circumstances make the diagnosis of CVD in women more challenging than in men. The clinician must weigh the likelihood of CVD based on vague symptoms and the unique risks of the woman. The effect of these disparities on women's outcomes after ACS is unknown.

6.3.2. Disease Findings

The notion that heart disease differs in men and women is partly attributed to anatomical and physiological variations between the sexes. It has only been recently possible to characterize the extent of sex-related disparities linked to coronary artery disease, and interventions that have the potential to significantly impact outcomes have not been implemented. Some of these differences have been better-understood thanks to the research conducted by the Women's Ischemia Syndrome Evaluation (WISE) study group, which was funded by the National Institutes of Health (NIH). When compared to men, women with ischemic heart disease have different coronary vasculature structures and functions. Women exhibit fewer obstructive lesions and more diffuse coronary disease at presentation. According to data from WISE, at the time of angiography, nonobstructive or nearly normal-looking arteries were present in nearly half of all women who presented with anginal pain.

Women who experienced chronic chest pain did not fare better than those who did not, even in the absence of flow-limiting disease in the epicardial coronary arteries. Women with persistent angina had a significantly higher combined end point of death, MI, stroke, and heart failure (14.4% vs. 8.5 percent) after four years. These women would typically be deemed low risk if they did not have obstructive disease, which would mean they might not receive aggressive primary preventive care or even stable angina. Nevertheless, at the 4-year follow-up in WISE, women with little to no obstructive disease showed a 9-percent absolute risk of MI or death upon angiography. WISE highlights a crucial clinical point: women with angina should be regarded as at-risk even in the presence of near-normal coronary angiographic findings.

Other distinctions include the observation that older women and men are more likely to present with plaque rupture, while younger women are more likely to experience plaque erosion (nonruptured erosions of plaque that contribute to thrombus formation). Intravascular ultrasound was performed on a subgroup of women participating in the WISE study, and the results showed that women had intramural atherosclerosis as opposed to the more common form of intracoronary lumenal plaque protrusion. More evidence of subendocardial myocardial ischemia in women has been obtained through magnetic resonance imaging. Women who do not have angiographic evidence of obstructive artery disease may experience angina-like chest pain due to endothelial dysfunction, inflammation-mediated atherosclerosis, or underlying microvascular disease. Based on these results, all women who are at risk must be identified and treated, which calls for a greater understanding of the various disease pathologies. Future studies should concentrate on how the pathophysiology of coronary artery disease differs in men and women, with a particular focus on endothelial and vascular dysfunction. Research in this area is critical because there are no sex-specific strategies available to reduce mortality (Hage and Oparil, 2013).

6.3.3. Diagnostic Testing Challenges

An affordable method that can be used to diagnose and assess coronary disease is noninvasive exercise testing. However, women are less sensitive to and specific from traditional tests (like the exercise tolerance test) that are used to detect signs of obstructive coronary disease. The test is less accurate for women with higher false-positive rates, even though the false-negative rate is similar to that of men. Fewer obstructive diseases, reduced exercise-induced pulse rate responses, and the impact of estrogen on the ST segment in women are some of the hypothesized explanations for the sex-related discrepancy in accuracy. Exercise testing is a common practice for women, regardless of accuracy rates. If this strategy is employed, it is important to take the pretest probability of disease into consideration. Although multiple studies have indicated that women with positive stress tests are examined less aggressively than their male counterparts, higher false positives from exercise testing may increase recommendations for needless invasive workups for women with a low probability of disease. In both men and women, the addition of scores from noninvasive coronary artery calcium screening improves the predictability of disease events over traditional risk factors alone; however, there is evidence to suggest that women are more likely than men to experience events at any given level of calcification. There exists a debate regarding the appropriate use of coronary artery calcium scoring data in treatment decisions, particularly with regard to the potential benefit of invasive strategies for patients with high calcium scores who do not exhibit any other symptoms.

6.3.4. Prognosis and Treatment Outcomes

Because of improvements in heart disease diagnosis and treatment, the rate of cardiovascular deaths has dropped by 35 to 50% over the last 20 years; however, the reductions in mortality rates for women have not kept pace with those for men. Statistics reveal that women have a generally worse prognosis than men when it comes to obstructive coronary disease. Women have higher short- and long-term MI mortality rates than men do, independent of age or comorbidity. Women are far more likely to have a subsequent MI, heart failure, and pass away. Compared to 18% of men, 23% of women 40 and older will pass away from MI within a year, according to 2009 AHA statistics. Women over 40 will die from MI at a rate of 43% within 5 years, compared to only 33% for men. According to registry data, the risk of death following an MI is the same for men and women over 75, but women under 75 make up a significant portion of the sex-related disparity in mortality. The sex-related difference is still noticeable in terms of morbidity; following an MI, a disproportionately high number of women will experience heart failure or a stroke. Even with a preserved ejection fraction, women are more likely to suffer from debilitating heart failure following an MI. Table 6.3 lists the numerous sex-specific variations in heart failure (Ferrara et al., 2003).

There are several factors that contribute to the different prognoses seen between men and women after experiencing ACS. Women tend to be older and have more comorbid conditions like diabetes and hypertension. They also have a higher risk of complications, such as reinfarction, death, heart failure, stroke, and needing transfusions, during their hospital stay compared to men. Referral bias and sex-based differences in disease pathophysiology play a role in the outcomes observed between the sexes. It is important to work on standardizing the use of life-saving ACS treatments and researching targeted therapeutic approaches based on gender to improve outcomes for both men and women.

Table 6.3. Sex-Specific Heart Failure Findings

Comorbidities and Disease Findings	Laboratory Findings	Medication Concerns
Women with heart failure are more likely to have hypertension Women with heart failure are more likely to have preserved left ventricular function Women with decompensated heart failure are more commonly found with thyroid disease Women with heart failure have a lower quality of life than men with heart failure Retrospective data from SOLVD suggest women are at increased risk of thromboembolic events associated with heart failure	B-type natriuretic peptide values > 500 pg/mL have been observed to be stronger predictors of mortality in women than in men	Most trials for heart failure caused by systolic dysfunction have not evaluated treatments in a sex-specific fashion Meta-analyses suggest mortality reductions in women treated with ACE inhibitors and β-blockers for systolic dysfunction

Source: https://www.accp.com/docs/bookstore/psap/p7b01sample03.pdf.

6.3.5. Treatment Disparity Among Men and Women

6.3.5.1. Interventional Therapies

6.3.5.1.1. Percutaneous Coronary Intervention

The underutilization of effective medical and interventional therapies for CVD in women is a global observation. Merely 33% of the 11.6 million percutaneous coronary intervention (PCI) surgical procedures carried out annually in the US involve women. Risk-adjusted analyzes of short- and long-term outcomes show that high-risk women benefit from PCI in a manner comparable to men, despite women using the procedure less frequently than men. This is a promising finding from a popular and highly effective intervention. However, women are more likely to experience bleeding and vascular complications, so when considering PCI, a thorough evaluation of the risk-benefit ratio of an invasive strategy must be done.

A meta-analysis of 12 PCI trials revealed that women experienced vascular complications like bleeding 1.5–4 times more frequently than men. The benefit of PCI in women with ACS may be restricted to the highest-risk women only due to the increased risk of morbidity from vascular complications (e.g, women with elevated troponin concentrations). In women with low-risk features, the 2007 Unstable Angina/ Non-ST-segment Myocardial Infarction (UA/NSTEMI) guideline supports a conservative approach; in women with higher risk, it advocates an earlier invasive strategy (i.e., positive indicators).

6.3.5.1.2. Coronary Artery Bypass Graft

In the US, approximately one-third of patients having coronary artery bypass graft surgery are female. Regretfully, following surgery, they experience less symptom relief and have fewer functional gains than men. The baseline comorbid conditions, referral patterns, procedural characteristics, and postoperative care of women undergoing coronary artery bypass graft differ from those of men; historically, women have been reported to be at higher risk of surgery than men. According to recent data, there are specific procedural factors that can improve long-term graft patency and survival, particularly for women. These consist of off-pump techniques and the use of internal thoracic artery grafts. Women are reported to have higher readmission rates than men following coronary artery bypass graft, and they also have significantly lower referral and attendance rates for cardiac rehabilitation. Research on the impact of sex on current outcomes following coronary artery bypass grafting ought to be conducted.

6.3.5.2. Pharmacotherapy

6.3.5.2.1. Use of Evidence-Based Pharmacotherapy

Compared to men, women with ACS have received less evidence-based medication therapy, which is similar to the underutilization of surgery and interventional procedures. Studies conducted prior to the availability of primary PCI for acute MI revealed that although women were less likely to receive fibrinolysis, those who did had a higher rate of side effects from the treatment. Unfortunately, the treatment of men and women still varies despite significant advancements in the field. Even when elevated troponin values are documented, women are less likely to receive heparin, an ACE inhibitor, or a glycoprotein IIb/IIIa inhibitor (GPI) at the time of admission, according to recent data from ACS registries in the United States. Moreover, women are less likely to receive an aspirin prescription at the time of discharge (87.5% vs. 90.4% of men) and statin medication (55.9% vs. 63.4% among males). This is true even though current guidelines suggest that statins, ACE inhibitors, β-blockers, aspirin, clopidogrel, and anticoagulants benefit women equally to men (Zelniker et al., 2019).

Women are prescribed less medication for chronic stable angina than men, despite the fact that women have a higher risk of cardiac events within a year. The Euro Heart Survey of Stable Angina revealed that women used statins at a statistically significant lower rate (45% vs. 51% of males. Additionally, women used aspirin at a lower rate (73% vs. 81% among males). These results showed that women were receiving much less medication, both at the time of the initial diagnosis and a year later. Surprisingly, women in this survey had twice the rate of nonfatal MI and death compared with their male counterparts at 1-year follow-up, even after controlling for age, heart failure, diabetes, disease severity, and pharmacotherapy differences. For women, adherence to guideline-based management may be improved by greater awareness and a lack of bias. Future research should focus on whether applying guideline-based therapies to women improves the clinical outcomes of coronary heart disease.

6.3.5.2.2. Medication-Related Adverse Events

Women experience more drug-related adverse events than men. The U.S. Food and Drug Administration, through its Adverse Event Reporting System, has noted that 53% of reported events from 1969 to 2002 concerned female patients, whereas only 35% were reported in male patients (12% did not report sex).

Variations in the side effects of cardiovascular medications in women may be explained by variations in body mass, volume of distribution, liver metabolism, and kidney function (Table 6.4). According to genomic research, there is a sex-based influence on gene expression that may account for variations in drug response and disease in men and women. Future research should concentrate on the clinical significance of these variations.

Table 6.4. Sex-Based Differences in the Pharmacokinetic Response of Cardiovascular Drugs

Drug Absorption	Drug Distribution	Drug Metabolism	Drug Elimination
Differences include: • A 25% increased absorption of verapamil in women • A 40% increased absorption of aspirin in women	General differences include: • A larger percentage of body fat is found in women (resulting in lower serum concentrations of lipophilic medications) • Women have a smaller body water compartment, intravascular volume, and muscle mass (resulting in higher serum concentrations of hydrophilic medications)	Sex-specific CYP alterations include: • Drugs processed by CYP3A4 (e.g., amiodarone, amlodipine, atorvastatin, simvastatin, gemfibrozil, verapamil) are metabolized 20% to 40% faster in women than in men • The CP450 1A2 enzyme is more active in men than in women, affecting drugs such as clopidogrel and propranolol • Sex-specific data are limited with respect to metabolism of drugs by CYP2D6 and CYP2C9 (e.g., carvedilol, metoprolol, losartan, irbesartan, warfarin, rosuvastatin) Glucuronidation of drugs during phase 2 metabolism occurs more rapidly in men, speeding inactivation of epinephrine, norepinephrine, and dopamine	Age-adjusted glomerular filtration is about 20% lower in women

Source: https://www.accp.com/docs/bookstore/psap/p7b01sample03.pdf.

Finally, the frequency of drug use in women compared to men should be carefully taken into account when assessing the risk of negative effects between men and women. Women are more likely to experience diuretic-induced hyponatremia and hypokalemia, while men are more likely to experience gout. Amlodipine produced more peripheral edema in women during clinical trials (14.6% vs. 5.6%among men). Compared to men, women are twice as likely to experience ACE inhibitor-induced angioedema, and they are three times more likely to experience an ACE inhibitor-related cough.

6.3.5.2.3. QT Prolongation

Women experience potentially fatal torsades de pointes more frequently than men do when taking medications that change cardiac repolarization. Women taking antiarrhythmics like quinidine, disopyramide, ibutilide, and sotalol as well as non-antiarrhythmics like haloperidol, erythromycin, thioridazine, and clarithromycin are more likely to experience drug-induced torsades de pointes. Even after accounting for weight and creatinine clearance, women still have dofetilide clearance rates that are between 12 and 18% lower than those of men. Making sure that serum potassium and magnesium concentrations are within normal limits and that the dosage has been appropriately adjusted for kidney cleared agents like dofetilide and sotalol are important clinical considerations because prescribing antiarrhythmic drugs to women carries a higher risk of torsades de pointes (Emdin et al., 2015).

The impact of sex hormones on cardiac myocytes may be one of the mechanisms underlying the sex-related variation in proarrhythmia risk. Men's corrected QT intervals shorten after puberty, while women's corrected QT intervals are longer and their cardiac repolarization occurs more slowly. Women have shown a greater QT prolongation during the first half of the menstrual cycle, when estrogen concentrations rise and peak just before ovulation, though this has not been consistent in all research. In the first half of the menstrual cycle, ibutilide causes the QT interval to prolong more than usual. Furthermore, estradiol has the ability to amplify drug-induced QT prolongation. Sex hormones have been shown in animal studies to modify the L-type calcium current, the transient outward potassium current, and the rapidly activating delayed rectifier potassium current. Another area that needs more investigation is how progesterone and/or estradiol affect these ion currents in humans.

6.3.5.2.4. Bleeding Complications

Women who receive anticoagulants or fibrinolytic therapy in the context of PCI are more likely to experience bleeding. Anticoagulant dosage in women should be carefully considered when PCI is planned, especially when using kidney cleared medications like GPIs and low-molecular-weight heparins. Data from the CRUSADE registry demonstrate that excessive dosing of GPIs was almost 3 times more common in women (46.4% vs. 17.2% in men). In general, women tend to be older, have a lower body weight, and have more comorbid conditions influencing kidney function. Without the proper assessment of kidney function by an estimation of creatinine clearance, excessive dosing is more likely to occur. Women had higher rates of major bleeding if treated with GPIs (15.8% vs. 7.3% in men) and even if a GPI was not given (8.5% vs. 5.4% in men). This suggests that the administration of drugs may have contributed to some, but not all, of the excess bleeding risk in women. In both genders, bleeding was considerably reduced upon receiving the appropriate dosage modification.

Evidence points to comparable outcomes for enoxaparin and fibrinolytics, with separately increased risks of bleeding complications and possibly even death when these drugs are administered to female patients. A more accurate description of the discrepancy and data on the effectiveness of alternative management techniques for women are essential to bridging this gender gap. It is crucial to enroll a sufficient number of women in clinical trials that are capable of identifying sex-based differences for this extremely important side effect. Researchers should adopt the alternative dosing strategy for the elderly found in the enoxaparin-prescribing information for STEMI as a model for obtaining sex-based dosing recommendations. This strategy could also be applied to other populations at high risk of bleeding with anticoagulant therapies. Future studies on doses based on estimated creatinine clearance and sex-specific factors could result in a better way to administer enoxaparin and other antithrombotic medications to women.

6.4. Evidence-Based Treatment Guidelines

More women being enrolled in clinical trials has made it possible to create evidence-based recommendations tailored to the needs of women. A scientific statement regarding PCI and adjunctive medication, an evidence-based guideline for CVD prevention, and a scientific statement detailing the function of noninvasive testing in the clinical evaluation of women with suspected coronary artery disease are the three sets of guidelines that are specifically focused on the care of women. In addition, sex-specific subsections are included in the 2007 UA/NSTEMI guideline from the AHA and the American College of Cardiology. Furthermore, the eighth edition of the American College of Chest Physicians Evidence-Based Clinical Practice Guideline on antithrombotic therapy and the U.S. Preventive Services Task Force Guideline have sex-specific discussions with respect to aspirin therapy (Table 6.5). The guidelines for treating and preventing CVD in women are largely the same as those for men, with very few exceptions. Nonetheless, due consideration is given to women's heightened risk of CVD-related morbidity and mortality, as well as the possibility of treatment disparities (Stanhewicz et al., 2018).

Table 6.5. Evidence-Based Guidelines Specific for Women

Guidelines	General Recommendations
Evidence-Based Guidelines for Cardiovascular Disease Prevention in Women: 2007 Update	Provides a risk stratification system specific for women Recommends against using drug classes (e.g., those that block the renin-angiotensin-aldosterone system) in pregnancy or in women who plan to become pregnant Recommends against the use of hormone therapy for primary and secondary prevention of CVD in women Recommends the use of aspirin for primary prevention as an age- and sex-based approach[a]
2008 CHEST Guidelines	Recommends the use of aspirin for primary prevention as an age- and sex-based approach[a]
2009 U.S. Preventive Services Task Force	Recommends the use of aspirin for primary prevention as an age- and sex-based approach[a]
Percutaneous Coronary Intervention and Adjunctive Pharmacotherapy in Women (2005)	Medication recommendations do not differ by sex; however, unique risks of PCI in women are highlighted
Role of Noninvasive Testing in the Clinical Evaluation of Women with Suspected Coronary Artery Disease (2005)	Notes no major differences between the recommendations for diagnostic testing between the sexes
ACC/AHA 2007 Guidelines for the Management of Patients with Unstable Angina/Non–ST-Elevation Myocardial Infarction	Recommends a noninvasive, conservative strategy for women who present with low-risk features Notes that GPIs may lack efficacy in women without elevated troponin concentrations

Source: https://www.accp.com/docs/bookstore/psap/p7b01sample03.pdf.

6.4.1. Sex-Specific Drug Therapy

Sex-specific drug therapy recognizes and addresses the biological and physiological differences between men and women that affect the efficacy, safety, and metabolism of medications. These differences arise from variations in body composition, hormonal levels, enzyme activity, and genetic factors, which can influence how drugs are absorbed, distributed, metabolized, and excreted. Understanding these differences is crucial for optimizing treatment outcomes and minimizing adverse effects in both sexes.

In cardiovascular therapy, for instance, women often respond differently to medications such as statins, beta-blockers, and anticoagulants. Women are more likely to experience statin-induced myopathy and may have different cholesterol-lowering responses, necessitating careful monitoring and dose adjustments. Similarly, women may experience more pronounced blood pressure reductions with certain antihypertensives, such as ACE inhibitors and angiotensin II receptor blockers (ARBs), which require tailored dosing to avoid hypotension.

Hormonal differences significantly impact drug therapy, especially in conditions like depression and anxiety, which are more prevalent in women. Women tend to have higher blood levels of certain antidepressants and may respond better to selective serotonin reuptake inhibitors (SSRIs) but are also more prone to side effects such as weight gain and sexual dysfunction. These variations necessitate personalized treatment plans and close monitoring for adverse effects.

Sex-specific differences also play a role in the pharmacokinetics and pharmacodynamics of drugs used in diabetes management. For example, women with diabetes are more susceptible to hypoglycemia, particularly when using insulin or sulfonylureas, highlighting the need for individualized dosing and monitoring strategies to prevent complications (Paduszyńska et al., 2021).

In oncology, sex differences in drug metabolism and hormone receptor status influence treatment efficacy and toxicity. Women often metabolize chemotherapy drugs differently, leading to variations in drug levels and side effects. For instance, women may have higher rates of adverse reactions to certain chemotherapeutic agents, necessitating dose modifications and supportive care measures.

Clinical trials have historically underrepresented women, leading to a gap in knowledge about sex-specific drug responses. Recent regulatory guidelines emphasize the importance of including both sexes in clinical research to better understand these differences and develop more effective, personalized therapies. This inclusion helps identify sex-specific dosing recommendations, potential side effects, and efficacy profiles, ultimately improving patient care.

Pharmacogenetics, the study of how genetic variations affect drug response, is an emerging field that further underscores the importance of sex-specific therapy. Genetic differences can influence drug-metabolizing enzymes, transporters, and receptors, leading to variations in drug response and toxicity. Incorporating pharmacogenetic testing into clinical practice can enhance personalized medicine, ensuring that both men and women receive the most effective and safe treatments based on their genetic makeup.

Healthcare providers must be aware of sex-specific differences in drug therapy to optimize treatment outcomes. This awareness includes understanding the unique pharmacokinetic and pharmacodynamic profiles of medications in men and women, considering hormonal influences, and recognizing the need for tailored dosing and monitoring. By incorporating sex-specific considerations into clinical practice, healthcare professionals can improve the efficacy and safety of drug therapies, ultimately enhancing patient care for both men and women.

6.4.1.1. Aspirin

The majority of information regarding aspirin use for primary prevention prior to the WHS came from five sizable trials with a preponderance of male participants. The evidence consistently demonstrated aspirin's effectiveness in preventing MI, but it showed no discernible impact on preventing strokes. The Physician's Health Study's opposite was discovered by the WHS in 2005; while aspirin therapy had no effect on MI in women, it did reduce the incidence of stroke. A subgroup analysis of women over 65 revealed that they had a lower risk of MI, which was comparable to the advantages men experienced. Three sets of evidence-based guidelines that provide sex-specific aspirin recommendations have been updated in light of these data. These suggestions are summarized in Table 6.6. The fact that no single trial provides meaningful numbers of direct comparisons between male and female participants is a limitation of the sex-specific aspirin recommendation. Because younger women have fewer MIs than men of the same age, patient risk may have affected the protective benefit of aspirin based on age. Moreover, the dosage administered in the WHS (100 mg every other day) differed from the dosage that has been demonstrated to lower cardiovascular events in males. Women have been found to be 2–4 times more likely to develop aspirin resistance, and one drawback of the WHS was that an appropriate aspirin dosage may not have been administered (Iorga et al., 2017). More research is needed to demonstrate that aspirin at comparable dosages is therapeutically equivalent in both sexes and to determine the dosages based on sex that produce the best results in each gender.

Table 6.6. Sex-Based Comparison of Recommendations for Aspirin use in the Primary Prevention of CVD

Guideline	Men	Women
2007 Evidence-Based Guidelines for Cardiovascular Disease Prevention in Women	N/A	High-risk women: 75–325 mg of aspirin daily unless contraindicated At-risk or healthy women ≥ 65: aspirin 81 mg daily or 100 mg every other day if blood pressure is controlled and benefit for ischemic stroke and MI prevention likely outweighs risk of GI bleeding or hemorrhagic stroke At-risk or healthy women ≤ 65: aspirin 81 mg daily or 100 mg every other day when benefit for ischemic stroke prevention is likely to outweigh adverse events
2008 CHEST Guidelines	Men at moderate risk of a coronary event (based on age and cardiac risk factor profile with a 10-year risk of a cardiac event > 10%): aspirin 75–100 mg daily is recommended	Women > 65 at risk of ischemic stroke or MI: aspirin 75–100 mg daily Women < 65 at risk of ischemic stroke; aspirin 75–100 mg daily
2009 U.S. Preventive Services Task Force Recommendation[a]	Men aged 45–79 in whom the potential MI benefit outweighs the potential harm caused by an increase in GI hemorrhage: aspirin 75 mg daily (as effective as higher doses) is recommended Men aged > 80[a]: no recommendation	Women aged < 54: aspirin is not recommended because of small benefits from reducing ischemic stroke and moderate evidence for harm Women aged 55–79: aspirin 75 mg daily (as effective as higher dosages) is recommended when the potential benefit from reduction in ischemic stroke outweighs the potential harm from GI hemorrhage Women > 80[a]: no recommendation

Source: https://www.accp.com/docs/bookstore/psap/p7b01sample03.pdf.

When determining whether aspirin therapy may benefit a woman, the risk of bleeding should be taken into account. There were 47 people in the WHS cohort over 65 who needed to be treated and 128 people who needed to be harmed. This risk-to-benefit ratio is generally favorable. The number of women in the 55–64 age range that needed to be harmed was 196, while 2001 needed to be treated. Given the minimal benefit in women under 65, aspirin therapy's bleeding risk is too great for it to be regularly advised. Aspirin therapy needs to be customized for each patient, taking into account their unique risks and benefits. Although most of the evidence for this claim comes from earlier secondary prevention trials that did not examine the risk/benefit of aspirin therapy in a sex-specific manner, current secondary prevention guidelines indicate that women benefit from aspirin in the same way that men do. Although few women were included in these trials, subgroup analysis revealed that both sexes benefited from the same treatments. Aspirin use is advised as a secondary preventive measure for CVD regardless of age or gender, even though it is specifically advised for women as the primary preventive measure (Iorga et al., 2017).

6.5. Management of Cardiovascular Risk in Perimenopausal Women with Diabetes

For women, the menopausal transition and postmenopause are times when their risk of CVD is higher. Growing older contributes to this increased risk: during the menopausal transition, blood pressure, glucose, and non-traditional risk factors all rise linearly with age. The hormonal changes associated with the transition may also contribute to an increased risk: levels of low-density lipoprotein cholesterol (LDL-C) rise sharply in the year preceding and following the final menstrual period (FMP). However, there is conflicting evidence regarding intermediate outcomes, and estrogen-based therapies do not seem to reduce CVD events during this window. These findings imply that while estrogen-based treatments may be used with caution to relieve menopausal symptoms, their potential to prevent chronic diseases is probably minimal. Therefore, the cornerstone of reducing the risk for CVD morbidity and mortality for women with diabetes continues to be close monitoring and management of blood pressure, lipids, and glucose during perimenopause and postmenopause.

6.5.1. The Menopausal Transition, CVD Risk Factors, and CVD Risk

Age at natural menopause, which is synonymous with age at the FMP, is the point at which a woman stops having periods if she has not had a hysterectomy or bilateral oophorectomy. The age at the FMP has risen gradually among Korean women over the past 50 years, most likely due to increases in life expectancy and standard of living. The age at FMP increased in younger cohorts among the 12,761 participants in the Korea National Health and Nutrition Examination Survey (KNHANES) who underwent natural menopause. The age at FMP for women born before 1930 was 47.9 years, while the age at FMP for women born between 1945 and 1949 was 50.05 years. Although the term "perimenopause" is often used imprecisely to refer to the years surrounding the first menstrual period, the International Stages of Reproductive Aging Workshop (STRAW) consortium defines it as irregular menstruation. Women enter perimenopause when their menses differ by more than seven days between successive cycles, according to the STRAW criteria. After a year without a menstrual period, women are categorized as postmenopausal.

These changes in menstruation are accompanied by changes in several organ systems, which raise the risk of CVD (Figure 6.1). Although weight gain is not linked to the menopausal transition per se, women experience a redistribution of body fat that leads to a comparatively higher level of visceral adiposity. This, in turn, causes unfavorable adipokine profiles, which in turn cause insulin resistance and dyslipidemia. Modified vascular reactivity and endothelial dysfunction are the consequences of abnormal endothelial factors and the activation of the renin-angiotensin system, which are caused by changes in sex hormone profiles. Healthy lifestyle practices that reduce the risk of CVD may be hampered by the elevated risk of depression during the menopausal transition and sleep disturbances brought on by vasomotor symptoms, though not all women who go through this phase experience these symptoms. Study of Women's Health Across the Nation (SWAN): This multicenter, longitudinal cohort of American women has evaluated sex steroid levels, symptoms during menopause, and serial CVD risk factors (Song et al., 2016). The levels of total cholesterol, LDL-C, and apolipoprotein B significantly rose in the year starting one year before the FMP and ending one year after the FMP. This implies that lipid levels may be adversely affected by changes in sex steroid levels that take place in the year before and after the FMP, especially drops in estradiol. On the other hand, non-traditional risk factors like inflammatory markers and blood pressure and glucose levels increased in a linear fashion around the FMP, indicating that these midlife risk factors were deteriorating due to chronologic aging. Few studies have looked specifically at how women with diabetes's CVD risk profiles change during the menopausal transition; one study of diabetic women hospitalized suggested that postmenopausal status was linked to higher CVD risk and worse CVD risk factors than premenopausal status, though it was unclear if this effect held true regardless of acute illness and chronological age.

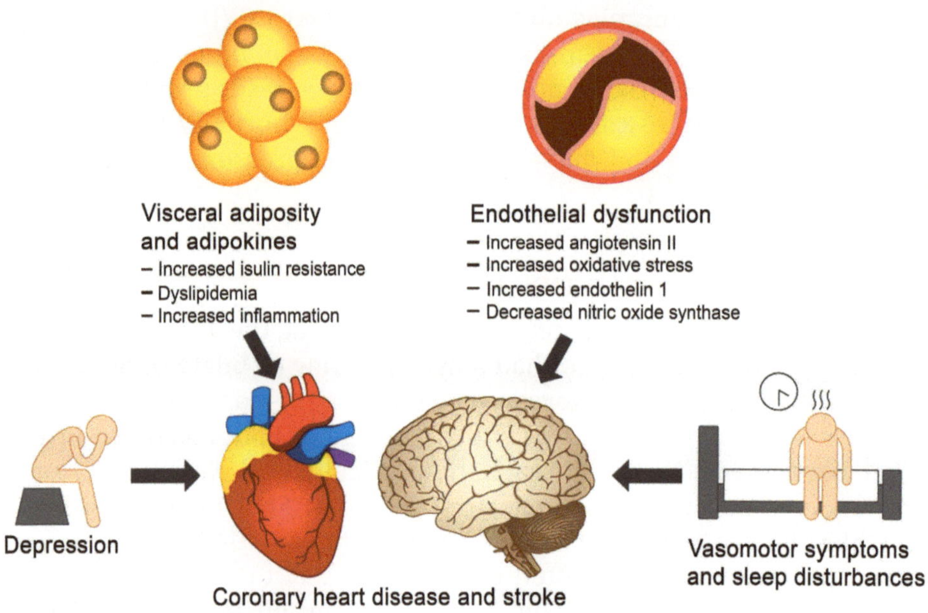

Figure 6.1. *Menopausal- and age-related changes in visceral adiposity and endothelial dysfunction, along with increased risk of depression, vasomotor symptoms and sleep disturbances, increase the risk of coronary heart disease and stroke in midlife women.*

Source: https://www.e-dmj.org/journal/view.php?number=2568.

Even when risk factor levels are below the cutoffs for diabetes, hypertension, and dyslipidemia, they are probably still harmful. The Emerging Risk Factors Collaboration found that even in people without diabetes, levels of fasting plasma glucose above 100 mg/dL were linearly associated with the risk of coronary heart disease (CHD). This association was observed by combining data from 102 prospective studies that collectively enrolled people across over 30 countries, including China and Japan but not Korea. In a similar vein, analyzes utilizing data from the UKPDS revealed an elevated risk of myocardial infarction in individuals with diabetes at all blood pressure and LDL-C levels, with no indication of a threshold effect. Women with diabetes already have an increased risk of atherosclerotic events; these perimenopausal changes probably make it worse. The prevalence of known coronary heart disease (CHD) among women with diabetes is less than 5% for both men and women under the age of 45, but it increases quickly and linearly after that point.

6.5.2. Trials of Estrogen Therapy

The use of estrogen supplements by postmenopausal and perimenopausal women has changed as well. Nowadays, vasomotor symptoms and/or symptoms related to vaginal atrophy are treated with estrogen therapy, which was formerly commonly used to prevent chronic diseases. Women who averaged roughly 63 years old at randomization participated in the Women's Health Initiative (WHI), a sizable randomized trial in the United States testing estrogen therapy (with and without progestin). Women with an intact uterus were assigned to conjugated equine estrogen plus medroxyprogesterone (n=8,506) versus placebo (n=8,102), while women who had undergone a hysterectomy were assigned to conjugated equine estrogen alone (n=5,310) versus placebo (n=5,429). Neither estrogen therapy alone nor estrogen plus progestin therapy appeared to decrease the risk of CHD events and risk of stroke was increased. After the study results were released in 2001, prescription of estrogen-based therapies declined to less than 10% in the United States (Song et al., 2016). More recent research has looked at whether using estrogen might be more beneficial if it is studied for a longer amount of time. Owing to the size of WHI, the results of a 2017 systematic review that looked at the long-term risks of estrogen therapy heavily weighted the follow-up data from the WHI. Over a decade after randomization, the risk of stroke remained elevated while the risk of myocardial infarction gradually decreased. The subgroup of diabetic women in the WHI study showed similar results, and oral estrogen was actually linked to a marginally lower risk of diabetes in the WHI. Notably, estrogen therapy is contraindicated in women with known CVD and may be especially dangerous in women with diabetes: women with abnormal glucose tolerance and angiographic CHD who were randomly assigned to estrogen use experienced worsening of their inflammatory risk profiles and atherosclerotic progression; additionally, estrogen use was linked to an increased risk of myocardial infarction in these women (Ferrara A, Quesenberry CP, Karter AJ, Njoroge CW, Jacobson AS, and Selby JV, et al 1995–1998).

According to the timing hypothesis, estrogen therapy might stop plaque from forming without promoting plaque regression. Thus, this theory suggests that beginning estrogen therapy during the perimenopause or the early postmenopausal stage may be beneficial for CVD. A subanalysis of WHI participants under 60 years old and of those randomly assigned to receive estrogen without progestin revealed that this particular population may have benefited from estrogen use in terms of CHD. But there wasn't enough statistical power in this subanalysis to find a benefit. Notably, a subanalysis of WHI participants under 60 years old who were randomly assigned to receive progestin and estrogen failed to find evidence of this benefit. Numerous other studies have looked at the effects of conjugated estrogen or estradiol on intermediate atherosclerotic markers in recently postmenopausal women, like cIMT and CAC. Both the Early Versus Late Intervention Trial with Estradiol (ELITE) and the Kronos Early Estrogen Prevention Study (KEEPS) found no differences in levels of CAC or cIMT between the estrogen-based therapy groups, nor did they find any effect of oral estradiol or randomization on CAC. Despite the fact that cIMT progression was slower in the estradiol group, there were insufficient events to determine the clinical significance of this finding. The effects of randomization to estradiol therapy versus. found a decreased risk of a composite outcome that included myocardial infarction, hospital admission for heart failure, and death when no therapy was used. But this trial has come under fire for using an outcome that wasn't predetermined and for not having a placebo (Song et al., 2016).

In conclusion, neither younger nor older populations seem to consistently benefit from estradiol supplementation when it comes to the prevention of CVD events. Nonetheless, these treatments don't seem to significantly raise the risk of CVD or overall mortality in younger perimenopausal and postmenopausal women with vasomotor symptoms. As a result, vasomotor symptoms and vaginal atrophy may be treated with estradiol, especially in transdermal formulations. Given that overweight and obese women are more likely to experience symptoms than non-obesity women, women with diabetes may be especially susceptible to them.

6.5.3. Risk Calculators for CVD and Breast Cancer

Women who are perimenopausal or recently postmenopausal, have diabetes, menopause symptoms, and a history of known cardiovascular disease (CVD), thromboembolic events, active liver disease, or estrogen-sensitive cancer, such as breast cancer, are more likely to experience adverse events from estrogen therapy. For women with these conditions, alternative therapies to estrogen are advised to relieve menopausal symptoms. These alternative strategies, which are covered in more detail in other reviews, include behavioral adjustments, gabapentin, selective serotonin or norepinephrine reuptake inhibitors. Risk calculators can help women who are not contraindicated for estrogen therapy make decisions. Numerous CVD risk engines and calculators, such as the Korean Risk Prediction Model (KRPM), were developed in the Korean Heart Study population and are based on large cohorts of people with decades of follow-up data. The UKPDS engine, the Pooled Cohort Equations risk engine, and the Prediction for ASCVD Risk in China (China-PAR) risk engine are a few more risk calculators that can be accessed for free online. As a result, each calculator has hypothetical benefits and limitations for risk estimation in Korean perimenopausal or newly menopausal women with diabetes. To the best of our knowledge, the accuracy of these calculators has not been compared for Korean women with diabetes specifically. The most people with type 2 diabetes mellitus are on the UKPDS calculator; multiple cohorts were pooled for the Pooled Cohort Equations risk calculator; East Asian populations were used to validate the China-PAR calculator; and additional Korean populations validated the KRPM calculator. The categorization of individuals as being at medium or high risk is fairly consistent across calculators, despite differences in the weighting of specific factors. Estrogen therapy should not be administered to women who have a high risk of cardiovascular disease events because of age, family history, or low levels of risk factors. This typically includes diabetic women who are over 60, have not menstruated in over ten years, and have elevated CVD risk factors. Similarly, risk engines that take into account a woman's family history of cancer as well as her reproductive history can be used to determine her risk of developing breast cancer. Estrogen therapy should not be administered to women whose family or reproductive history has resulted in a markedly increased risk of breast cancer. A recent summary of these breast cancer risk models' benefits and drawbacks for Korean women was published in 2020. Chronologic age, family history of breast cancer, age at menarche and menopause, history of pregnancies and abortions, breastfeeding practices, breast biopsy history and histology, use of oral contraceptives, and physical activity levels are all taken into account by these engines, albeit to differing degrees. Gail created the most widely validated model for predicting breast cancer, and a redesigned version called the Breast Cancer Risk Assessment Tool (BRCAT) is accessible online. AUC of 0.546 (95% confidence interval, 0.500 to 0.594) indicates that the test cannot distinguish between people with and without the condition, whereas AUC >0.7 is typically thought to be useful for risk prediction. Nevertheless, discriminatory accuracy in Korean women has been limited. Notably, adjustments to this model based on Korean women's populations likewise had suboptimal AUC, indicating that historical data is not as reliable for predicting breast cancer in general. As a result, women thinking about estrogen therapy should also be open to getting regular follow-up and mammograms (Song et al., 2016).

Transdermal or oral estradiol therapy can be started if diabetic women are found to be at low risk for CVDor cancer using these calculators, and if they are interested in the limited use of estrogen therapy for symptom relief. Since oral estradiol may more severely impact thromboembolic risk, coagulation profiles, and inflammation than transdermal estradiol, transdermal estradiol is typically recommended. Oral estradiol should be avoided by women at moderate or high risk, and if it is started, the 10-year CVD risk should be minimal. In general, progesterone should be administered at the lowest possible dosage to relieve symptoms and lower the risk of uterine cancer in women who have uteruses.

6.5.4. Healthy Lifestyle Behaviors

The foundation of managing diabetes complications in both men and women with the disease is the promotion of healthy lifestyle behaviors. Table 6.7 provides an overview of these suggestions. There is a wealth of epidemiologic data supporting the advantages of leading a healthy lifestyle. However, the impact of such behaviors in well-controlled randomized trials is limited, partly because of the compelling epidemiologic evidence and partly because it is challenging to implement and sustain such changes in behavior over the duration of time required to influence the incidence of chronic diseases. Women with diabetes who smoke have a significantly higher risk of CHD events; conversely, quitting smoking lowers that risk. Lowering sodium intake (<2,300 mg/day and <1,500 mg/day in hypertensive individuals), consuming more fruits and vegetables, and abstaining from excessive alcohol use are all linked to lower risk of CVD. Additional observational studies conducted on individuals with diabetes highlight the benefits of increased physical activity in preventing CVD events and overall and CVD mortality.

Table 6.7. Recommendations for Reducing Cardiovascular Risk in Peri- and Newly Postmenopausal Women with Diabetes

Lifestyle Behaviors	Additional Considerations
Smoking cessation	Limited data from randomized studies
Weight reduction	Limited data from randomized studies
Physical activity at least 30 minutes a day	Limited data from randomized studies
Restrict sodium intake <2,300 mg/day	<1,500 mg/day if hypertension
Fruit and vegetable consumption of 10 servings/day	Limited data from randomized studies
Alcohol consumption ≤1 serving per day	Limited data from randomized studies
Glycemia	Higher A1c if limited life expectancy or morbidity from therapy
A1c <7%, with lower targets if tolerated for microvascular disease	
Consider SGLT-2 inhibitor or GLP-1 receptor agonist for women with CVD	
Blood pressure	Higher BP if limited life expectancy or morbidity from therapy
Blood pressure <140/90 mm Hg, with lower SBP and DBP if tolerated	Contraindicated in pregnancy
Consider ACE inhibitor or angiotensin receptor blocker	
Cholesterol	No or moderate statin if low CVD risk
Statin use for women with CVD	Contraindicated in pregnancy
Anti-platelet therapy	No use if low CVD risk
Aspirin use for women with CVD	Clopidogrel if aspirin allergy

SGLT-2, sodium glucose co-transporter 2; GLP-1, glucagon-like peptide 1; CVD, cardiovascular disease; SBP, systolic blood pressure; DBP, diastolic blood pressure; ACE, angiotensin converting enzyme; BP, blood pressure.

Source: https://www.e-dmj.org/journal/view.php?number=2568.

Randomized trials have produced less conclusive evidence about the positive effects of physical activity on weight loss in people with diabetes. To lower cardiovascular morbidity and mortality, men and women with diabetes were randomized to an intensive lifestyle intervention in the Action for Health in Diabetes (also known as Look AHEAD) trial. Orlistat or more aggressive weight loss techniques were started if weight loss objectives were not met in six months. These weight loss objectives were met by upping physical activity levels and implementing a low-calorie diet that contained less than 30% fat in the diet. The randomization arm did not show any decreases in CVD morbidity or death. Reasons for the lack of significance have included the challenge of maintaining a relatively large amount of weight loss over an extended period of time, the gradual loss of weight in the placebo arm, the generally good control of risk factors, and the low risk of

CVD events relative to non-randomized populations. Yet, losing weight is still highly advised for diabetics due to the simultaneous improvements in hemoglobin A1c, blood pressure, functioning, and quality of life (Song et al., 2016).

6.5.5. Antiplatelet and Statin Therapy

It is advised that all diabetic women with known cardiovascular disease take aspirin. Diabetes increases the risk of cardiovascular disease in perimenopausal women, even if they do not yet have a known CVD. However, gastrointestinal bleeding may be more likely to occur for these women than cardiovascular disease, especially in younger patients. To ascertain whether the risk of CVD may be greater than the risk of gastrointestinal bleeding, one can utilize the CVD risk calculators discussed in the preceding section. As a general rule, the risk of gastrointestinal bleeding is higher in women with diabetes under 50 years of age than it is in men, and women may benefit less from aspirin in terms of reducing the risk of CVD. On the other hand, women who are over 50 years old and have diabetes along with one or more major risk factors (such as smoking, dyslipidemia, hypertension, family history of premature ASCVD, chronic kidney disease, or albuminuria) but are not at higher risk of bleeding (e.g., renal illness, anemia, and advanced age). When discussing aspirin therapy for primary prevention, shared decision-making should be taken into account. This involves carefully weighing the benefits to the cardiovascular system against the relatively comparable increase in risk of bleeding.

People with diabetes who are in their midlife often have lipid disorders, and statin use is advised for all women with diabetes who have established cardiovascular disease. Statin use should be taken into consideration for all women with diabetes, as they offer benefits for preventing CVD risk in addition to lipid levels. However, the benefits of statin therapy are not as well-established for women with type 1 diabetes mellitus or perimenopausal diabetes without known CVD as they are for older women with type 2 diabetes mellitus. The addition of a statin may be postponed until risk increases occur if younger women, based on the previously mentioned risk calculators, have CVD risk levels less than 5% and are actively managing other risk factors such as blood pressure, glycemia, and lifestyle modification.

6.5.6. Glycemic Control

Hemoglobin A1c <7% targets are advised for people with diabetes in general, with more stringent targets for particular groups, like expectant mothers. Significant macrovascular benefits have not been observed in randomized trials for individuals assigned to intensive glycemic reductions. Reductions in risk for microvascular disease were noted in a 2013 meta-analysis of such trials, which included 18,717 participants randomized to intensive glycemic control versus 16,195 participants to conventional control. However, reductions in CVD events or mortality were not observed. To lower microvascular disease, strict control of A1c to levels <7% can be tried. A1c targets can be raised for women whose reduced life expectancy or comorbidity from intensive glycemic therapy take precedence over the reduction of CVD risk. In addition to the degree of glycemia, the use of particular hypoglycemic medications may be beneficial for reducing the risk of CVD. The pros and cons of each of these therapies are too complex to cover in detail in this article on the menopausal transition, but I will mention here that glucagon-like peptide 1 (GLP-1) receptor agonists and sodium glucose co-transporter 2 (SGLT-2) inhibitors have been linked to a lower risk of CVD events in people with diabetes, especially in those who have a history of the disease (Zelniker et al 2019).

6.5.7. Blood Pressure

The ideal blood pressure goals for diabetics differ based on the risk of CVD and the burden of comorbidities. Individuals with diabetes in general have lower risk of CVD and mortality when their blood pressure is less than 140/90 mm Hg. In a meta-analysis of 49 trials involving 73,738 diabetes participants, lower blood pressure was actually linked to a higher risk of CVD. However, other meta-analyzes indicate that more intensive lowering to targets <130 mm Hg is linked to a lower risk of CVD. The main source of benefit is not overall CVD events or death, but rather the decreased risk of stroke. Women who are perimenopausal or have recently gone through menopause tend to be younger than the general population of people with diabetes and hypertension. These younger women might be more resilient to blood pressure drops of less than 130 mm Hg than older populations, whose pulse pressures are typically much wider and who are more likely to experience medication side effects. Nowadays, most organizations advise aiming for a blood pressure of at least 140/90 mm Hg, with more intense targets as tolerated. Angiotensin converting enzyme (ACE) inhibitors can be used as first-line therapy in diabetics because they prevent nephropathy and may also protect diabetic patients from cardiovascular disease (CVD). The majority of the benefits of lowering blood pressure are not agent-specific if ACE-inhibition is intolerable (Emdin, Rahimi, Neal, Callender, Perkovic, Patel et al., 2015). Alternative treatments for these women include the use of calcium channel blockers, diuretics, and angiotensin receptor blockers (Oppermann et al., 2019).

A Closer Look

Woman's Heart Matters

Woman's heart matters immensely because CVD is the leading cause of death among women worldwide, yet it remains under-recognized and often undertreated compared to CVD in men. Women exhibit unique risk factors, symptoms, and disease progressions that necessitate specialized attention and tailored medical approaches. Understanding and addressing these differences can significantly improve diagnosis, treatment, and outcomes for women suffering from heart disease.

Firstly, hormonal influences play a significant role in women's cardiovascular health. Estrogen, which provides protective cardiovascular effects before menopause, helps maintain healthy blood vessels and favorable lipid profiles. However, the decline in estrogen levels post-menopause increases the risk of CVD sharply. Pregnancy-related complications such as preeclampsia, gestational diabetes, and preterm birth are unique to women and elevate the risk of future cardiovascular events. Women with polycystic ovary syndrome (PCOS) also face increased cardiovascular risk due to associated metabolic issues.

Secondly, women often present with different and atypical symptoms of heart disease compared to men. While men typically report chest pain as a primary symptom, women are more likely to experience non-specific symptoms such as fatigue, shortness of breath, nausea, and pain in the back, neck, or jaw. These atypical presentations can lead to misdiagnosis or delayed diagnosis, resulting in worse outcomes. Additionally, women are more susceptible to microvascular disease, where the small arteries are affected, which standard diagnostic tools designed for larger vessel disease may not detect effectively.

*Third*ly, lifestyle and mental health factors significantly impact women's cardiovascular health. Women are more prone to depression and anxiety, which are recognized risk factors for CVD. These conditions can exacerbate cardiovascular risk by increasing physiological stress and promoting unhealthy behaviors such as poor diet, physical inactivity, and smoking. Despite lower overall smoking rates among women, the relative risk of developing CVD from smoking is higher in women than in men.

Furthermore, sex-specific differences in drug metabolism and responses necessitate tailored treatment approaches. Women may experience different side effects and efficacy profiles from cardiovascular medications, such as statins and antihypertensives, which require careful monitoring and dose adjustments. Invasive procedures like percutaneous coronary intervention (PCI) and coronary artery bypass grafting (CABG) also have varying outcomes in women, emphasizing the need for gender-specific treatment plans (Maas et al., 2021).

Addressing these issues through increased awareness, research, and education is crucial. Healthcare providers must be trained to recognize the unique aspects of cardiovascular disease in women and adopt gender-specific diagnostic and treatment strategies. More inclusive clinical research is essential to develop evidence-based guidelines that consider the specific needs of women. Public health campaigns should focus on educating women about their unique risks and promoting proactive heart health management.

Summary

- CVDs include disorders like coronary heart disease, cerebrovascular disease, rheumatic heart disease, arterial disease, peripheral arterial disease, congenital heart disease, deep vein thrombosis and pulmonary embolism.
- The evaluation of cardiovascular symptoms in women remains challenging due to the atypical nature of presentation. In addition, the use of 'typical' angina symptoms in the assessment of females may be imprecise due to the transposition of symptoms derived from male cohorts.
- Dyslipidemia and cholesterol accumulation are more common during menopause, which may be associated with an estrogen deficiency.
- Sex steroids have a great effect on the risk of coronary heart disease. Loss of ovarian hormones leads to an increase in LDL-C, triglycerides, and a decrease in high density lipoprotein cholesterol (HDL-C).
- Hypertension is one of the risk factors for cardiovascular disease. Hypertension affects an increasing proportion of the world population and is one of the leading causes of morbidity and mortality worldwide.
- Transition to postmenopausal status is associated with a worsening coronary heart disease (CHD) risk profile in women, conveying the same degree of cardiovascular risk as being males.
- An emerging risk factor for CVD of unique significance to women is a history of pregnancy-related problems. The presence of hypertension and diabetes in pregnancy may indicate a higher risk of CVD as women age.
- Anatomic and physiologic differences between the sexes contribute to the idea that heart disease is different in women and men. The degree of sex-related disparities associated with coronary artery disease has only recently been characterized and has yet to be addressed in a significant manner that affects outcomes.
- Cardiovascular death rates have decreased by 35% to 50% during the past 20 years because of advances in the diagnosis and treatment of heart disease, yet the reductions obtained in women do not match those in men.

References

1. Anagnostis, P., Paschou, S. A., Katsiki, N., Krikidis, D., Lambrinoudaki, I., & Goulis, D. G. (2019). Menopausal hormone therapy and cardiovascular risk: Where are we now? *Current Vascular Pharmacology, 17*(6), 564–572. https://doi.org/10.2174/15701611166661904221238.
2. de Villiers, T. J., Hall, J. E., Pinkerton, J. V., Perez, S. C., Rees, M., Yang, C., et al. (2016). Revised global consensus statement on menopausal hormone therapy. *Maturitas, 91*, 153–155. https://doi.org/10.1016/j.maturitas.2016.05.016.
3. Emdin, C. A., Rahimi, K., Neal, B., Callender, T., Perkovic, V., & Patel, A. (2015). Blood pressure lowering in type 2 diabetes: A systematic review and meta-analysis. *JAMA, 313*(6), 603–615. https://doi.org/10.1001/jama.2015.0356.

4. Ferrara, A., Quesenberry, C. P., Karter, A. J., Njoroge, C. W., Jacobson, A. S., Selby, J. V., et al. (2003). Current use of unopposed estrogen and estrogen plus progestin and the risk of acute myocardial infarction among women with diabetes: The Northern California Kaiser Permanente Diabetes Registry, 1995-1998. *Circulation, 107*(1), 43–48. https://doi.org/10.1161/01.CIR.0000053108.79248.C6.

5. Guthrie, J. R., Dennerstein, L., & Dudley, E. C. (1999). Weight gain and the menopause: A 5-year prospective study. *Climacteric, 2*(4), 205–211. https://doi.org/10.3109/13697139908999356.

6. Hage, F. G., & Oparil, S. (2013). Ovarian hormones and vascular disease. *Current Opinion in Cardiology, 28*(4), 411–416. https://doi.org/10.1097/HCO.0b013e3283628716.

7. Hodis, H. N., Mack, W. J., Henderson, V. W., Shoupe, D., Budoff, M. J., Hwang-Levine, J., et al. (2016). Vascular effects of early versus late postmenopausal treatment with estradiol. *New England Journal of Medicine, 374*(13), 1221–1231. https://doi.org/10.1056/NEJMoa1600677.

8. Hong, S. C., Yoo, S. W., Cho, G. J., Kim, T., Hur, J. Y., Park, Y. K., et al. (2007). Correlation between estrogens and serum adipocytokines in premenopausal and postmenopausal women. *Menopause, 14*(5), 835–840. https://doi.org/10.1097/gme.0b013e318033a69c.

9. Iorga, A., Cunningham, C. M., Moazeni, S., Ruffenach, G., Umar, S., & Eghbali, M. (2017). The protective role of estrogen and estrogen receptors in cardiovascular disease and the controversial use of estrogen therapy. *Biology of Sex Differences, 8*(1), 33. https://doi.org/10.1186/s13293-017-0142-2.

10. Maas, A., Rosano, G., Cifkova, R., et al. (2021). Cardiovascular health after menopause transition, pregnancy disorders, and other gynecologic conditions: A consensus document from European cardiologists, gynecologists, and endocrinologists. *European Heart Journal, 42*(10), 967–984. https://doi.org/10.1093/eurheartj/ehaa951.

11. Manson, J. E. (2013). The Kronos Early Estrogen Prevention Study by Charlotte Barker. *Women's Health (London), 9*(1), 9–11. https://doi.org/10.2217/whe.12.36.

12. Matthews, K. A., Gibson, C. J., El Khoudary, S. R., & Thurston, R. C. (2013). Changes in cardiovascular risk factors by hysterectomy status with and without oophorectomy: Study of Women's Health Across the Nation. *Journal of the American College of Cardiology, 62*(2), 191–200. https://doi.org/10.1016/j.jacc.2013.02.069.

13. Moreau, K. L., Hildreth, K. L., Meditz, A. L., Deane, K. D., & Kohrt, W. M. (2012). Endothelial function is impaired across the stages of the menopause transition in healthy women. *Journal of Clinical Endocrinology & Metabolism, 97*(12), 4692–4700. https://doi.org/10.1210/jc.2012-2251.

14. Oppermann, K., Colpani, V., & Spritzer, P. M. (2019). Risk factors associated with coronary artery calcification in midlife women: A population-based study. *Gynecological Endocrinology, 35*(10), 904–908. https://doi.org/10.1080/09513590.2019.1610903.

15. Paduszyńska, A., Banach, M., Maciejewski, M., Dąbrowa, M., & Bielecka-Dąbrowa, A. (2021). The outcomes of hypertension treatment depending on gender in patients over 40 years of age. *Przegląd Menopauzalny, 19*(4), 174–178. https://doi.org/10.5114/pm.2021.112123.

16. Park, C. Y., Lim, J. Y., & Park, H. Y. (2018). Age at natural menopause in Koreans: Secular trends and influences thereon. *Menopause, 25*(4), 423–429. https://doi.org/10.1097/GME.0000000000000952.

17. Song, Y., Wang, E. S., Xing, L. L., et al. (2016). Follicle-stimulating hormone induces postmenopausal dyslipidemia through inhibiting hepatic cholesterol metabolism. *Journal of Clinical Endocrinology & Metabolism, 101*(1), 254–263. https://doi.org/10.1210/jc.2015-3014.
18. Stanhewicz, A. E., Wenner, M. M., & Stachenfeld, N. S. (2018). Sex differences in endothelial function important to vascular health and overall cardiovascular disease risk across the lifespan. *American Journal of Physiology: Heart and Circulatory Physiology, 315*(6), H1569–H1588. https://doi.org/10.1152/ajpheart.00363.2018.
19. Tchernof, A., Desmeules, A., Richard, C., Laberge, P., Daris, M., Mailloux, J., et al. (2004). Ovarian hormone status and abdominal visceral adipose tissue metabolism. *Journal of Clinical Endocrinology & Metabolism, 89*(7), 3425–3430. https://doi.org/10.1210/jc.2003-031307.
20. Zelniker, T. A., Wiviott, S. D., Raz, I., Im, K., Goodrich, E. L., Furtado, R. H., et al. (2019). Comparison of the effects of glucagon-like peptide receptor agonists and sodium-glucose cotransporter 2 inhibitors for prevention of major adverse cardiovascular and renal outcomes in type 2 diabetes mellitus. *Circulation, 139*(15), 2022–2031. https://doi.org/10.1161/CIRCULATIONAHA.118.038419.

Chapter 7

UROGENITAL HEALTH

Contents

Introduction

The urogenital system comprises the reproductive organs and the kidneys, ureters, bladder, and urethra of the urinary tract.

The entire group of organs involved in reproduction, urine formation, and release is called the female urogenital tract. It consists of the uterus, fallopian tubes, kidneys, ureters, bladder, urethra, ovaries, and vagina. Infections of the female urogenital tract include vaginal infections, pelvic infections, urinary tract infections (UTIs), infections following gynecologic surgery, and pelvic inflammatory disease (PID). Bacterial colonization of the urinary tract can lead to infectious processes, and if these bacterial infections are not treated, they can lead to involvement of the bladder, urethra, ureters, and kidney. Women are more likely to suffer from UTIs because of the short urethra, which facilitates the spread of bacteria. An important factor contributing to urinary tract infections, in addition to anatomy, is an imbalance in the normal vaginal flora, which is why it is important to individually analyze all the risk factors in a patient with a urinary tract infection, especially in the context of menopause (Oros et al., 2020).

Orientation and Directional Terms

Term	Definition	Illustration
Vaginal flora	Vaginal flora are the microorganisms that colonize the vagina.	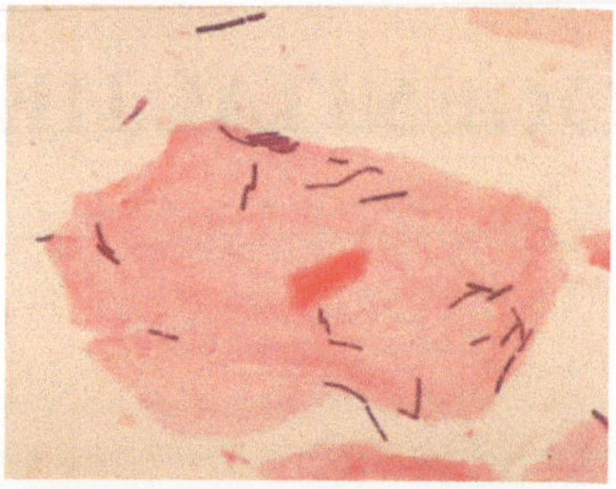
Microbiome	The microbiome is the collection of all microbes, such as bacteria, fungi, viruses, and their genes, that naturally live on our bodies and inside us. Although microbes are so small that they require a microscope to see them, they contribute in big ways to human health and wellness.	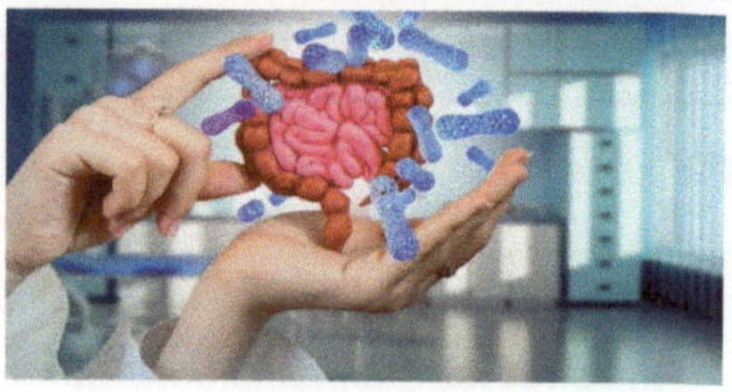
Amplicon sequence variant (ASV)	An amplicon sequence variant (ASV) is any one of the inferred single DNA sequences recovered from a high-throughput analysis of marker genes.	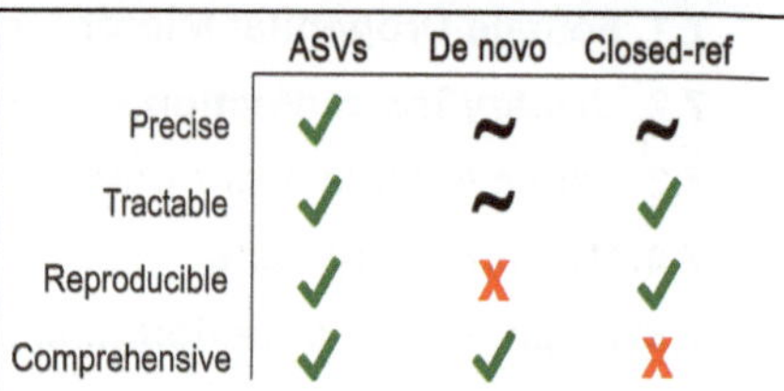
Probiotics	Probiotics are live microorganisms that are intended to have health benefits when consumed or applied to the body. They can be found in yogurt and other fermented foods, dietary supplements, and beauty products.	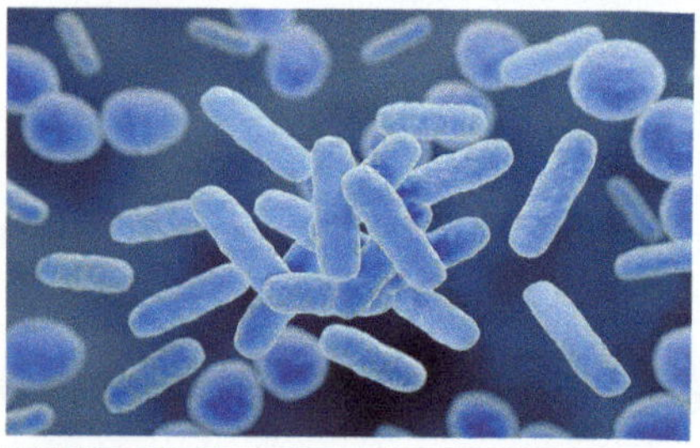
Galacto-oligosaccharides (GOS)	Galacto-oligosaccharides (GOS) are prebiotics made up of plant sugars linked in chains. They're found in dairy products, beans, and certain root vegetables.	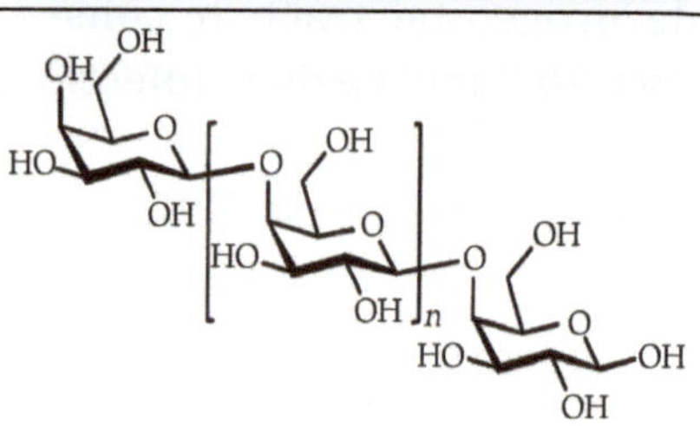

7.1. Female Urogenital Microbiome

The urogenital microbiota is made up of microorganisms that constitute the normal flora in the female genital tract.

It is now widely accepted that healthy individuals have a significant amount of microbiota in their urinary system, which varies by individual and gender.

The vagina and the gut are the two closest niches inhabited by residual/native microbiota, they are not the same as the urinary microbiota, although there are some similarities between the two.

According to current theories, urinary microbiota may originate from the gut microbiota, the vaginal microbiota (in women), and the environment, among other places. Research indicates that there may be the possibility of bacterial migration from the gut to the urinary tract because the composition and diversity of the gut and urinary microbiomes are similar. Furthermore, because some bacteria found in the vagina can also be found in urine, research has indicated that vaginal microbiota may influence urinary microbiota in women. Finally, the composition of the urinary microbiota can also be influenced by environmental factors, such as exposure to bacteria from the outside world.

The majority of the composition of the healthy vaginal microbiota in the population is dominated by the Lactobacillus genus, which lowers the pH of the vagina and affects epithelial cells and the host immune system, protecting the vagina from pathogen colonization. This makes the healthy vaginal microbiota unique compared to the rest of the human body sites that harbor native microbiota. Four species (Lactobacillus iners, L. crispatus, L. gasseri, and L. jensenii) have been recognized as distinct in attempts to classify vaginal microbiota types, all of which are dominated by lactobacilli. These species are found in varying amounts as major components of the female microbiota worldwide. A smaller percentage of women have a balanced vaginal microbiota composed mainly of facultative and obligate anaerobes, belonging mainly to the genera Gardnerella, Atopobium and Prevotella. This microbiota is not dominated by lactobacilli. This type of vaginal microbiota profile is linked to a higher risk of infections and unfavorable health outcomes due to the low presence of lactobacilli. More than 20 years of research on the vaginal microbiota have supported the observed protective role of this microbiota, which is characterized by low diversity and a predominance of Lactobacillus spp. This contrasts with the popular belief that a microbiota with a high diversity is necessarily "healthy."

Ultimately, we are still developing our understanding of the composition of a healthy urinary microbiota, how it contributes to our overall well-being, and how it affects our vulnerability to different diseases and conditions. Interactions with adjacent sites harboring native microbiota, such as the genital and digestive systems, influence urinary tract dynamics. Therefore, it is critical to differentiate between microorganisms that are native to the urinary tract and those that are temporarily transferred from surrounding body niches to understand their role in promoting health or disease. Urinary tract infections (UTIs) are one of the most common infections diagnosed globally and have a serious impact on patients' lives and healthcare systems. For this reason, it would be useful to identify protective factors and fully understand the role played by microbiota in the onset of UTIs.

7.1.1. Urogenital Microbiome

Accurately identifying microorganisms present in the urinary microbiota is essential for discussions about the microbiota and its impact on the host. To achieve this, preliminary procedures, including sample preparation and collection, are crucial. Urine sample collection can be problematic because the most popular and noninvasive method, midstream urine sampling, can be contaminated by surrounding skin, genital tract, and urethral areas. This can result in a genitourinary/urogenital microbiota for microbial communities obtained from urine samples from women, and may lead to unreliable or contaminated taxonomic profiles (Bukavina et al., 2023).

It must be acknowledged that the composition of commensal urinary microbiota remains unclear, as does the case for more thoroughly studied microbial niches like gut microbiota. The issue is further complicated by the absence of an accurate definition of bladder health. The current body of knowledge regarding the makeup of the urogenital microbiota is derived from a relatively small number of publications that favorably portray women. The phylum Firmicutes, which makes up between two thirds and three-quarters of the total phyla composition, dominates the urinary microbiota in both males and females. Actinobacteria, Bacteroidetes, and Proteobacteria are the next most prevalent phyla. Most commonly found genera in the urinary microbiota of healthy adults are members of Lactobacillus, Gardnerella, Prevotella and Streptococcus, as well as some members of Escherichia, Enterococcus, Corynebacterium, Staphylococcus and Proteus.

Attempts to define universal "urotypes" or "community structure types," bacterial communities dominated by single taxa, have so far not resulted in consensus, but have confirmed previously identified genera as major contributors to the composition of urinary microbiota. A research project by Ugarcina Perovic and colleagues. had found significantly higher species-level diversity within the female urinary microbiota, highlighting differences in the techniques used to characterize the bacterial composition of the female urinary microbiota and suggesting that the bacterial diversity of the previous studies was underestimated. It is important to remember that each person's urogenital microbiota is unique and can be impacted by a variety of factors, including age, sex, nutrition, and overall health. Modifications in the endogenous urinary microbiota's composition have been linked to kidney stones, incontinence, bladder cancer, prostate inflammation, and cancer, among other conditions, in addition to the common association with urinary tract infections. Since the majority of this knowledge is derived from high-throughput DNA sequencing projects, conclusions have been made based on DNA fragments rather than actual microorganisms. Thus, when discussing urinary microbiota, it is more accurate to refer to it as the microbiome, or more precisely, the "urobiome." Urobiome has been identified as a contributing factor to the incidence and prevalence of UTIs, one of the most common infections among humans. The etiology of urinary tract infections (UTIs) remains unclear; it could be that bacteria from other bodily niches colonize the urinary tract as a result of disruptions in the urinary microbiota that lead to dysbiosis, or that these are just two sides of the same coin. Thus far, research suggests that uropathogenic *Escherichia coli* (UPEC) is the primary cause of UTIs, accounting for 80% of all cases. Its presence cannot, however, be regarded as the only sign of infection because it can also be found in commensal urinary flora and gut microbiota (Price et al., 2016).

As of right now, the most convincing theory explaining the increase in pathogenicity of E. coli appears to be the crosstalk or interaction between bacteria. coli and additional sly urinary microbiota members. These additional gut microbiota members, *Klebsiella* pneumoniae, *Staphylococcus saprophyticus*, Enterococcus faecalis, and *Proteus mirabilis,* are frequently associated with the etiology of UTIs. It has been proposed that the relative abundance of all these opportunistic pathogens in the gut is a risk factor for UTI development. As the gut is the most prevalent microbiota niche and is strongly associated with UT, it is crucial to enumerate the key distinctions between the two microbial niches, as Table 7.1 below does.

Table 7.1. Key Differences Between Urogenital and Gut Microbiota

Feature	**Characteristics**
Composition	• The urobiome has been observed in several urotypes, usually dominated by a single species or genus. Most common are urotypes dominated by *Lactobacillus*, but identified were also ones dominated by bacteria such as *Gardnerella*, *Prevotella* and *Streptococcus* or without dominant taxa. The urogenital microbiome was also described in several subtypes following similar distribution and composition as the urobiome. • The gut microbiome is significantly more complex, without a single species dominating.
Location	• The urogenital microbiome is found in the female reproductive tract and in the male and female urinary tracts. • The gut microbiome, on the other hand, is found in the gastrointestinal tract.
Function	• The urogenital microbiome plays a critical role in maintaining a healthy vaginal pH and preventing infections, such as urinary tract infections and bacterial vaginosis. • The gut microbiome, in contrast, is involved in digestion and absorption of nutrients, as well as immune system regulation.
Diversity	• Urobiome is less diverse than its intestinal counterpart. It is usually dominated by a single species or genus. • The gut microbiome is much more diverse, with hundreds of different species of microorganisms living in the gut. This diversity is important for maintaining overall health, as disruptions to the gut microbiome have been linked to a variety of health conditions, such as inflammatory bowel disease and obesity.

Source: Čeprnja M, Hadžić E, Oros D, Melvan E, Starcevic A, Zucko J. Current viewpoint on female urogenital microbiome—the cause or the consequence? Microorganisms. 2023; 11(5):1207. https://doi.org/10.3390/microorganisms11051207.

The most notable mechanisms of interaction and virulence factors that can transform commensal bacteria in the urinary tract into pathogenic ones are listed in Table 7.2.

Table 7.2. Five Most Common Examples of Virulence Factors and/or Mechanisms of Interaction That can Turn Otherwise Harmless Urinary Tract Bacteria into Potential Pathogenic Ones

Factor	Characteristics
Adhesion and colonization	Pathogenic bacteria can adhere to and colonize the urinary tract by using surface structures called pili and fimbriae to bind to specific receptors on the epithelial cells that line the urinary tract. This allows the bacteria to establish a foothold in the urinary tract and avoid being flushed out by urine flow.
Biofilm formation	Once pathogenic bacteria have colonized the urinary tract, they can form biofilms, which are dense aggregates of bacteria encased in a matrix of extracellular polymeric substances. Biofilms can protect the bacteria from the host immune system and antimicrobial agents, making them more difficult to eradicate.
Production of toxins	Pathogenic bacteria can produce a range of toxins that can cause damage to host cells and tissues. For example, some strains of E. coli produce hemolysins, which can cause lysis of red blood cells and damage to epithelial cells in the urinary tract.
Type III secretion system	Pathogenic bacteria can also use a type III secretion system (T3SS) to inject effector proteins into host cells, altering their function and contributing to pathogenesis. The T3SS is a specialized protein secretion system that allows the bacteria to directly manipulate host cell signaling pathways, leading to changes in cell morphology, cytokine production and other immune responses.
Antibiotic resistance	Some pathogenic bacteria have acquired resistance to multiple antibiotics, making them more difficult to treat and increasing the risk of recurrent infections.

Source: Čeprnja M, Hadžić E, Oros D, Melvan E, Starcevic A, Zucko J. current viewpoint on female urogenital microbiome—The cause or the consequence? Microorganisms. 2023; 11(5):1207. https://doi.org/10.3390/microorganisms11051207.

7.1.2. Microbial Dynamics in Response to Change in Conditions

Over time, microbial communities undergo changes in response to environmental conditions and internal processes. They adjust their dynamics by altering their composition or modifying gene expression. While system dynamics provides valuable insights, longitudinal studies are essential for a comprehensive understanding of microbiota stability and variability. Limited research has been done on the changes in urogenital microbiota over time, revealing higher variability compared to gut microbiota. These studies have confirmed the dynamics and resilience of the urobiome, identifying menstruation and vaginal intercourse as key factors influencing these changes (Brubaker et al., 2021).

The urobiome's vital role in human health is becoming better understood overall, but its dynamic nature is still unknown. The primary reason for this is that the well-established culture-dependent techniques, which are mostly employed in clinical settings and involve bacterial culture and antibiotic sensitivity testing, are unable to offer the "motion picture" perspective required to document changes in the composition of the microbiome. It is critical to begin utilizing culture-independent techniques in addition to culture-dependent ones, such as 16S rRNA amplicon sequencing and whole-genome shotgun metagenomic sequencing, to completely comprehend the diversity and functionality of this niche microbiome. These techniques help us identify bacteria that are challenging to cultivate with conventional microbiological methods and track changes in the overall composition of the microbiome over time. Next-generation sequencing (NGS) platforms can be used to sequence variable 16S rRNA gene regions by isolating collective DNA from urine samples using specialized purification kits. After that, downstream analysis can be carried out using bioinformatics tools like QIIME2, and taxonomic classification can be carried out using mathematical techniques like the naive Bayes taxonomy classifier against specialized rRNA databases like Silva or Greengenes. The variation seen in biological data that avoids clustering based on distance-based thresholds is represented by the resulting amplicon sequence variants (ASV), which are used as a proxy for taxonomic diversity. It is also feasible to model the dynamics of a microbial community connected to a health problem if several of these analyzes are carried out over time on the same patient samples.

The study of microbiota dynamics has demonstrated the value of mathematical models, and in recent years, several modeling techniques, such as network-based models that deduce species interactions from abundance data, have been put forth to further our comprehension of these dynamics. Cross-sectional co-occurrence data or experimental time series data from microbial communities can be used to infer these interactions. The generalized Lotka-Volterra model (GLVM) is a widely used method for simulating interactions between biological entities. Ordinary differential equation (ODE) systems, such as general linear population models (GLVMs), are useful for simulating pairwise species interactions, including competition, amensalism, and predator-prey dynamics. Using first-order differential equations for predictive and dynamic modeling (e.g., GLVMs) are becoming more common and have given important insights into the dynamics and interactions of microbes. However, the wider application of such methods is limited by the requirement for massive datasets and dense longitudinal sampling (since the number of parameters grows quadratically with the number of species). Since there aren't many longitudinal study data because of funding constraints, moral dilemmas, and other issues, generalized Lotka-Volterra models can be fitted to cross-sectional data from several communities by making a few more assumptions. However, these techniques continue to have statistical and biological drawbacks. Statistically speaking, the relative abundances of species deduced from microbiome sequencing data are not normally distributed and, contrary to initial assumptions, do not take measurement error into account when extrapolated to actual microbiota abundances. From a biological perspective, the suggested methods may incorrectly infer competitive interactions among pairs of taxa when none exist because the negative correlations are not taken into consideration. A Bayesian approach should be used to infer the GLVM parameters from cross-sectional data to resolve these problems (Ravel et al., 2011).

7.1.3. Factors Affecting Microbiota and Host Interactions

The urinary tract's low-biomass community, known as the urinary microbiota, is influenced by both exogenous and UT physiological parameters on bacterial colonization and growth (Figure 7.1).

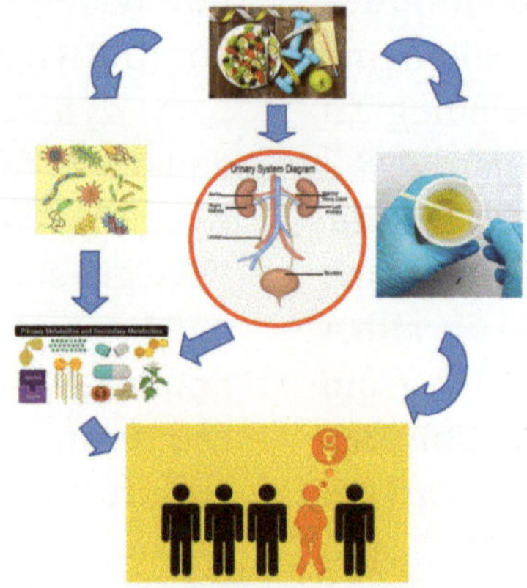

Figure 7.1. *An illustration of interconnected relations between microbiota and host-mediated through host-modifiable parameters such as diet, exercise, hormones, habits and microbiota modifiable parameters such as excreted metabolites and virulence factors, which make a difference between healthy and diseased urotype.*

Source: Čeprnja M, Hadžić E, Oros D, Melvan E, Starcevic A, Zucko J. Current viewpoint on female urogenital microbiome—The cause or the consequence? Microorganisms. 2023; 11(5):1207. https://doi.org/10.3390/microorganisms11051207.

7.1.3.1. Host Part of the Equation

The pH range of urine is normally between 4.5 and 8, with the tendency to be slightly acidic due to metabolic activity. Urine that is more alkaline is associated with diets richer in fruits and vegetables and lower in meat; urine that is more acidic is associated with diets high in proteins and acidic fruits. Oxygen tension: The availability of oxygen is a critical factor in the growth of microorganisms and influences the ecology of the urinary tract microbiota. Recently, there has been a correlation found between the urinary microbiota's composition and the subsequent clinical variables and bladder urine oxygen tension. Urine's specific gravity serves as a gauge for an individual's level of hydration. Research has demonstrated that consuming more water can be a useful preventive measure against recurrent cystitis in premenopausal women who consume low amounts of fluid on a daily basis. The movement of urine through the urinary tract has the ability to flush out bacteria that are either non-attached or weakly adherent, thereby preventing colonization. Urinary tract obstructions, catheterization, and bladder function are some of the factors that can affect urine flow. It is assumed that resident microbes receive nutrients from the flow of fresh urine. Urine composition: By altering the availability of nutrients and other elements that bacteria require to survive and flourish, urine composition, including the presence of urea, electrolytes, and other compounds, can have an effect on bacterial growth and colonization. Numerous soluble substances, such as electrolytes, osmolytes, amino acids, and carbohydrates, are found in human urine. More than 2600 metabolites found in human urine are listed in the Urine Metabolome Database. Urine composition analysis tailored to the patient's needs may be included in a customized combination therapy with antibiotics, antimetabolites, and dietary changes that impact urine composition. Food ingredients that aren't completely digested or absorbed by the body can pass through the urine and have the ability to impact the microbiota in the urine. Here are some examples: Polyphenols—they belong to a group of plant compounds that are found in many foods, including fruits, vegetables, tea, coffee and red wine. Some polyphenols, such as cranberry proanthocyanidins, have been shown to have antimicrobial effects against bacteria in the urinary tract (Ravel et al., 2011).

Food preferences played a major role in the large variations of 34 dietary polyphenols in urinary excretion in the European population. Fructooligosaccharides (FOS), prebiotic fibers, can be found in a variety of foods, such as artichokes, onions, and garlic. Because FOS are not completely broken down by the body, they can enter the colon undigested and encourage the development of good bacteria. Fructooligosaccharides (FOS), galacto-oligosaccharides (GOS), xylo-oligosaccharides (XOS), and lactulose are examples of common prebiotics. Urine may contain a trace amount of FOC. Compounds related to cranberries: Studies have demonstrated the antimicrobial properties of proanthocyanidins and flavonoids against bacteria in the urinary tract. It has been demonstrated that cranberry juice lowers the risk of UTI.

D-mannose is a kind of sugar present in cranberries, peaches, and apples, among other fruits. It has been demonstrated that D-mannose possesses antimicrobial properties against *E. coli*, which is the most frequent cause of mild UTIs. The presence of D-mannose in urine is thought to stop *E. coli* from attaching to the urothelium and thereby preventing infection. Over the past ten years, there has been a general consensus that D-mannose, either by itself or in conjunction with other therapies, may help treat the symptoms of cystitis and UTIs. Probiotics are live microorganisms that have demonstrated potential as innovative treatments for the management and avoidance of urinary tract infections. While more research, particularly clinical trials, is necessary to thoroughly and impartially evaluate their efficacy in treating urological disorders, preliminary findings suggesting the positive impact of multiple Lactobacillus and Bifidobacterium species are heartening. Questions about probiotic strain selection, dosage, administration method, duration of therapy, and interactions with an individual's urotypic still require further investigation (Barrons and Tassone, 2008).

Lastly, sex hormones and secretory immunoglobulins, such as secretory IgA (SIgA), also affect urinary health. The primary role of the antibody SIgA is immune exclusion at mucosal surfaces. This mechanism keeps neutralized antigens from interacting with the epithelium. Controlling the commensal-host symbiotic relationship and preserving the homeostatic regulation of urogenital mucosal epithelia is one of SIgA's other key roles. Sex hormones have been demonstrated to have a significant, if indirect, impact on the dynamics of the urinary microbiota and the microbiota in general. Postmenopausal women have been found to have a higher incidence of rUTIs, as well as a relative decrease in Lactobacillus species abundance and an increase in alpha diversity. These findings may be related to a decrease in estrogen levels both during and after menopause. Hormone replacement therapy was administered to women to treat a variety of urinary symptoms, but it was stopped after its negative effects were discovered. Although using hormonal contraception was linked to a markedly lower risk of bacterial vaginosis, its effect on urinary tract infections is less evident. Furthermore, reports of alterations in microbiota dynamics throughout the menstrual cycle have been made. In conclusion, dietary components like probiotics, polyphenols, fructose, cranberry compounds, D-mannose, and D-mannose have the ability to modify the urinary microbiota and provide positive health outcomes for the host. The endocrine and immune systems of the host also have a significant impact, but more research is required to fully support their use as an alternative treatment for UT disorders.

7.1.3.2. Microbiota Part of the Equation

The urinary microbiota has been found to secrete several molecules that may have health-related effects. For instance, certain bacteria in the urinary tract produce short-chain fatty acids (SCFAs), which can have immune-modulating and anti-inflammatory properties. Research has indicated that the presence of urinary SCFAs may be linked to a lower incidence of UTIs and other UTI-related conditions. SCFAs are crucial for gut health. The migration of immune cells, the synthesis of cytokines, and the preservation of cellular homeostasis are all facilitated by SCFAs. Additionally, there is mounting evidence that SCFAs influence the interaction between the intestinal microbiota and urinary tract infections (UTIs) and play a significant role in the gut-bladder and gut-vagina-bladder axis crosstalk (Bukavina et al., 2023).

7.1.4. Bladder as a Bioreactor

The bladder is similar to a bioreactor in that it performs a simplified function similar to that of a vessel used to temporarily store urine before being voided and refilled. All of those need to be in the ideal range for the urinary tract to operate normally and preserve homeostasis. Similar conditions apply to bioreactor settings: proper temperature, nutrient supply, and oxygenation are necessary for the growth of microorganisms or cells. Contaminant microorganisms or undesirable, hazardous substances can have an impact on both a bioreactor and a bladder. Pathogenic bacteria in the bladder can lead to infections and other disorders of the urinary tract, while impurities in a bioreactor can hinder the growth and function of the material being processed. One must highlight the two in terms of their design, function, and relationship to the surroundings (Figure 7.2).

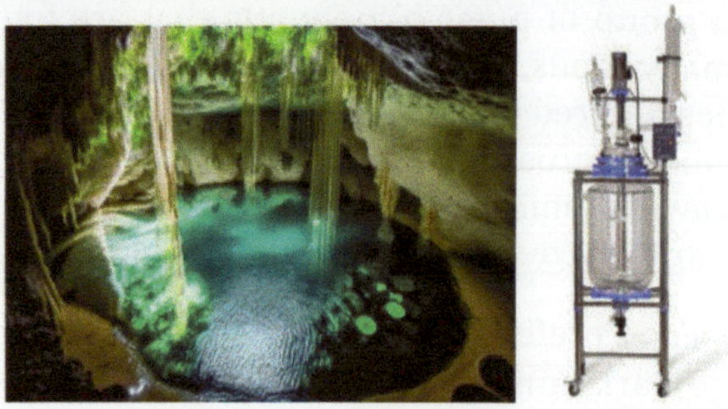

Figure 7.2. *An AI-made illustration of a natural phenomenon—a Cenote, surface connection to subterranean water bodies, usually represented by small sheltered sites with no surface exposed water containing small numbers of bacteria, next to a stirred jacket glass bioreactor.*

Source:Čeprnja M, Hadžić E, Oros D, Melvan E, Starcevic A, Zucko J. Current viewpoint on female urogenital microbiome—the cause or the consequence? Microorganisms. 2023; 11(5):1207. https://doi.org/10.3390/microorganisms11051207.

Although the bladder is a naturally occurring organ and a component of the human body, a bioreactor is an artificial apparatus made for a particular use that includes simulating the bladder. While a bioreactor is usually isolated from the outside world and built to reduce interference from outside sources, a bladder is subject to biological processes and interactions, contained within the host organism, and as such, much harder to isolate from the surrounding tissues. In terms of function, we have to concede that a bioreactor has a wider range of applications. The goal of developing a bioengineered bladder reactor is to eventually replace the human bladder with one that is fully functional. Systems akin to those created for the human gut microbiota may one day be developed and used to reveal the dynamics of the residential urobiome, its interactions with the vaginal and gut microbiota, and its function in defense against urinary tract infections and other urinary conditions. This is conceivable given the advancements in technology and tissue engineering. Urinary system microbiota presents unique challenges for in vitro systems due to its low biomass and single species prevalence in composition. However, if successful, these efforts may provide insights into the real-time dynamics of the urobiome in relation to exogenous and endogenous conditions, as well as better solutions for a healthy urinary system (Brubaker et al., 2021).

7.1.5. Food and Drugs Administration in Relation to Urinary Health

7.1.5.1. Probiotics and Urogenital Microbiota

Probiotics have a variety of therapeutic benefits, depending on the strain. Probiotic bacteria have an impact on several health issues, including immune system modification, cholesterol reduction, lactose intolerance relief, Crohn's disease relief or even remission, diarrhea prevention, and urogenital infection prevention. At the genus level, Lactobacillus is the most prevalent urotype, followed by Gardnerella, Corynebacterium, Streptococcus, and Staphylococcus. These are all Gram-positive bacteria, as opposed to the Gram-negative bacteria that cause most acute, mild urinary tract infections. Changes in the distribution of the urogenital microbiota bacteria can result in infections, but lactobacilli, the predominant bacteria of the vaginal flora, have antimicrobial qualities that regulate other urogenital microbiota. It is proposed that the restoration of the urogenital microbiota through the application of probiotics, especially those lactobacilli-based ones, has the potential to prevent and stop urinary tract infections because lactobacilli predominate in the urogenital flora of healthy women and play a protective role. Probiotic strains *Lactobacillus rhamnosus* GR-1 and *Lactobacillus reuteri* RC-14 (formerly known as Lactobacillus fermentum RC-14) appear to have promise for the treatment and prevention of urinary tract infections (UTIs), according to research conducted over the past 20 years. Furthermore, research has demonstrated the efficacy of *Lactocaseibacillus casei* Shirota and *L. crispatus* CTV-05 in a small percentage of instances.

Research suggests that probiotics like *L. rhamnosus* GR-1 and *L. reuteri* may be effective in preventing or treating bacterial vaginosis, vulvovaginal candidiasis, and urinary tract infections in women. Studies have shown that oral administration of *Lacticaseibacillus rhamnosus* GR-1 and *Limosilactobacillus fermentum* RC-14 for 60 days had no harmful effects and helped restore a healthy vaginal microbiota. Additionally, probiotics have been found to establish a healthy urogenital microbiota in up to 90% of participants, but the correct dosage is crucial. Probiotics have been shown to have a significant impact on urinary system health by reducing the colonization of potentially harmful bacteria and fungi in the vagina. Lactobacilli may achieve this by producing lactic acid, lowering the pH of the environment, adhering to the vaginal epithelium to prevent pathogen attachment, and competing for nutrients to limit pathogen growth (Pendharkar et al., 2013).

7.1.5.2. Prebiotics and Urogenital Microbiota

There is currently a dearth of research on the direct effects of prebiotics on urogenital tract health, and the only way to establish a connection with a healthy urogenital microbiota is indirectly, through prebiotics' influence on gut-dwelling beneficial bacteria. Prebiotic supplementation with the goal of increasing lactobacilli abundance in the gut may benefit the urinary tract because the presence of Escherichia and Enterococcus in the gut is a risk factor for the development of UTIs.

Combining synergistic probiotics and prebiotics would be the other, more direct way to boost the number of lactobacilli in the gut. *LimosiLactobacillus reuteri* metabolizes glycerol into the antimicrobial compound 3-HPA or reuterin, which inhibits pathogens like *Salmonella typhimurium*, *Escherichia coli*, and *Clostridium difficile*. The concentration of glucose affects the excretion of reuterin in addition to the availability of glycerol. Arabinose, cellobiose, esculin, ribose, sorbitol, and sucrose are examples of a synergistic effect involving a prebiotic that promotes the growth of *Lacticaseibacillus rhamnosus*, which subsequently produces the L-lactic acid isomer and ferments carbohydrates. In this instance, prebiotics are carbohydrates that the host is unable to digest and that intestinal probiotics can enzymatically break down. Although it is well known that the two most researched prebiotics, galacto-oligosaccharides (GOS) and inulin, promote the growth of a variety of lactobacilli, more recent research also suggests that prebiotics should be customized.

7.1.5.3. Antibiotics and Urinary Tract Infections

Numerous antibiotics, including Amoxicillin, Ceftriaxone, Cephalexin, Ciprofloxacin, Fosfomycin, Levofloxacin, Nitrofurantoin, and Trimethoprim/sulfamethoxazole, are prescribed for the treatment of urinary tract infections. The length of antibiotic treatment ranges from 3 to 14 days, depending on how serious the infection is. More and more studies are being conducted to determine the benefits and drawbacks of shorter vs. extended treatment periods, probiotic supplementation, and the potential replacement of antibiotics with probiotics. According to some research, there are no appreciable differences between taking antibiotics for three to six days or for seven to fourteen days. Reduced native lactobacilli are a common indicator of vaginal infections, and antimicrobial therapy frequently falls short of fully curing cystitis symptoms. Research has validated the theory that probiotics, such as *Lactobacillus rhamnosus* GR-1 and Liposo *Lactobacillus reuteri* RC-14, can increase the cure rate and function as an adjuvant to antibiotic therapy. In a different study, each participant group received a probiotic and a placebo in addition to the antibiotic treatment. In contrast to the group receiving an antibiotic and placebo, which had a cure rate of 50%, the experimental group taking probiotics along with antibiotics experienced an 87.5% cure rate. According to a study, probiotic lactobacilli can also make pharmaceutical agents more effective in fighting fungal infections when used to treat urogenital disorders.

7.1.5.4. Nutrition and Healthy Urogenital Microbiota

Certain foods can help prevent or lessen UTI symptoms, even though antibiotics are typically prescribed to treat UTIs. Among these foods are cranberries and cranberry juice. Studies have demonstrated that by stopping bacteria from sticking to the bladder walls, cranberries and cranberry juice can help prevent and treat UTIs. It might be beneficial to take cranberry supplements or drink only pure cranberry juice. By boosting the quantity of good bacteria in the stomach, probiotics can aid in gastrointestinal and urinary tract health. Probiotic-rich foods include kefir, yogurt, sauerkraut, and kimchi. UTIs can be avoided by taking even easy steps, like drinking lots of water, which helps wash out bacteria from the urinary tract. Some spices, like garlic, have antibacterial qualities that can aid in the treatment of bacterial infections. To avoid UTIs, including garlic in the diet or taking supplements may be helpful. Additionally, certain vitamins, like vitamin C, can help urine become more acidic, which can inhibit the growth of bacteria. Vitamin C-rich foods include bell peppers, oranges, strawberries, and kiwi fruit. It is crucial to remember that although these foods might aid in preventing or treating UTIs, they shouldn't be used in place of medical care. Eating a diet high in nutrients and adhering to the healthy diet pyramid is advised for the urinary tract's well-being. Other than cranberries and other fruits high in vitamin C and other antioxidants, a general recommendation seems to be to eat whole grains, sweet potatoes, and similar foods high in fiber that support the control of insulin resistance, as well as leafy vegetables for supporting vaginal moisture and probiotics in particular. Examples of foods that support probiotics, particularly Lactobacillus, include yogurt with live cultures, pickles and sauerkraut, Kimchi (a traditional Korean dish of pickled vegetables and sauerkraut), Miso (a Japanese seasoning made from fermented soybeans), Tempeh (a traditional Indonesian dish made from fermented soy and starter culture), and Kombucha (a Chinese tea made through yeast fermentation).

7.2. Urinary Tract Infection in Women

One of the most common infections that affect women at different stages of life is urinary tract infections, or UTIs. Because of the anatomy of the female lower urinary tract and its close proximity to the reproductive organs, women are far more susceptible to UTIs than men. Because the female urethra is shorter than the male, bacteria cannot enter the body as far. It also opens into the vestibule of the vulvar, i.e., an organ that, considering the frequency of vulvar vestibulitis and vaginitis, is also highly susceptible to infections. In this instance, the natural vaginal microbiome is frequently interfered with by sexual activity and excessive use of personal hygiene products. Conversely, the close proximity of the anus promotes the colonization of the reproductive organs and the distal urinary tract by Streptococcus species, Enterococcus fecalis, and Escherichia coli. Other distinctive periods that are characterized by recurrent UTIs are pregnancy and the perinatal period. An additional risk factor is the rise in perioperative catheterizations and cesarean sections. Falling estrogen levels during the postmenopausal era disrupt the vaginal epithelium, causing it to gradually atrophy, while a lack of glycogen lowers the number of lactic acid bacteria. Because of this, other bacteria, mostly *Escherichia coli*, frequently colonize the post-menopausal vagina, which has the potential to spread and infect the urinary tract. Frequent UTIs are also associated with urinary incontinence and pelvic organ prolapse. It is estimated that between 30 and 50% of women over 50 are impacted by these. Every other woman is expected to have experienced at least one UTI in her lifetime, with 10–60% of all women reporting symptoms at some point. As people age, their risk of infection rises (Ikäheimo et al., 1996).

7.2.1. Diagnosis

All cases of UTI can be categorized as either asymptomatic or symptomatic. Asymptomatic UTIs are identified through urinalysis results, with precise sample collection being vital due to the position of the external urethral opening in women. The number of leukocytes is the primary factor in UTI diagnosis; a count exceeding 10 leukocytes/mm3 indicates an infection, while in pregnant patients, the threshold is higher at 20 leukocytes/mm3. Contamination of the sample by vaginal secretions can lead to inaccurate diagnoses such as multiple mucus threads and abundant bacterial growth in urine sediment, or even a false diagnosis of proteinuria due to mucus presence. Menstruation, postpartum bleeding, or other uterine bleeding can contaminate the sample with red blood cells, necessitating a thorough patient history and a carefully conducted repeat analysis. Urinalysis findings without corresponding symptoms are insufficient to start treatment; a urine culture may be required to confirm or rule out a UTI. The culture sample should be collected in a sterile container, preferably from the first morning urine, to prevent contamination. A UTI is confirmed by the presence of ≥ 105 colony-forming units per milliliter (CFU/mL), and an antibiogram can help assess the effectiveness of a specific treatment.

Treatment should start if there are elevated leukocyte values in the urine sediment and clinical symptoms. Due to the higher risk of premature birth linked to UTIs and the limited number of antibiotic treatment options that are safe to use while pregnant, it is advised to obtain a culture sample from the patient at the beginning of treatment. Even so, typical symptoms will point to the need for medical attention. In up to 90% of young women, the presence of typical UTI symptoms—such as burning in the vulvar vestibule and abnormal vaginal discharge—leads to the confirmation of infection. 15% of cases have elevated leukocyte counts in the urinalysis, but the urine cultures come back positive.

7.2.2. Characteristic Patient Groups

The primary causes of the higher incidence of UTIs in perimenopausal and postmenopausal women are aging connective tissues (pelvic organ prolapse, urinary incontinence) and hormonal changes (estrogen insufficiency). Urinary incontinence, which makes it difficult to maintain good hygiene, atrophy of the vaginal mucous membranes, which raises the possibility of vaginal infections spreading to the urinary tract, and anterior vaginal prolapse, which prevents full bladder voiding, are all risk factors for UTIs during the perimenopausal stage. In contrast to 10.5% in premenopausal women, the prevalence of asymptomatic bacteriuria rises in the peri- and postmenopausal era, reaching levels of 4–19%. Urinary incontinence and urinary tract infections can both be associated with estrogen deficiency in women going through menopause and beyond. It has been demonstrated that topical application of estrogens to the vagina (but not the systemic body) significantly lowers the risk of bacteriuria (OR = 0.3; 95% CI: 0.13–0.68). Guidelines released by research associations also advise topical estrogen use as a preventative measure against UTIs in perimenopausal and postmenopausal patients (Anger et al 2019).

For postmenopausal women, diabetes is a major risk factor for UTIs. Research involving 256,725 females with type 2 diabetes revealed that UTI diagnoses were much more common beginning in the 45–49 age range. The difference was as high as 100% in this age range and an additional 80% in the 50–54 age range. In another study, 901 diabetic patients and 913 controls, two groups of women aged 55 to 75 who had been diagnosed with an acute UTI, were compared. Diabetes was found to double the risk of UTI in postmenopausal women (OR = 2.2; 95% CI: 1.5–3.1). Type 2 diabetes (OR = 2.2) and oral medication or insulin therapy (OR 2.8 and 2.7, respectively) were significant factors. Glycated hemoglobin HbA1c levels, which measure the duration of the disease and the control of glycemia, did not show any significant correlation. Having surgery is another risk factor for UTIs in patients who are 57 years of age or older.

Uncontrolled diabetes mellitus, in particular, increases the risk of urinary tract infections as well as infections of the reproductive tract (vulva, vulvar vestibule, and/or vagina). UTIs are diagnosed in 23% of women with type 2 diabetes and 14% of women with type 1 diabetes. The two most important risk factors in this group are glycosuria and glucose regulation. Additionally, perimenopausal patients with longer disease duration have higher rates of infections. Increased prevalence was found for acute cystitis (OR = 1.46; 95% CI: 1.10–1.95; $p = 0.001$), acute vaginitis (OR = 1.20; 95% CI: 1.01–1.42; $p = 0.044$), and acute vulvitis (OR = 2.12; 95% CI: 1.56–2.90; $p < 0.001$) in a well-documented trial with 1357 female patients with type 1 diabetes. The most important risk factors for symptomatic infections in a group of 241 type 1 diabetic women were microangiopathy, oral contraceptive use, and sexual activity. Another possible contributing factor could be urinary incontinence, which is more common in female diabetics than in the general population (OR = 1.64; 95% CI: 1.19–2.26; $p = 0.001$). Asymptomatic bacteriuria is more common in type 2 diabetes patients than in healthy controls (17.5% vs. 10%, with $p = 0.015$). In 20% of cases, asymptomatic bacteriuria may develop into a symptomatic UTI within six months. Another study that included 348 women with type 2 diabetes found that the main risk factor for getting a symptomatic infection was also asymptomatic bacteriuria. Decreased renal function could also result from it. Based on the information that is currently available, it is advised that diabetic patients, especially those with type 2 diabetes, have regular urine cultures.

Patients with epilepsy were also found to need more frequent treatment for UTIs than people in general; approximately 58% of women and 42% of people with epilepsy were affected by the issue ($p < 0.0001$). Anti-epileptic medications were found to be the primary factor contributing to the higher incidence of UTIs in this group after a thorough investigation of the causes. Patients taking phenytoin (OR = 1.78; 95% CI: 1.24–2.55; $p = 0.001$), primidone (OR = 1.73; 95% CI: 1.21–2.49; $p = 0.002$), carbamazepine (OR = 1.61; 95% CI: 1.33–1.96; $p < 0.0001$), and valproate (OR = 1.52; 95% CI: 1.28–1.82; $p < 0.0001$) experienced a higher frequency of urinary tract infections. This is likely because these medications have immunomodulating effects. According to the aforementioned research, patients with epilepsy who experience recurrent UTIs should have their therapies carefully planned.

Patients who require intermittent self-catheterization or who have an indwelling urinary catheter are another group at increased risk for urinary tract infections. In that group of patients, UTIs affect 15% to 86% of them more than once a year; use of antiseptic products likely lowers the risk.

Urinary tract infections could also be more common during the perioperative phase. Additional risk factors in this case include age above 57–60 years, diabetes, immunosuppressant therapy, obesity, and iatrogenic blood transfusions. When patients with a diagnosis of asymptomatic bacteriuria are catheterized for surgery, the risk of a symptomatic infection developing is significantly decreased when antibiotics are administered preventatively (RR = 0.20; 95% CI: 0.13–0.31). Because of the anatomy of their reproductive systems, most surgeries involving female patients require catheterization. After block anesthesia, the catheter may remain in place for a few hours in the case of cesarean sections, but it usually remains in place for about 24 hours during gynecological procedures. However, surgical corrections of pelvic organ prolapse are an exception, sometimes necessitating a two- to three-day catheter stay (Zhou et al., 2007).

Pregnancy is associated with several risk factors for UTIs, including more basic urine, increased risk of urine flow obstruction (particularly toward the end of pregnancy), proteinuria, diabetes, and anemia. Urinalysis sample collection is more challenging, especially during the third trimester, when vaginal secretions often contaminate the sample with bacteria and proteins that do not necessarily indicate an infection. While protein may come from mucus contamination, it also indicates proteinuria, a sign of preeclampsia, in hypertensive patients. If an elevated leukocyte count is not present along with multiple bacteria in the field of view during urine sediment analysis, the bacteria are most likely lactic acid bacteria. This is important information for making a differential diagnosis of urinary tract infection (UTI) in pregnant patients. UTIs that cause no symptoms affect 2–8% of expectant mothers. Other sources state that up to 50–60% of pregnant women are diagnosed with UTIs, making them the most common infections during pregnancy. The findings of the study point to a higher incidence of preterm birth linked to asymptomatic bacteriuria. Due to the higher diagnosis rate of UTI in women with gestation-induced hypertension, there is a correlation between the illness and a higher risk of intrauterine growth restriction, preterm birth, and cesarean delivery. But keep in mind that a diagnosis of UTI does not automatically require a particular kind of obstetric intervention. One in four pregnant women with UTIs have recurrent infections, and in 4–5 of those cases, pyelonephritis develops. 30% of pregnant women who had UTIs also had a significant risk of their child getting UTIs as well. 68.8% (OR = 5.9% at 95% Confidence Interval: 1.9%–18.3%; p = 0.001).

7.2.3. Bacteria Identification Key to Therapy Selection

Research examining the types of pathogens responsible for UTIs in individuals without diabetes had *Escherichia coli* (69%), *Enterococcus* sp. 10%), bacteria *Klebsiella* sp. (4 percent), *Proteus* sp., and *Pseudomonas aeruginosa* (4 percent). 4%), along with *Staphylococcus* species. (2 percent) as the bacteria that are most common. *Escherichia coli* (71%), *Klebsiella* spp. (6 percent), *Staphylococcus* spp. (5 percent), and *Enterococcus* spp. (4 percent) were the most common pathogens found in diabetic patients. Urinary tract infections in pregnant women are typically caused by the bacteria *Escherichia coli* (30–90%), Staphylococcus bacteria (4–32%), *Proteus mirabilis* (10.2%), *Enterococcus faecalis* (1–8.1%), and *Klebsiella pneumoniae* (6.1–9.1%). The most prevalent pathogens in infants were *Staphylococci* (9.8%), *Escherichia coli* (65.9%), and *Klebsiella* (14.6%).

7.2.4. Antibiotic Treatment

Antibiotic dosages proposed by international associations are included in the Table 7.3.

Table 7.3. Proposed Antibiotic Dosage

Indication	Antibiotic	Dosage	Treatment Duration
Prophylaxis in asymptomatic bacteriuria; continuous treatment	Trimethoprim	100 mg 1 × a day	
	Trimethoprim + sulfamethoxazole	40–200 mg 1 × a day 40–200 mg 3 × a week	
	Nitrofurantoin	50–100 mg a day	

	Cephalexin	125–250 mg 1 × a day	
	Fosfomycin	3 γ every 10 days	
Prophylaxis in asymptomatic bacteriuria; periodic treatment	Trimethoprim + sulfamethoxazole	40/200 mg 80/400 mg	
	Nitrofurantoin	50–100 mg	
	Cephalexin	250 mg	
Uncomplicated cystitis	Fosfomycin	3 g	For 1 day
	Nitrofurantoin	50–100 mg a day	For 5 days
	Extended-release nitrofurantoin	100 mg 2 × a day	For 5 days
	Pivampicillin	400 mg 3 × a day	For 3–5 days
	Cephalosporins	500 mg 2 × a day	For 3 days
	Trimethoprim + sulfamethoxazole	80/400 mg 2 × a day	For 3 days
	Trimethoprim	100 mg 2 × a day	For 3–5 days
Complicated cystitis	Ciprofloxacin	500–750 mg 2 × a day	For 7 days
	Levofloxacin	750 mg a day	For 5 days
	Trimethoprim + sulfamethoxazole	160/800 mg 2 × a day	For 14 days
	Cefpodoxime	200 mg 2 × a day	For 10 days
	Ceftibuten	400 mg a day	For 10 days
Pyelonephritis, parenteral therapy 1st line of treatment	Ciprofloxacin	400 mg 2 × a day	
	Levofloxacin	750 mg a day	
	Cefotaxime	2 γ 3 × a day	

	Ceftriaxone	1–2 γ a day	
Pyelonephritis, parenteral therapy 2nd line of treatment	Cefepime	1–2 γ 2 × a day	
	Piperacillin/ tazobactam	2.5–4.5 γ 3 × a day	
	Gentamycin	5 mg/kg a day	
	Amikacin	15 mg/kg a day	

Source: https://www.ncbi.nlm.nih.gov/pmc/articles/PMC8077804/table/T1/?report=objectonly.

Pregnant patients who exhibit asymptomatic bacteriuria should receive targeted treatment, which necessitates a urine culture antibiogram before starting any medication. Treatment should start in acute cases while the results of the culture are being obtained. For pregnant patients, cephalosporins are the recommended medication. Kashif along with others advise exercising extra caution when administering augmentin (fetal tissue necrotizing enterocolitis has been reported in the third trimester), trimethoprim (folic acid antagonist), and nitrofurantoin to expectant mothers due to the possibility of hemolytic disease of the fetus. To ensure that the treatment is working, a follow-up urine culture should be taken seven to ten days after the end of the course. An effective substitute for treatment is single-dose fosfomycin. Its efficacy was demonstrated to be comparable to other antibiotics in a 2020 meta-analysis, and it was found to be highly safe for both pregnant and non-pregnant patients (Barrons et al., 2008).

Research by Malmartel and colleagues examined the frequency of bacteria that are resistant to antibiotics and cause UTIs. Table 7.4 displays data indicating that patients with diabetes had a slightly higher resistance to ofloxacin and cefixime.

Table 7.4. Percentage of Strains Resistant to Selected Antibiotics

Antibiotic	**Percentage of Resistant Strains**	
	In Study by Malmartel	**According to NICE Guidelines**
Ofloxacin	10.8%	–
Cefixime	3.8%	9.9%
Trimethoprim, sulfamethoxazole	16.8%	30.3%
Nitrofurantoin	4.05%	2.5%
Fosfomycin	3.2%	–
Pivampicillin	–	7.5%

Source: https://www.ncbi.nlm.nih.gov/pmc/articles/PMC8077804/table/T2/?report=objectonly.

7.2.5. Non-Antibiotic Prophylactic Treatment – Immunomodulation

The medication OM-89 is immunomodulatory. It works well against *Escherichia coli* infections, which account for 70–80% of urinary tract infections. After receiving OM-89 treatment for six months, women with recurrent UTIs had a twofold lower chance of subsequent recurrence (67.3% vs. 32.7%). On the other hand, uncontrolled diabetes greatly diminished the effectiveness of treatment. Following a 3-month initial treatment course and a 10-day booster course of OM-89, a 34% reduction in urinary tract infections was noted in a multi-center, double-blind study involving 453 women. In a retrospective analysis of 79 patients, the primary pathogen was found to be *Escherichia coli* in 49% of the cases, despite the same treatment regimen being used. 53% of the total population and 63% of individuals with *Escherichia coli* infections responded well to treatment.

Menopausal women who participated in the study also confirmed the effectiveness of OM-89. A group of patients, average age 66, participated in a clinical trial. After the immunomodulatory treatment, the group's recurrent infection rate decreased by 65%, from 3.4 to 1.8.

The European Association of Urology (EAU) and the Polish Association of Urology both advise OM-89 oral immunomodulatory treatment for the prevention of recurrent urinary tract infections in women with simple UTIs. The course of treatment lessens the likelihood of antibiotic resistance, patient symptoms, and the frequency of recurrent infections. For a duration of ninety days, OM-89 is taken once daily, prior to meals, to prevent recurrent UTIs. Due to the medication's ability to strongly stimulate the immune system against both E. coli and other pathogens that cause urinary tract infections, it can be used in conjunction with antibiotic therapy during the acute phase of an infection without the need for prior urine culture results (Ikäheimo et al., 1996).

The strongest level of evidence of any non-antibiotic strategy for preventing UTIs is associated with OM-89.

7.2.6. Other Non-Antibiotic Methods of Prevention

Cranberry juice has been demonstrated in vitro experiments to decrease the adherence of *Escherichia coli* bacteria to the vaginal epithelium and urinary tract. The symptoms that the patients were experiencing due to bacterial irritation should therefore be alleviated. However, decreased symptom levels do not mean that the infection has been eradicated. There was no statistically significant difference in the prevalence of urinary tract infections (UTTIs) diagnosed by urine cultures between the groups that drank cranberry juice and the placebo in prospective randomized trials involving women between the ages of 18 and 45. A Cochrane analysis released in 2012 came to similar conclusions.

An additional difficulty is treating persistent UTIs and avoiding future recurrences. It was discovered that D-mannose effectively inhibits the adherence of bacteria to the urinary tract epithelium, thereby preventing recurrent UTIs. A meta-analysis with eight papers in total was published in 2020, but the final conclusions relied on data from only sixteen three patients. Although the results are encouraging, more research is required to establish the ideal dosage and length of treatment.

7.2.7. Antibiotic Prophylaxis

For women who have recurrent UTIs, some physicians advise long-term prophylactic antibiotic use. Positive results of prophylactic antibiotic use were shown by a Cochrane meta-analysis in young women with recurrent UTIs. Findings released by Ahmed et al., however, indicate that patients 65 years of age and older who received long-term antibiotic prophylaxis only saw favorable results when the treatment lasted longer than two years. Trimethoprim, cephalexin, or nitrofurantoin were given to the patients. Treatment decreased the need for additional antibiotic prescriptions (OR = 0.61; 95% CI: 0.59–0.62) and the frequency of recurrent symptomatic urinary tract infections (OR = 0.57; 95% CI: 0.55–0.59). Simultaneously, there was a slight but statistically significant rise in UTI-related hospitalizations (OR = 1.16; 95% CI: 1.05–1.28).

7.3. Pelvic Inflammatory Disease (PID)

An infection of one or more of the upper reproductive organs, such as the uterus, fallopian tubes, and ovaries, is known as pelvic inflammatory disease (PID). If left untreated, the reproductive tract may develop abscesses—pockets of infected fluid—and scar tissue that could be permanently damaging.

Symptoms of pelvic inflammatory disease can range from subtle to mild, with some women not experiencing any symptoms at all. This means that you may not be aware of the condition until you face difficulties with fertility or suffer from persistent pelvic discomfort.

7.3.1. Symptoms

Pelvic inflammatory disease can have subtle, hard-to-diagnose signs and symptoms. Some women exhibit no symptoms at all. When signs and symptoms of pelvic inflammatory disease (PID) are present, they most often include:

- Pain—ranging from mild to severe—in your lower abdomen and pelvis
- Unusual or heavy vaginal discharge that may have an unpleasant odor
- Unusual bleeding from the vagina, especially during or after sex, or between periods
- Pain during sex
- Fever, sometimes with chills
- Painful, frequent or difficult urination

7.3.2. Causes

PID can be caused by a wide variety of bacteria, but gonorrhea or chlamydia infections are the most prevalent. Most often, these bacteria are picked up through unprotected sex.

Less frequently, bacteria can enter your reproductive tract whenever the cervix's natural barrier is compromised. This may occur throughout the menstrual cycle, following childbirth, miscarriage, or abortion. In rare cases, bacteria can also enter the reproductive system through any medical procedure that involves putting instruments inside the uterus, such as the implantation of an intrauterine device (IUD), a long-term birth control method (Anger et al., 2019).

7.3.3. Risk Factors

Several factors might increase your risk of pelvic inflammatory disease, including:

- Being sexually active and younger than 25 years old
- Having multiple sexual partners
- Being in a sexual relationship with someone who has more than one sex partner
- Having sex without a condom
- Douching regularly, which upsets the balance of good versus harmful bacteria in the vagina and might mask symptoms
- Having a history of pelvic inflammatory disease or a sexually transmitted infection

After the implantation of an intrauterine device (IUD), there is a slight increase in the risk of PID. Usually, this risk is limited to the first three weeks following insertion.

7.3.4. Complications

If pelvic inflammatory disease is left untreated, the reproductive tract may develop scar tissue and pockets of infected fluid, or abscesses. These have the potential to permanently harm reproductive organs.

Complications from this damage might include:

- **Ectopic Pregnancy:** This is caused by scar tissue in the fallopian tubes, causing the fertilized egg to not be able to pass through the tube and implant in the uterus.
- **Infertility:** This is caused by direct damage to the reproductive organs. The likelihood of infertility increases with the number of episodes of PID the patient has.
- **Chronic Pelvic Pain:** This can persist for several months or even years. Pain during ovulation and sexual activity can be the result of scarring of the fallopian tubes and other pelvic organs.
- **Tubo-Ovarian Abscess:** These can form in the uterus or other pelvic organs, but usually affect the ovaries and fallopian tubes. If an abscess is not treated, a life-threatening infection can result.

7.3.5. Prevention

To reduce the risk of pelvic inflammatory disease:

- Practice safe sex.
- Talk with health care provider about contraception.
- Get tested.
- Test partner
- Don't douche

7.4. Bacterial Vaginosis

An overabundance of the normal vaginal flora leads to the illness known as bacterial vaginosis. The most typical clinical presentation for this is increased, fishy-smelling vaginal discharge. Usually, the discharge is thin and appears white or gray. Patients who have been diagnosed with bacterial vaginosis are more likely to contract STIs, and pregnant patients may experience an earlier delivery risk. *Gardnerella vaginitis*, the previous name for bacterial vaginosis, was used to attribute the illness exclusively to Gardnerella bacteria. On the other hand, the term "bacterial vaginosis" more correctly refers to the possible proliferation of different anaerobic bacteria within the vaginal environment. Bacterial vaginosis is primarily caused by this imbalance. The fact that it is now called bacterial vaginosis emphasizes the knowledge that various naturally occurring bacteria in the vagina may multiply excessively, resulting in this illness.

Bacterial vaginosis is usually caused by an overabundance of anaerobic bacteria in the vagina and a decrease in lactobacilli that produce hydrogen peroxide. But the exact cause of bacterial vaginosis, which is caused by the growth of anaerobic bacteria like Gardnerella, is still unknown. Although *Gardnerella vaginalis* is not usually thought to be contagious, it is still unknown how widely it can spread. Sexual activity-related transmission of this bacteria could upset the normal bacterial balance in the vagina. This unbalance fosters the unchecked development of opportunistic anaerobic bacteria, such as *G. vaginalis*, which may lead to bacterial vaginosis (Popa et al., 1996).

Up to 50% of asymptomatic women had *G. vaginalis* found in their vaginal tracts, according to studies, indicating that it is probably a normal part of the vaginal flora. Numerous factors, such as frequent bathing, douching, smoking, having multiple sexual partners, using over-the-counter intravaginal hygiene products, being under a lot of stress, and having more frequent sexual activity, can lead to the development of bacterial vaginosis. It has been noted that females who mate with other females may transfer *G. vaginalis* through shared sex toys or direct contact of the mucous membranes. It has been demonstrated that a woman who has a female sexual partner increases her risk of bacterial vaginosis by 60%.

7.4.1. History and Physical

Many women with bacterial vaginosis experience smelly vaginal discharge, which can worsen after sex. Other symptoms may include painful urination, painful intercourse, and vaginal itching. However, some women may not show any symptoms. It's important for the healthcare provider to ask about risk factors such as vaginal douching, multiple sexual partners, recent antibiotic use, smoking, and the use of an intrauterine device when assessing a history of bacterial vaginosis infections (Deese et al, 2018).

To identify the features of the vaginal discharge and rule out other conditions that could present similarly, such as vaginal candidiasis, cervicitis, chlamydia, gonorrhea, herpes simplex virus, and trichomoniasis, a comprehensive physical examination should include a pelvic exam. Furthermore, HIV, other STIs, pelvic inflammatory disease, and other obstetric disorders are all at risk due to bacterial vaginosis. To rule out the more serious conditions that are still on the differential diagnosis list, it is crucial to check for fever, pelvic pain, and a history of sexually transmitted infections.

It is possible to send cervical swabs to test for gonorrhea or chlamydia infection. Cervical friability and cervical motion tenderness should also be evaluated. Self-collected swabs and swabs taken without a speculum exam have shown to be unreliable in the diagnosis of bacterial vaginosis and ought to be avoided. Similarly, pap smears, culture, and history by themselves are not accurate ways to diagnose bacterial vaginosis and ought to be avoided.

The vaginal discharge can be examined under a microscope because clue cells are a dependable diagnostic indicator of bacterial vaginosis. This diagnostic procedure can also aid in ruling out the existence of trichomonads or yeast. It is crucial to remember that a lot of these illnesses can coexist, so even if another pathology is discovered initially, the entire specimen needs to be examined for clue cells. The diagnosis of bacterial vaginosis can also be aided by testing the pH of the vaginal fluid.

7.4.2. Evaluation

A vaginal discharge swab is usually used to suggest the diagnosis of bacterial vaginosis, which is then confirmed by developing a wet mount slide that can be examined under a microscope. A positive whiff test result, clue cells on a wet mount, and a higher than normal vaginal pH (>4.5) may all be signs of bacterial vaginosis in the swab sample. pH paper can be used to measure the vaginal pH and compared to color controls. To find clue cells, a drop of sodium chloride (NaCl) solution is applied to the wet mount slide. To see the distinctive clue cells, the slide is examined under a microscope after being covered with a cover slip. Clue cells are cervix epithelial cells that have rod-shaped bacteria embedded in them.

To conduct the whiff test, a tiny amount of potassium hydroxide (KOH) is added to the microscopic slide that holds the vaginal discharge. If a distinct fishy smell is detected, the whiff test is positive. The presence of the distinctive discharge combined with two of these positive tests is usually sufficient to confirm the diagnosis of bacterial vaginosis. To make the diagnosis, all three of these requirements must be met if there is no discharge (Toh et al., 2017).

In clinical settings, the Amsel criteria are frequently used to diagnose bacterial vaginosis. To confirm the diagnosis, at least three of the four findings must be present. A thin white to yellow discharge, homogenous discharge, clue cells on microscopy, a pH of vaginal fluid greater than 4.5, and the release of a fishy odor upon adding an alkali solution (10% KOH) to the specimen are all considered Amsel criteria. Only two of the aforementioned factors are acceptable under the modified Amsel criteria, and studies have shown that this is equally diagnostic. The Amsel criteria has a sensitivity of 70% and a specificity of 94%.

As an alternative, the predominant strain of bacteria in the vaginal fluid can be examined using a gram stain. This methodology is known as the Nugent process. The Nugent scoring system uses gram-stain analysis and microscopic inspection to assess the presence of vaginal bacteria and assigns a numerical score between 0 and 10. An increased score denotes a more noteworthy existence of bacteria linked to bacterial vaginosis. Research is the main field in which Nugent score is applied. Although data indicate that this method has an 83% specificity and an 89% sensitivity, it is not often employed in clinical practice.

7.4.2.1. Amsel Criteria

Three out of 4 criteria must be present to diagnose bacterial vaginosis. Amsel criteria indicators that collectively aid in the accurate assessment of the condition include the following:

- Homogenous, thin, grayish-white vaginal discharge that coats the vaginal walls evenly
- Detection of ≥20% clue cells on a wet mount
- Vaginal pH >4.5
- Positive whiff test result

Because point-of-care tests can be expensive, they are typically not used in clinical settings. As an alternative, commercial molecular diagnostic assays are frequently used by clinical practitioners for evaluation. These assays allow for the measurement of bacteria and show sensitivity values between 90.5 and 96.7% and specificity values between 85.8 and 95%. It is now feasible to isolate 91.4% of Gardnerella strains using a micro method involving starch, raffinose fermentation, and Hippurate hydrolysis since the rapid identification method was introduced in 1982.

7.4.3. Management

It is estimated that 30% of cases of bacterial vaginosis resolve on their own without medical intervention. Gardnerella colonization that shows no symptoms does not require treatment. As of right now, there is not enough evidence to support the idea that treating asymptomatic bacterial vaginosis improves patient outcomes. Nonetheless, it is advised to seek treatment with oral or vaginal medication if a patient feels distressed by the symptoms of bacterial vaginosis. One of the two available treatments for bacterial vaginosis is metronidazole or clindamycin. When applied vaginally or taken by mouth, both of these drugs work well. Both can be used safely on expectant patients. First-line therapy for bacterial vaginosis is quite effective; cure rates in less than a month usually fall between 80 and 90%.

Bacterial vaginosis can recur in up to 80% of women within 9 months of initial treatment. Approximately 10–15% of women do not see improvement after the first round of antibiotics and may need further treatment. If symptoms return, a second course of antibiotics is typically recommended. A 2009 Cochrane review provided limited evidence on the effectiveness of probiotics for treating and preventing bacterial vaginosis. It is important to note that there is no clear, universal definition of recurrent bacterial vaginosis.

There is no risk of the infection spreading between partners because bacterial vaginosis is not regarded as a sexually transmitted infection (STI). Therefore, partners do not need to be treated. High-quality evidence was discovered in a 2016 Cochrane review indicating that treating a female patient's sexual partner did not impact the patient's symptoms, clinical prognosis, or risk of recurrence.

According to certain research, to lower the risk of preterm labor, pregnant patients exhibiting symptoms of bacterial vaginosis should receive treatment before 22 weeks of gestation. To avoid negative consequences like preterm birth, there isn't a clear agreement on whether screening for or treating bacterial vaginosis in the general population is a good idea. As of right now, testing and treatment for females who exhibit symptoms are indicated but screening for bacterial vaginosis in asymptomatic individuals is not advised.

2017 saw the U.S. approve secnidazole. S. FDA for oral medication administered as a single dose to treat bacterial vaginosis. The next-generation 5-nitroimidazole secnidazole has a long history of use in the treatment of bacterial and parasitic infections.

A single-dose clindamycin vaginal gel was approved by the FDA in 2021 to treat bacterial vaginosis in females 12 years of age and older. The introduction of a therapy with a single dose was welcomed due to its ease of use and favorable effects on patient adherence.

7.4.4. Prognosis

With treatment, the majority of simple cases of bacterial vaginosis go away. Recurrences, however, are not unusual because antibiotic therapy frequently fails to return the vagina to its normal Lactobacillus-dominant state. The barrier that the Gardnerella bacteria's biofilms form helps stop metronidazole from entering. 80% of women may relapse with bacterial vaginosis within three months of finishing treatment. A rising number of reports over the last ten years have mentioned strains of bacterial vaginosis that are resistant to standard therapies (Lavigne et al., 2008).

A powder containing the naturally occurring live strain Lactobacillus crispatus CTV-05 was used in a recent randomized controlled trial. Women used the intravaginal powder to lessen the recurrence of bacterial vaginosis after receiving metronidazole treatment. The powder was to be used four times a day for the first week of the regimen and then twice a week for the remaining ten weeks. Up to 24 weeks following the start of metronidazole treatment for bacterial vaginosis, the recurrence rate was considerably reduced by using lactobacilli powder. Notably, the FDA has not yet approved this strategy. To lower the rates of bacterial vaginosis recurrence, several substitute vaginal products are presently being researched.

An elevated risk of acquiring sexually transmitted infections (STIs), such as gonorrhea, chlamydia, trichomoniasis, herpes, human papillomavirus (HPV), and HIV, has been linked to bacterial vaginosis. Gardnerella increases the risk of HPV infection at the same time that it damages the vaginal epithelium. Furthermore, although a causal link has not yet been established, bacterial vaginosis may be a factor in tubal infertility and challenges conceiving using assisted reproductive technologies. It has also been suggested to use intravaginal boric acid to treat recurrent bacterial vaginosis. The evidence currently available supports the safety of intravaginal boric acid use in non-pregnant females, despite the regimen's lack of FDA approval. As a preventative measure against bacterial vaginosis, women should take 600 mg of intravaginal boric acid twice a week. During pregnancy, it is best to avoid using boric acid vaginal suppositories and to avoid taking it orally.

7.4.4.1. Complications

Numerous complications can arise from bacterial vaginosis, highlighting the significance of prompt diagnosis and treatment. The complications associated with bacterial vaginosis include the following:

- Increased risk of endometritis and salpingitis
- Increased risk of acquiring STIs
- Elevated risk of postsurgical infections
- Adverse pregnancy outcomes include premature labor, premature rupture of membranes, and postpartum endometritis
- Development of pelvic inflammatory disease
- Increased risk of neonatal meningitis

7.5. Vaginal Yeast Infection

Thrush, or vaginal yeast infections, can result in burning, itching, and abnormal vaginal discharge. There may also be an impact on the labia ("lips") and the vaginal opening. There are instances when the infection shows no symptoms at all.

When an overgrowth of yeast occurs in the vagina, it can lead to a vaginal yeast infection, causing inflammation. Yeast is a type of fungus that, along with bacterial infections like bacterial vaginosis, is a common cause of inflammation in the vagina and outer female genital area.

Vaginal yeast infections are more common in women during specific life stages, such as pregnancy. Additionally, taking specific medications and having a compromised immune system increase their risk.

After a brief course of treatment with vaginal suppositories or creams, yeast infections frequently go away. Taking tablets can be a wise decision at times (Stapleton et al., 2012).

7.5.1. Symptoms

Itching, a burning sensation, and pain are the usual signs of a vaginal yeast infection. The white coating and reddening of the vaginal membranes occur. A few days prior to the onset of your period, the symptoms might get worse. The labia ("lips") may be red and swollen if the inflammation has extended to the external genitalia.

A white-yellow discharge from the vagina is frequently the result of vaginal yeast infections. It resembles cottage cheese or curdled milk and can be chunky or watery. Having a yeast infection can make having sex uncomfortable. Peeing hurts more if the urethra, the tube through which urine is expelled, is also inflamed.

7.5.2. Causes and Risk Factors

Candida albicans is the type of yeast that typically causes vaginal yeast infections. This yeast is known to thrive in the mucous membranes that line the genitalia. However, it usually only occurs in trace amounts, so there are no issues.

However, there are situations when the normal balance of microorganisms (germs) in the membranes is upset, such as during pregnancy or when taking medication.

During pregnancy, the body has elevated levels of estrogen which can disrupt the balance and make it more likely for a woman to develop a vaginal yeast infection. Similarly, taking the contraceptive pill can impact hormone levels in a manner akin to pregnancy, increasing the risk of developing thrush in women who use it.

Certain diseases, like diabetes, can heighten the likelihood of developing vaginal yeast infections by weakening the immune system. Additionally, certain medications, like antibiotics and steroids, as well as lifestyle factors such as stress and wearing tight clothing, can increase the risk of these infections. Using non-breathable feminine hygiene products and washing the genital area with soap also contribute to the growth of yeast, which can cause inflammation.

If a significant amount of yeast enters the vagina from the outside, such as through intercourse with a man who has a yeast infection on the head of his penis, women may occasionally contract the infection from someone else.

7.5.3. Prevalence and Outlook

Bacterial infections are the most frequent cause of vaginal inflammations, with yeast infections coming in second. At some point in their lives, up to 75 out of 100 women will experience a vaginal yeast infection. Women who are fertile are most likely to contract these infections. Women who take medication containing estrogen hormones after menopause may develop yeast infections as a result.

Symptoms of yeast infections are typically mild or absent. Severe symptoms are rare, but if present, more aggressive treatment is required. In some cases, frequent infections or those caused by a compromised immune system may warrant intensified treatment (Deese et al., 2018).

7.5.4. Effects

The symptoms can worsen if the vaginal membranes are inflamed or if scratching the itchy skin in the outer genital area allows other bacteria to grow more easily. Additionally, the inflammation is easily transmissible to adjacent tissue, including the urethral opening.

Serious side effects are extremely uncommon and typically stem from compromised immune systems, as in the case of AIDS or cancer therapy. After that, the inflammation may worsen and extend.

Vaginal infections during pregnancy may somewhat raise the chance of complications like early labor, miscarriage, or early birth. Babies may also contract vaginal yeast infections during childbirth. For example, this may result in an inflammation of the membranes lining the newborn baby's mouth or diaper rash, also known as "nappy rash."

It is common for people who have genital health issues to be embarrassed to discuss them. Women may therefore delay treating a yeast infection or choose not to disclose it to their partner. This may lengthen the infection more than is necessary and raise the possibility of spreading the infection to others.

7.5.5. Diagnosis

Most often, vaginal yeast infections can be diagnosed by observing symptoms and examining the vaginal lining. If there is uncertainty, a doctor may collect a sample of vaginal discharge for further investigation to confirm the presence of yeast.

If a woman experiences severe symptoms or recurrent yeast infections, additional testing may be necessary to determine whether she has a weakened immune system or other risk factors. It could be a good idea to get your partner checked out by a doctor if you both have recurrent yeast infections (Roberts et al., 2015).

7.5.6. Prevention

Antifungal drugs, also called antimycotics, are sometimes prescribed to people with compromised immune systems to prevent fungal infections. As a precaution, some women take antifungal medication in addition to antibiotics. However, there isn't enough solid research to determine if this aids in the prevention of vaginal yeast infections. Women who are in good health don't require any additional precautions. It's advisable to avoid having sex with your partner again until the yeast infection has cleared up, as you could contract it from them (Farhan et al., 2019).

The question of whether probiotic-containing special products can prevent yeast infections is not well-researched. These are either inserted into the vagina or swallowed, depending on the kind of product. Restoring or fostering a balanced population of microorganisms in the vagina (healthy vaginal flora) is the goal. Certain products are more harmful than beneficial. For example, vaginal douches and feminine hygiene products, should not be used by women. These goods increase the risk of infections by upsetting the normal balance of germs.

7.5.7. Treatment

Usually, a single course of treatment is sufficient. This involves applying a cream or suppository inside the vagina with an applicator to make contact with the afflicted tissue lining the vagina. The suggested length of treatment varies based on the product being used. However, it usually only takes a day or two. As a side effect, the treatment itself may cause burning or itching (Denning et al., 2018).

Certain medications can also be taken as a single tablet and swallowed orally. But that may result in adverse effects like nausea, diarrhea, or headaches, as well as interactions with other medications. Oral antifungal medications are not recommended for use by expectant mothers.

Seeking medical advice from a doctor can be a good idea if you have severe symptoms, recurrent infections, or an increased risk of complications, such as weakened immune system. After that, you might require a more intensive course of therapy, like taking antifungal tablets for a few months. Generally speaking, treating your partner is not required. They are only treated for this if they also have a genital yeast infection.

Additionally, probiotics—capsules or suppositories containing live lactic acid bacteria—can be used. The goal of these therapies is to preserve and replenish the vagina's natural flora, or balance of microorganisms. Insufficient data currently exists to determine their efficacy.

Some women also put tampons soaked in tea tree oil or garlic cloves into their vagina. Some people use natural yogurt to increase the vagina's pH, which makes it more acidic. However, little research has been done to determine the efficacy or safety of these kinds of home remedies. Allergic reactions or irritated mucous membranes are among the potential risks (Yano et al., 2019).

A Closer Look

Lactobacilli As Good Probiotics for Prevention of Urogenital Infections

A focus on lactobacilli has resulted from their dominance in the urogenital microflora of healthy women and their obliteration in patients who develop a UTI, BV, and many other genital infections [apart from candidiasis]. Gram-positive rods known as lactobacilli are mostly facultative or strict anaerobes with a strict growth requirement. By generating lactic and other acids, they both contribute to and prefer an acidic environment. For more than a century, lactobacilli have been considered nonpathogenic members of the intestinal and urogenital flora and have not been linked to any illnesses.

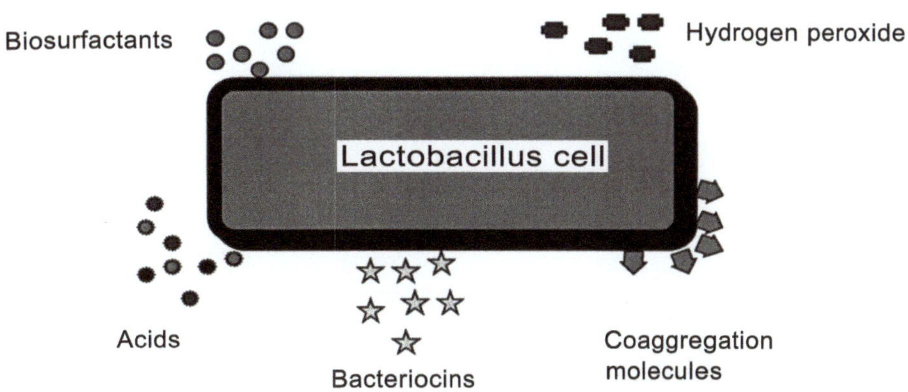

The dairy and agricultural sectors have long been interested in lactobacilli, but over the past century, research on their effects on human health has been inconsistent and frequently inconclusive. There are a few instances where lactic acid bacteria have been used, with varying degrees of success, to treat or prevent infections of the genital and intestinal tracts. The ideal lactobacilli dosage, duration, and mode of delivery have not been found, nor has the inclusion of a placebo in the study. Nevertheless, it has been unsuccessful to pinpoint the characteristics of lactobacilli that are necessary for the prevention and treatment of disease. Research has not been able to properly identify, recover, or document lactobacilli or demonstrate their mechanisms of action (Donders et al., 2017).

Reliability is another issue with probiotic treatments. This was demonstrated in one study by the fact that some health food products' contents differed from what was listed on the labels and were inconsistent. More recently, we found that Lactobacillus plantarum is present in US and

Canadian products, even though the food label does not mention it, and that some health food products in Canada seem to contain ≥1 common Lactobacillus strain, which is apparently identical to ATCC strain 21052.

Probiotics in general and lactobacilli in particular have drawn more attention recently as an inexpensive, natural, and alternative treatment to preserve and improve health. Two strains of Lactobacillus, i.e., Lactobacillus GG (ATCC 53103) and Lactobacillus rhamnosus GR-1, seem to be useful in colonizing and guarding against microbial infection in the intestine and urogenital tract, respectively.

Summary

- Urogenital health encompasses the health and well-being of the urinary and genital systems. These systems include the kidneys, ureters, bladder, and urethra in the urinary tract, as well as the reproductive organs.
- The urogenital microbiota is the community of microorganisms that natively resides in the urinary and the genital tract.
- The urinary microbiota is distinct from two closest niches inhabited by residual/native microbiota—gut and vagina—but still shares similarities with both of them.
- The urinary microbiota and its more famous counterpart, the gut microbiota, are two distinct microbial communities that play important roles in human health.
- With time, all microbial communities change as a response to variations in environmental conditions or endogenous processes within microorganisms themselves.
- Urinary microbiota is a low biomass community located within the urinary tract where bacterial growth and colonization are affected by UT physiological parameters in combination with exogenous factors.
- Probiotic bacteria affect modification of the immune system, reduction of cholesterol, alleviation of lactose intolerance, alleviation or even remission of Crohn's disease, prevention of diarrhea and prevention of urogenital infections.
- Urinary tract infections (UTIs) in women are one of the most prevalent infections occurring at various stages of life.
- The main reasons behind the increased prevalence of urinary tract infections in peri- and postmenopausal women include hormonal changes (estrogen insufficiency) and connective tissue aging (urinary incontinence, pelvic organ prolapse).
- Pelvic inflammatory disease (PID) is an infection of one or more of the upper reproductive organs, including the uterus, fallopian tubes and ovaries.
- Bacterial vaginosis is a condition caused by an overgrowth of normal vaginal flora. Most commonly, this presents clinically with increased vaginal discharge that has a fish-like odor.
- Vaginal yeast infections occur when too much yeast grows in the vagina, leading to an inflammation. Yeast is a type of fungus. Along with bacterial infections (bacterial vaginosis), yeast infections are among the most common causes of inflammation in the vagina and on the outer part of the female genitals.

References

1. Anger, J., Lee, U., Ackerman, A. L., et al. (2019). Recurrent uncomplicated urinary tract infections in women: AUA/CUA/SUFU guideline. *Journal of Urology, 202*(2), 282–289. https://doi.org/10.1097/JU.0000000000000339.
2. Barrons, R., & Tassone, D. (2008). Use of Lactobacillus probiotics for bacterial genitourinary infections in women: A review. *Clinical Therapeutics, 30*(3), 453–468. https://doi.org/10.1016/j.clinthera.2008.03.001.

3. Brubaker, L., Gourdine, J. P. F., Siddiqui, N. Y., Holland, A., Halverson, T., Limeria, R., Pride, D., Ackerman, L., Forster, C. S., Jacobs, K. M., et al. (2021). Forming consensus to advance urobiome research. *mSystems, 6*(5), e01371–20. https://doi.org/10.1128/mSystems.01371-20.

4. Bukavina, L., Isali, I., Ginwala, R., Sindhani, M., Calaway, A., Magee, D., Miron, B., Correa, A., Kutikov, A., Zibelman, M., et al. (2023). Global meta-analysis of urine microbiome: Colonization of polycyclic aromatic hydrocarbon-degrading bacteria among bladder cancer patients. *European Urology Oncology, 6*(2), 190–203. https://doi.org/10.1016/j.euo.2023.01.002.

5. Deese, J., Pradhan, S., Goetz, H., & Morrison, C. (2018). Contraceptive use and the risk of sexually transmitted infection: Systematic review and current perspectives. *Open Access Journal of Contraception, 9*, 91–112. https://doi.org/10.2147/OAJC.S162869.

6. Denning, D. W., Kneale, M., Sobel, J. D., & Rautemaa-Richardson, R. (2018). Global burden of recurrent vulvovaginal candidiasis: A systematic review. *Lancet Infectious Diseases, 18*(11), e339–e347. https://doi.org/10.1016/S1473-3099(18)30471-4.

7. Donders, G. G. G., Ravel, J., Vitali, B., Netea, M. G., Salumets, A., & Unemo, M. (2017). Role of molecular biology in diagnosis and characterization of vulvo-vaginitis in clinical practice. *Gynecological Obstetric Investigation, 82*(6), 607–616. https://doi.org/10.1159/000477568.

8. Farhan, M. A., Moharram, A. M., Salah, T., & Shaaban, O. M. (2019). Types of yeasts that cause vulvovaginal candidiasis in chronic users of corticosteroids. *Medical Mycology, 57*(6), 681–687. https://doi.org/10.1093/mmy/myz013.

9. Ikäheimo, R., Siitonen, A., Heiskanen, T., et al. (1996). Recurrence of urinary tract infection in a primary care setting: Analysis of a 1-year follow-up of 179 women. *Clinical Infectious Diseases, 22*(1), 91–99. https://doi.org/10.1093/clinids/22.1.91.

10. Lavigne, J. P., Bourg, G., Combescure, B., et al. (2008). *In vitro* and *in vivo* evidence of dose dependent decrease of uropathogenic *Escherichia coli* virulence after consumption of commercial Vaccinium macrocarpon (cranberry) capsules. *Clinical Microbiology and Infection, 14*(4), 350–355. https://doi.org/10.1111/j.1469-0691.2008.01926.x.

11. Oros, D., Ceprnja, M., Zucko, J., Cindric, M., Hozic, A., Skrlin, J., Barisic, K., Melvan, E., Uroic, K., Kos, B., et al. (2020). Identification of pathogens from native urine samples by MALDI-TOF/TOF tandem mass spectrometry. *Clinical Proteomics, 17*(1), 25. https://doi.org/10.1186/s12014-020-09263-1.

12. Pendharkar, S., Magopane, T., Larsson, P. G., de Bruyn, G., Gray, G. E., Hammarström, L., & Marcotte, H. (2013). Identification and characterization of vaginal lactobacilli from South African women. *BMC Infectious Diseases, 13*, 43. https://doi.org/10.1186/1471-2334-13-43.

13. Popa, G., Lauber, K. D., Rothe, H., & Rugendorff, E. (1996). Rezidivierende Harnwegsinfektionen in der Postmenopause. Wirksamkeit einer oralen Immuntherapie mit E. coli-Fraktionen. *Münchener Medizinische Wochenschrift, 138*(18), 713–716. https://doi.org/10.1007/BF08445715.

14. Price, T. K., Dune, T., Hilt, E. E., Thomas-White, K. J., Kliethermes, S., Brincat, C., Brubaker, L., Wolfe, A. J., Mueller, E. R., & Schreckenberger, P. C. (2016). The clinical urine culture: Enhanced techniques improve detection of clinically relevant microorganisms. *Journal of Clinical Microbiology, 54*(5), 1216–1222. https://doi.org/10.1128/JCM.03409-15.

15. Ravel, J., Gajer, P., Abdo, Z., Schneider, G. M., Koenig, S. S. K., McCulle, S. L., Karlebach, S., Gorle, R., Russell, J., Tacket, C. O., et al. (2011). Vaginal microbiome of reproductive-age women. *Proceedings of the National Academy of Sciences USA, 108*(Suppl. S1), 4680–4687. https://doi.org/10.1073/pnas.1007619107.

16. Roberts, C. L., Algert, C. S., Rickard, K. L., et al. (2015). Treatment of vaginal candidiasis for the prevention of preterm birth: A systematic review and meta-analysis. *Systematic Reviews, 4*, 31. https://doi.org/10.1186/s13643-015-0023-7.

17. Stapleton, A. E., Dziura, J., Hooton, T. M., et al. (2012). Recurrent urinary tract infection and urinary *Escherichia coli* in women ingesting cranberry juice daily: A randomized controlled trial. *Mayo Clinic Proceedings, 87*(2), 143–150. https://doi.org/10.1016/j.mayocp.2011.11.007.

18. Toh, S. L., Boswell-Ruys, C. L., Lee, B. S. B., et al. (2017). Probiotics for preventing urinary tract infection in people with neuropathic bladder. *Cochrane Database of Systematic Reviews, 9*, CD010723. https://doi.org/10.1002/14651858.CD010723.pub2.

19. Yano, J., Sobel, J. D., Nyirjesy, P., Sobel, R., Williams, V. L., Yu, Q., Noverr, M. C., & Fidel, P. L. (2019). Current patient perspectives of vulvovaginal candidiasis: Incidence, symptoms, management, and post-treatment outcomes. *BMC Women's Health, 19*(1), 48. https://doi.org/10.1186/s12905-019-0724-x.

20. Zhou, X., Brown, C. J., Abdo, Z., Davis, C. C., Hansmann, M. A., Joyce, P., Foster, J. A., & Forney, L. J. (2007). Differences in the composition of vaginal microbial communities found in healthy Caucasian and Black women. *ISME Journal, 1*(2), 121–133. https://doi.org/10.1038/ismej.2007.12.

Chapter

MENTAL HEALTH AND COGNITIVE FUNCTION

8

Contents

Introduction

The endocrine axis aging naturally, ovarian excision, or medical interventions that block ovarian endocrine function can all contribute to menopause-related declines in function. Nevertheless, several the classic symptoms of menopause—such as mood swings, hot flashes, insomnia, and forgetfulness—also indicate that menopause is a neurological alteration. Therefore, in women, there is an inextricable link between ovarian and brain health (Amin et al., 2006).

Reduced estrogen causes alterations in nerve cell morphology, quantity, and interactions, as well as in gene expression and glucose metabolism. Low levels of estrogen have been associated in female animal models with the build-up of the aberrant protein amyloid-beta (Aβ), which is well known for causing plaques to form in brain tissue in AD patients, as well as occasionally in healthy individuals.

Orientation and Directional Terms

Term	Definition	Illustration
Neurosteroids	Neurosteroids are steroids synthesized within the brain and modulate neuronal excitability by rapid non-genomic actions.	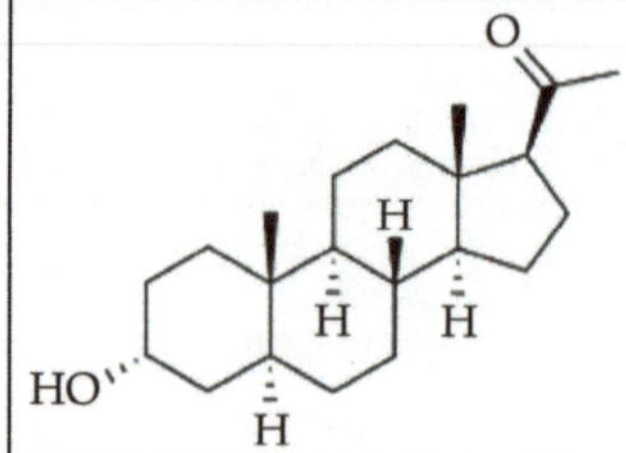
Progestogens	Progestogens, also sometimes written progestagens or gestagens, are a class of natural or synthetic steroid hormones that bind to and activate the progesterone receptors. Progesterone is the major and most important progestogen in the body.	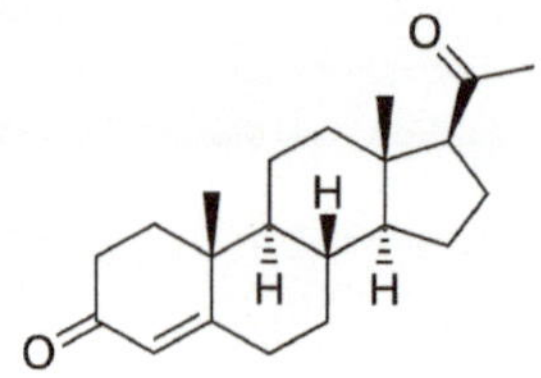
Estrogens	Estrogens are a group of hormones that play an important role in the normal sexual and reproductive development in women.	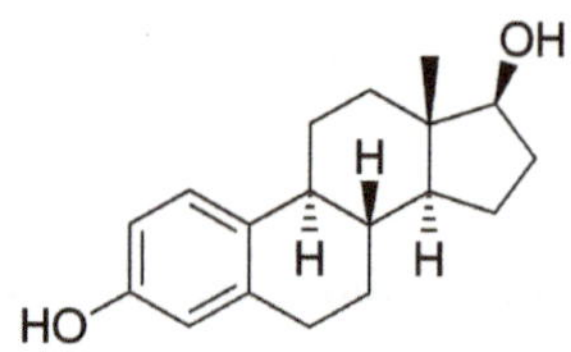
Adenosine triphosphate	Adenosine triphosphate is a nucleotide that provides energy to drive and support many processes in living cells, such as muscle contraction, nerve impulse propagation, and chemical synthesis.	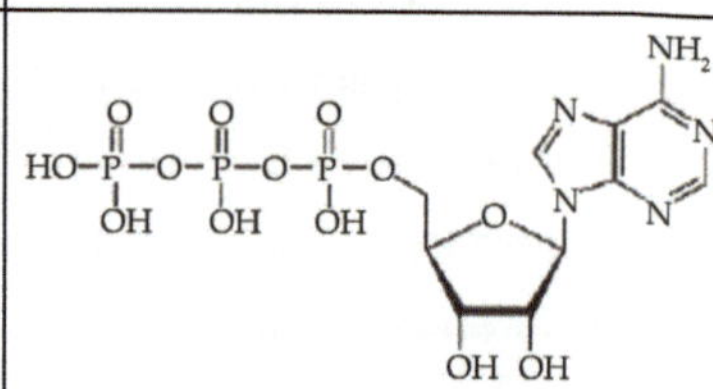
Oligodendrocytes	Oligodendrocytes are the myelinating cells of the central nervous system (CNS). They are the end product of a cell lineage which has to undergo a complex and precisely timed program of proliferation, migration, differentiation, and myelination to finally produce the insulating sheath of axons.	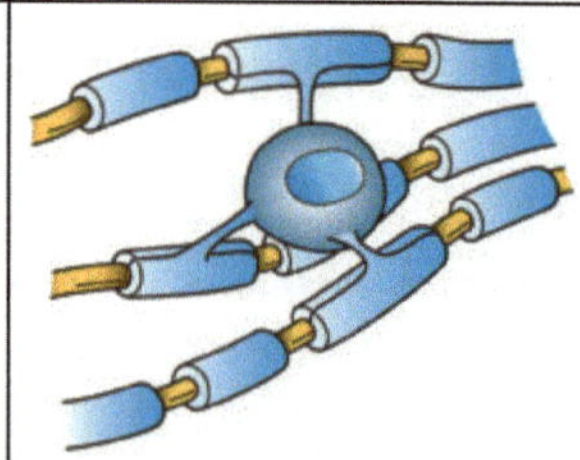
Allopregnanolone	Allopregnanolone is a naturally occurring neurosteroid which is made in the body from the hormone progesterone.	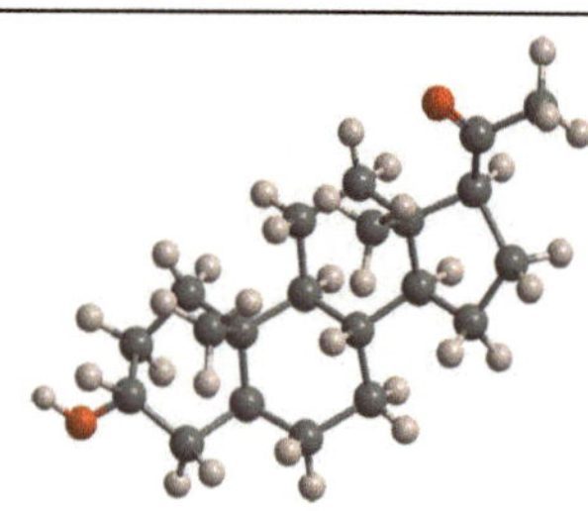

8.1. Impact of Menopause on Mood and Cognition

Middle-aged women undergo a progressive change in ovarian activity and a physiologic deterioration of the hypothalamic-pituitary-ovarian axis function associated with fluctuating hormone levels during the menopausal transition, which starts four to six years before the cessation of menses. Women may experience menopause symptoms during this time, including hot flashes, sleep disturbances, mood swings, memory problems, and dry vagina. Women going through menopause frequently complain about neurological symptoms like mood swings, sleep disturbances, and "brain fog," which can have a serious negative influence on their physical and mental well-being as well as their quality of life and productivity.

8.1.1. Sexual Steroids and Central Nervous System: Biologic Aspects

Women's levels of the sexual hormones androgens, progesterone, and estradiol fluctuate dramatically throughout their lives as they go through the various stages of life, from menarche to menopause. These variations can cause changes in behavior, thought, and mood. They also have a substantial effect on the central nervous system (CNS) and the entire body.

Sex steroids act via both genomic and non-genomic pathways on cortical and subcortical brain structures. Numerous molecular and cellular processes are believed to be involved in determining changes in the structure and function of neural systems through both gene expression modulation and activation of signaling pathways, despite the fact that the majority of the evidence in this field is based on non-human studies. Sex steroids can alter several bodily processes, such as behavior, mood, pain, memory, sleep, and coordination. Through receptors in the nuclei as well as along the membranes at the synapsis, spine, and mitochondria, they carry out their function. Additionally, they have been discovered in glia, where they may play a part in demyelinating diseases and regulate the formation of myelin.

Neurosteroids are steroid hormones that have CNS activity. They can be produced peripherally and have the ability to cross the blood-brain barrier, or they can be synthesized by neurons and glial cells in the central and peripheral nervous systems, either by local metabolism of intermediate steroids produced in the periphery or by de novo synthesis from cholesterol. Since steroid hormones can cross the blood-brain barrier, measuring their plasma levels is crucial for understanding their role in CNS activity, even though their levels in peripheral blood differ from those in the central nervous system (Barrett-Connor and Goodman-Gruen, 1999).

Different hormones can regulate the brain in ways that are specific to a particular sexual orientation. For example, estrogens have been shown to have neuroprotective effects on brain tissue, whereas androgens appear to be more active in helping men recover from demyelinating events. Progesterones, on the other hand, appear to be more effective in helping men reduce abnormal proliferation and apoptosis following trauma or stroke (Zárate et al., 2017).

Estrogen receptors (ERs) are widely distributed in the central nervous system (CNS) and are found in brain regions related to memory and executive function. Whereas magnocellular cholinergic neurons of the basal forebrain are primarily represented in ERα signaling, the ER isoform ERβ is primarily expressed in the cerebral cortex and hippocampus. Estradiol has been shown to mediate neurotransmitter interactions in the prefrontal cortex, which is relevant to executive functions, and to induce a trophic effect in the basal forebrain and the hippocampus, which is fundamental for memory and executive functions. Additionaly linked to an increase in dentate gyrus neurogenesis are estrogens. Numerous neurotransmitter systems, including acetylcholine, serotonin, noradrenaline, and glutamate, are involved in the function of estrogens. The cholinergic neurotransmitter system is particularly important for memory functions. Estrogen affects the brain through a variety of mechanisms, including neurotrophic and neuroprotective ones that improve hippocampal neurogenesis, neurite growth, and synaptic plasticity while guarding against apoptosis and neural injury. Moreover, estrogen appears to enhance mitochondrial respiration and adenosine triphosphate (ATP) synthesis, both of which are critical processes in an organ with a high energy requirement like the brain. Additional ways that estrogen functions in the brain include repairing DNA and enhancing antioxidant activity. Additionally, estrogen has been connected to higher levels of the inflammatory marker C-reactive protein, which has been connected to decreased cognitive function.

Progesterone is a strong regulator of neurogenesis, cell survival, and bioenergetic systems, much like estrogen. When administered together, they have no synergistic effect and produce a smaller response than when administered alone. Progesterone functions through two distinct pathways. The first involves binding to its receptors, PRα and PRβ, and regulating gene transcription. The other pathway, which it shares with dihydroprogesterone (DHP) and allopregnanolone, activates different signaling cascades and regulates the transcription of multiple genes. The two pathways have major effects on neuronal cell proliferation, bioenergetic regulation, and the promotion of anti-apoptotic and cell survival effects. Additionally, progesterone acts on glial cells, primarily enhancing the activity and proliferation of oligodendrocytes. The production of progesterone by oligodendrocytes is capable of converting progesterone from the bloodstream into DHP and allopregnanolone, which in turn modulates GABA-A receptors and myelination.

It is thought that progesterone, and particularly allopregnanolone, has an anti-anxiety effect akin to benzodiazepines by promoting the GABAergic system and inhibiting synaptic transmission. Antidepressant medications can detect and increase allopregnanolone, a metabolite that is linked to depression in humans. The effect of exogenous progestin administration on the cognitive performance of healthy women in working memory tests is explained by the GABAergic role of progesterone in the hippocampus. Progesterone and allopregnanolone have the ability to affect the dopaminergic systems, and when progesterone levels are higher during the menstrual cycle, there is an observed improvement in motor sensory functions. Depression and drug abuse may also be impacted by allopregnanolone's positive modulation of dopamine release (Davis et al., 2015).

Furthermore, independent of the gonads, the brain has the capacity to locally produce the androgen dihydrotestosterone. It has been shown that androgens can cause spine synapses and neurogenesis in the hippocampal region in the animal model. Additionally, androgens have neuroprotective properties just like estrogens do. It appears that testosterone in particular may increase serotonergic tone (also through its conversion to estradiol) and the effect of noradrenergic anti-depressant agents, despite the fact that there are fewer studies on the relationship between androgens and neurotransmitters. Dehydroepiandrosterone (DHEA) appears to have antioxidant, neuroprotective, and anti-glucocorticoid effects, though much is still unknown. It can alleviate anxiety, cognitive impairments, psychotic and depressive symptoms, and cognitive deficits through these mechanisms.

8.1.2. The Influence of Menopausal Transition and Menopause Hormone Therapy on Cognition

8.1.2.1. Menopausal Transition and Cognition

Many women experience memory issues during the menopausal transition, including "brain fog," difficulty pronouncing words, and forgetfulness (Sullivan Mitchell E., Fugate Woods N, 2001), implying that menopausal hormone changes could be the cause of cognitive alterations. It also seems that older women are more likely than older men to develop age-related dementia, pointing to gender disparities in dementia that may not be entirely explained by longevity (Rocca et al., 2014).

However, compared to age-matched men, women in their early midlife performed better on detailed memory tasks in a recent cross-sectional study (Rentz et al., 2017). The years following menopause saw a reduction in these sex differences. Within the Rents et al. study. greater levels of plasmatic estradiol were linked to improved outcomes. Higher levels of estradiol were linked to lower cognitive impairment in women who were already experiencing cognitive decline, according to a different study (Lui et al, 2003). Other research found no connection between estrogen levels and cognitive issues or cognition (Barrett-Connor and Goodman-Gruen, 1999).

There are few longitudinal studies examining the effects of the menopausal transition on memory and cognitive abilities. Two long-term studies found modest declines in cognitive function: an 18-month follow-up of premenopausal women in the Kinmen Women-Health Investigation (KIWI) revealed no evidence of significant cognitive decline, except for verbal fluency (Fuh et al., 2006). According to the Study of Women's Health Across the Nation (SWAN), there is a decline in cognitive function, primarily in learning abilities, during the menopausal transition. However, after menopause, these abilities recover to pre-menopausal levels (Greendale et al., 2009). We anticipate that in the coming years, the SWAN study, which has been monitoring 3,302 women during the entire menopausal transition since 1996, will offer a unique perspective on the long-term consequences of hormonal changes in middle-aged women.

It should be mentioned that hormonal processes throughout life as well as events during the menopausal transition appear to be important for cognition. Improved verbal memory was linked to a longer fertile period, defined as later age at natural or surgical menopause, according to a recent observational study involving 1,315 women. However, a longer fertile period was not linked to a lower risk of dementia in another observational study involving 3,602 women.

8.1.2.2. Menopause Hormone Therapy and Cognition

8.1.2.2.1. *In Women without Dementia*

There is conflicting evidence regarding the relationship between menopause hormone therapy (MHT) and its neuroprotective effects, despite medical literature emphasizing the close relationship between estrogen and cognitive function. Although several observational studies have demonstrated a positive effect of hormone therapy on Alzheimer's disease (AD) (Tang et al., 1996; Waring et al., 1995; Zandi et al., 2002), MHT being associated with a 29% reduction in AD in the meta-analyzes of observational studies (Yaffe, Sawaya, Lieberburg, and Grady, 1998), large clinical trials such as the Women's Health Initiative (WHI) and Women's Health Initiative Memory Study (WHIMS) did not support those findings (Morgan et al., 2018).

The first extensive, long-term study to address the cognitive effects of MHT (0.625 mg of conjugated equine estrogen (CEE) plus 2.5 mg of medroxyprogesterone acetate) in the prevention of AD was WHIMS, a randomized, placebo-controlled clinical trial that involved 4,532 post-menopausal women (over 65) who were enrolled in the larger WHI study. The Modified Mini-Mental State Examination (MMSE) total scores declined significantly and clinically significant when compared to placebo after a mean follow-up of 4.2 years, according to the results. Additionally, MHT was not able to reverse general cognitive decline.

The mean MMSE scores in the estrogen group were significantly lower than those in the placebo group, according to a subsequent analysis of 2,947 WHIMS estrogen-alone treated women (aged 65–79). Women with lower baseline cognitive function were more severely affected by estrogens.

The Nurses' Health Study, a prospective cohort of over 13,807 women aged 70 to 81, was the source of the data used in the analysis. It was discovered that there was minimal difference in cognitive decline between current hormone users and those who had never used them. In most cognitive tests, those who have used estrogen or estro-progestin for a prolonged period of time (at least 5–10 years) were more likely to experience a significant decline. The impairment was more pronounced in women who began taking hormones later in life. Further investigation revealed that MHT users who carried the apolipoprotein E (APOE) E4 allele had more severe cognitive impairment.

According to a 2008 meta-analysis of clinical trials examining MHT (estrogen or estrogen-progestin therapy) in postmenopausal women (over 60), MHT does not shield normal women from the decline in cognitive function.

It should be noted that the so-called "timing hypothesis" was not taken into account in studies involving older women (the WHIMS was over 65). In fact, additional research has indicated that estrogen may only be neuroprotective if taken soon after the onset of menopause, much like the cardiovascular risk. According to certain epidemiologic studies, the use of MHT in the early stages of postmenopause is associated with a lower risk of dementia, while its use later in life is not, supporting the "critical window hypothesis."

Findings from the Cache County Study indicated that women who started hormone therapy soon after menopause had a lower risk of Alzheimer's disease compared to those who did not use hormone therapy. Research by Whitmer et al. also suggested that starting hormone therapy during midlife could have a positive impact on cognitive health in post-menopausal women, while initiating therapy later in life may have negative consequences. However, other studies have not definitively linked hormone therapy use near menopause to improved cognitive function or decreased risk of dementia in later years.

Additional small-scale clinical trials have also been conducted on the relationship between early MHT and later-life cognitive function. In the WHIMS-Young (WHIMSY) trial, 326 postmenopausal women aged 50 to 55 were randomly assigned to receive either a placebo or MHT (CEE with or without 2.5 mg of medroxyprogesterone acetate over a mean of 7.0 years). When CEE-based therapies were given to postmenopausal women between the ages of 50 and 55, there was no overall sustained benefit or risk to cognitive function. Cognitive testing done on people up to the age of 67 did not reveal any long-term advantages of MHT over a placebo. These studies reassure us that hormone therapy does not negatively impact cognition in young postmenopausal women, even though they do not support the theory of cognitive improvement in MHT users.

8.1.2.2.2. In Women with Dementia

Dementia and cognitive decline are becoming more common public health issues. One potentially concerning symptom of the very early stages of Alzheimer's disease (AD) or other types of dementia is the inability to recall information, which is known as impaired episodic memory. The most common cause of dementia is AD, which affects women more often than men. Some authors have suggested that the incidence of AD varies depending on a person's sex. This illness is marked by a progressive loss of cognitive function and episodic memory, which leads to language and visuospatial impairment. Behavioral disorders like depression, aggression, and apathy are frequently present as well.

Given the importance of this illness, there has been a great deal of interest from the scientific community and the general public in this area of study. Estrogen's role in treating and/or preventing AD has been studied in addition to maintaining cognitive function in women without dementia. Preliminary data both in vitro and in vivo point to the possibility that estrogen prevents amyloid deposition. It has been demonstrated that estradiol reduces tau hyperphosphorylation, reduces amyloid b deposition, and ameliorates the inflammatory consequences of amyloid b.

A prospective study of incident dementia among 1,357 men (mean age 73.2 years) and 1889 women (mean age 74.5 years) was conducted in the Cache County Study. The results showed that women who used MHT had a lower risk of AD compared to non-users (adjusted HR 0.59). However, there were no apparent benefits associated with current MHT use unless it had been used for more than 10.

The relationship between exogenous estrogens and dementia risk has been the subject of several sizable epidemiologic studies. Even with some methodological limitations of the studies, the first meta-analysis of these observational studies from 2001 suggested that MHT users had a lower risk of dementia. However, a second meta-analysis of prospective studies did not find any correlation between MHT and AD or all-cause dementia (Devi, 2018).

Transdermal 17-beta estradiol therapy has been associated with a reduction in amyloid-beta deposition on neuroimaging studies, especially in apolipoprotein E (APOE) E4 carriers, according to recent findings from the Kronos Early Estrogen Prevention Study (KEEPS).

Recently, information from Savolainen-Peltonen et al. revealed that people using systemic hormone therapy had a higher risk of AD than people using vaginal estradiol. Long-term use of systemic hormone therapy may also be associated with a globally increased risk of AD, which is independent of the age at which the therapy is started. Both estradiol-only users and estrogen-progestogen users exhibited a similar risk of AD, and among the former, no particular progestogen (norethisterone acetate, medroxyprogesterone acetate, or other progestogens) was linked to increased risk. It is noteworthy that individuals who began estrogen therapy or estrogen plus progestin therapy prior to the age of 60 did not have an increased risk of AD for shorter treatment durations.

The idea of treating female Alzheimer's patients with estrogen has been explored in several small, randomized clinical trials.

Estrogen administration for a year (conjugated equine estrogens 0.625 mg or 1.225 mg vs placebo) did not slow the disease's progression or improve overall, cognitive, or functional outcomes in the largest study, which included 120 women. Similar results were reported by a subsequent meta-analysis encompassing seven trials.

We think those studies shouldn't change the way we currently practice medicine or how we make decisions about MHT. In fact, it's important to keep in mind that multiple randomized clinical trials have confirmed the safety profile of MHT on cognition in the early stages of menopause, despite the fact that some observational studies have produced contradictory and mixed results.

Overall, MHT is beneficial for young menopausal women who are not contraindicated for it and whose quality of life is compromised due to vasomotor symptoms, night sweats, or disturbed sleep. Multiple studies have confirmed that MHT does not negatively impact these women's cognitive abilities. On the other hand, it should be mentioned that, following guidelines, women without AD symptoms or those who are unwilling to begin hormonal treatment should not be prescribed MHT purely to prevent memory loss or AD.

Future research on this topic should concentrate on the long-term risks of MHT on cognition and AD, as well as the distinct effects of different types of molecules on cognitive outcomes, despite the abundance of data currently available.

8.1.3. The Influence of Menopausal Transition and Menopause Hormone Therapy on Mood

8.1.3.1. Mood Disorders During Menopausal Transition

Women who are going through menopause are more likely to experience emotional distress, anxiety, stress, and depression. Numerous investigators have endeavored to investigate the rationale behind women's heightened vulnerability to depression during specific phases of their lives. We can pinpoint specific times in a woman's life—like the menstrual cycle's phases, her pregnancy and postpartum, or the menopausal transition—when she is biologically vulnerable. There are certain windows of vulnerability for depression or episodes of depression related to reproduction. For example, some women are more sensitive to hormonal changes that occur during the luteal phase of their cycles, the postpartum period, and the menopause transition. It is likely that sleep issues (insomnia, nighttime awakenings, or early wakefulness) and depression are related and require separate treatment (Fuh et al., 2006).

Many other factors may also have a major impact on mood, according to longitudinal studies. These specifically include psychosocial, demographic, and health-related traits like being unemployed, having little education, being Black, Japanese, or Hispanic, having little social support, smoking, having chronic illnesses, having a history of anxiety, having a history of postpartum depression symptoms, being nulliparous, having VMS, going through stressful life events, losing a partner, having a high body mass index (BMI), and having low self-esteem. For women in their midlife, body dissatisfaction may be common. There is proof that the severity of menopause symptoms is positively correlated with age and BMI, as well as with modifications to lifestyle factors (e.g., physical activity), which can subsequently impact the mood of women. Anxiety and depression are directly correlated with self-esteem. Low self-esteem in particular has been linked to women's health, perceived stress, and mood during this time of life, and can predict the occurrence of distress in relation to menopause symptoms, such as hot flashes.

With varying degrees of success, some research have looked at the relationship between depression and hysterectomy, whether or not an oophorectomy was performed. An increased risk of depressive symptoms was found in a study by the Australian Longitudinal Study on Women's Health, which included 5336 women. The risk was found to be 20% higher in women who had a hysterectomy and ovarian conservation and 44% higher in women who had a hysterectomy without ovarian conservation when compared to controls (women who had not had a hysterectomy).

Even though the precise role of low or declining levels of estradiol in the onset of perimenopausal depression (PMD) is still unknown, the role of estrogens should be taken into account when analyzing the causes of mood changes during the menopausal transition. Serotonin, dopamine, and norepinephrine are the three classical neurotransmitters linked to depression. Estradiol (E2) controls their synthesis, metabolism, and receptor activity. It has been shown by researchers that the brain contains a large distribution of estrogen receptors. Estrogen activity detected in areas known to be related to mood and cognitive control (e.g., evidence for the idea that this hormone may have mediating effects on mood (and potentially therapeutic effects as well), including the hippocampus and prefrontal cortex. Serotonin (5-hydroxytryptamine, or 5-HT) synthesis and availability are both increased by E2, and these effects are generally considered to be beneficial to mood. Specifically, following E2 administration, there has been evidence of a decrease in the activity of monoamine oxidases (MAOs) A and B, which limits the breakdown of 5-HT. The rate-limiting enzyme for the synthesis of serotonin, tryptophan hydroxylase, is also encouraged to increase as a result of this. In addition to increasing mitochondrial respiratory efficiency, estrogens also help to prevent the production of oxygen free radicals, which have been shown to have a detrimental effect on mitochondria energetics in depression (Gleason et al., 2015).

By decreasing monoamine oxidases (MAOs) and increasing the activity of tyrosine hydroxylase, the rate-limiting enzyme in the synthesis of catecholamines, estrogen effects also increase the availability of noradrenaline (NE). The hydroxylation of dopamine to form NE is catalyzed by acute E2 administration, which also stimulates the transcription of the dopamine b-hydroxylase (DBH) gene. Finally, because estrogen stimulates brain-derived neurotrophic factor (BDNF), a crucial neuroprotective and growth factor agent that has been shown to be deficient in depression, it may also have an antidepressant effect.

Longitudinal studies are a better approach to evaluate the possible relationship between depression and the menopause transition stage, as well as the direction of that relationship, than cross-sectional studies. The purpose of the SWAN was to track clinical depression over a 13-year period of time. According to their study's findings, about 30% of the participants who experienced depression during the follow-up saw their persistency or recurrence of depression worsen. The results were validated in individuals with recently diagnosed depression as well. Similar findings have been noted in other sizable, longitudinal studies, including the Seattle Midlife Women's Health Study, the Australian Longitudinal Study of Women's Health (ASWH), and the Harvard Study of Midlife Mood and Cycles. These studies all show an increased risk for depressive symptoms during the menopausal transition. However, the Penn Ovarian Aging Study (POAS) hypothesis was that, in relation to the final menstrual period (FMP), the risk of higher depressive symptoms increased in the years prior to menopause and decreased in the years following menopause. During a 14-year follow-up, the study assessed 203 premenopausal women who had naturally entered menopause. Women in the menopause transition had a significantly higher risk of depressive symptoms prior to FMP, and a lower risk following FMP (Gordon et al., 2016).

Despite the overwhelming evidence of a higher incidence of major depressive disorder (MDD) during the menopausal transition, the existence of menopause-associated depression has been a contentious topic among clinicians. However, since several hormonal and metabolic variables may conflate the effects of estradiol withdrawal in perimenopausal women, it is impossible to define a "estradiol withdrawal hypothesis." Moreover, contradictory approaches employed in different studies to evaluate mental disorders or characterize reproductive staging introduce confusion into the issue at hand. Notable methodological variations include the menopausal state (peri-menopause versus. post-menopause), state determination (age has been used as a proxy measure in previous studies), baseline symptomatology (asymptomatic vs. depression signs as opposed to. depression syndromic), the method of hormone delivery (transdermal vs. oral), as well as measuring symptoms or syndromes. Due to these factors, a large portion of the research on women's mental health examines the menopausal transition from the perspective of disease risk. In keeping with this idea, Gordon et al. highlighted how a person's variability and sensitivity to changes in reproductive hormones determine when MDD starts, not the absolute levels of hormones.

8.1.3.2. Menopause Hormone Therapy and Mood

8.1.3.2.1. In Non-Depressed Women

One randomized controlled trial evaluated the mood of eighty-three non-depressed perimenopausal women during six months of hormone therapy. The women received CEE for two weeks, followed by CEE plus medroxyprogesterone acetate (MPA) for another two weeks. There were no notable effects on mood. A recent study that evaluated 38 non-depressed perimenopausal women found no appreciable changes in their mood.

One randomized trial evaluated the role of estrogen administration in preventing depressive symptoms in perimenopausal and early postmenopausal transition. Transdermal E2 (0.01 mg/d) plus intermittent oral micronized progesterone (200 mg/d for 12 days every three months) or placebo was administered to 172 women in a randomized fashion. Compared to women receiving a placebo, those receiving estrogens plus progesterone had a significantly lower likelihood of experiencing depressive symptoms after a year (32.3% vs. 17.3%), with women in the early stages of perimenopause showing a greater manifestation of this effect (Grady et al., 2002).

Studies evaluating the mood effects of hormone therapy in post-menopausal non-depressed women have shown that there are no appreciable effects of estrogens on mood in this population. Haines, among others. didn't detect any change in mood following a year of oral estradiol treatment (1 or 2 mg) compared to a placebo; likewise, Girdler et al. found no evidence of a significant change in mood between MHT users (CEE 0.625 mg/d or CEE 1 MPA, 10 mg/d) and those on a placebo. According to Almeida et al. also found that following 20 weeks of oral E2 treatment as opposed to placebo, there were no appreciable changes in mood symptoms. An additional extensive study involving 412 post-menopausal women with a mean age of 71 years verified that hormone therapy did not significantly impact mood symptoms in healthy women.

The Heart and Estrogen/Progestin Replacement Study (HERS), the Women's Health Initiative Study of Cognitive Aging (WHISCA), and the Women's International Study of long Duration Estrogen after the Menopause (WISDOM) did not find a significant effect of MHT on mood, despite the KEEPS study showing a positive effect of oral CEE versus transdermal E2.

Therefore, MHT should not be recommended to asymptomatic, non-depressed perimenopausal women to prevent or treat mood disorders. Certain subpopulations that are susceptible to depressive symptoms during the menopausal transition appear to benefit from estrogen.

8.1.3.2.2. In Depressed Women

There is some evidence that when given to depressed perimenopausal women, hormonal therapy may have an antidepressant effect akin to that of traditional antidepressant medications. Estrogen therapy (ET) is still not widely accepted as a therapeutic option for depression, despite the previously mentioned E2 antidepressant qualities. Soares et al. recently published a review. Aimed to categorize the effectiveness of estrogen-based depression treatments, illuminating the various clinical effects of MHT on mood depending on whether it was administered to post-menopausal or peri-menopausal women, and specifically if these women had a history of depression (Greendale et al., 2009).

Earlier findings from Gordon et al. support the "critical timing hypothesis," which proposes that the positive effects of estradiol are only seen when it is given close to the end of ovarian function. Estrogen therapy is not effective in treating depression in women who have gone through menopause.

Menopausal hormone therapy may have a neutral or positive impact on mood, according to additional results from trials including recently post-menopausal women with depression and several sizable observational studies, including women starting MHT soon after menopause. Four small studies evaluated the use of MHT (estradiol valerate 2 mg plus dienogest 2 mg, estradiol 1 mg/day plus medroxyprogesterone 10 mg/day for 2 weeks, and transdermal 17 -estradiol 0.05 mg/day) in postmenopausal women with depressive disorders and showed some improvements or no mood changes. Two of the studies showed the effectiveness of E2 for the management of depressive disorders during the perimenopause.

In contrast to women without a history of premenopausal depression (PMD), Schmidt and colleagues sought to ascertain whether women with a history of PMD had a different reaction to estradiol withdrawal (Schmidt P. J. along with others. 2015). Three weeks of transdermal E2 (100 mg/d) administration under open-label conditions were planned for this study. Following this time, participants were double-blindly randomized to receive E2 or matched placebo skin patches for a further three weeks (Greendale et al., 2011).

Even though depression is associated with menopause in only a small percentage of women, it is imperative to accurately investigate the cause of depression symptoms to identify women who had a history of depression prior to the menopause transition and those whose onset occurred during the menopausal transition. For patients who have had depression in the past, antidepressants continue to be the first line of treatment for depression. When treating women with mild mood disorders, physicians should take into account both non-pharmacologic (i.e., a healthy diet, regular exercise, dietary supplements, and/or hormonal methods).

More investigation is required to fully comprehend the mechanisms underlying the windows of vulnerability throughout distinct stages of a woman's reproductive life, as well as the connection between hormonal fluctuations and perimenopausal depression. Estradiol, progesterone, and androgens are sexual hormones that women experience dramatic fluctuations in during the menopausal transition. These fluctuations may be the cause of changes in behavior, mood, sleep patterns, and cognitive function.

The following short summary provides key concepts regarding MHT in menopause and perimenopause:

- **Cognitive Function and Cognitive Disorders:** although there is a strong correlation between estrogen and cognition, there is still conflicting evidence about the connection between hormone replacement therapy and neuroprotective effects. In women over 65 without underlying dementia, several studies have disproved any cognitive benefits of estrogen or combined estrogen-progestin therapy. Young women going through menopause who are not contraindicated for MHT and whose quality of life is compromised due to vasomotor symptoms, night sweats, or disturbed sleep are good candidates for MHT, and multiple studies have shown that MHT does not negatively impact these women's cognitive function.
- **Mood and Depressive Symptoms:** MHT should not be recommended to non-depressed perimenopausal women to prevent mood symptoms, despite some data suggesting a possible positive effect on mood. Because estrogens may enhance the response to antidepressants, they should be taken into consideration in menopausal women who also have other coexisting conditions, such as vasomotor symptoms.

8.2. Management of Depression and Anxiety

For some women, the period known as perimenopause, which precedes menopause, is a physically and psychologically taxing time. Hormonal changes can cause a variety of symptoms, including hot flashes, insomnia, mood swings, and even depression, which are associated with the so-called "change of life." Mental health experts say that women who experience abrupt hormonal changes, such as those associated with puberty, perimenopause, postpartum, or even their monthly cycle, are more likely to experience depression. In general, the condition affects women twice as often as it does men (Henderson and Sherwin, 2007).

8.2.1. Recognizing the Symptoms of Depression

It is normal to occasionally identify feelings of sadness, however, it is important for patients to be clear about the additional signs of depression:

- Irritability, frustration, or angry outbursts

- Anxiety, restlessness, or agitation
- Feelings of guilt or worthlessness
- Loss of interest in activities you used to enjoy
- Trouble concentrating or making decisions
- Lapses in memory
- Lack of energy
- Sleeping too little or too much
- Changes in your appetite
- Unexplained physical pain

8.2.2. Understanding the Risks of Depression

Changes in hormone levels related to menopause can affect both mental and physical well-being. In addition, mood may not be affected solely by the abrupt decrease in estrogen. In addition, the likelihood of experiencing anxiety or depression during menopause may be increased by the following factors:

- Diagnosis with depression before menopause
- Negative feelings toward menopause or the idea of aging
- Increased stress, either from work or personal relationships
- Discontent about your work, living environment, or financial situation
- Low self-esteem or anxiety
- Not feeling supported by the people around you
- Lack of exercise or physical activity
- Smoking

8.2.3. Treating Depression Through Lifestyle Changes

Treatment for depression during menopause is basically the same as for depression at any other stage of life. Therapy, medication, lifestyle modifications, or a combination of these are recommended. It is important to rule out any physical causes of the symptoms, such as thyroid problems, before linking depression to menopause. After a diagnosis, the following lifestyle changes may be suggested to see if they naturally alleviate anxiety or depression (Henderson et al., 2016).

- Adequate Sleep
- Regular Exercise
- Relaxation Techniques
- Quit Smoking
- Seek Support Groups

8.2.4. Treating Depression Through Medications and Therapy

Can be consider alternative treatments if altering the lifestyle doesn't alleviate the symptoms. For instance, talk therapy, antidepressant drugs, or hormone replacement therapy might be suggested.

- **Low-Dose Estrogen Replacement Therapy:** Can be recommend estrogen replacement therapy as a skin patch or pill. According to research, estrogen replacement therapy may help with menopause's emotional and physical symptoms. However, blood clots and breast cancer may also become more likely as a result of estrogen therapy.
- **Antidepressant Drug Therapy:** Should hormone replacement therapy not be a viable option, the physician may recommend conventional antidepressant drugs. These could be needed for a longer amount of time.
- **Talk Therapy:** Menopausal depression is a condition that can

be treated. It's crucial to keep in mind that there are a variety of treatment options available that may aid in symptom relief and offer adaptation techniques.

8.3. Cognitive Decline and Dementia

While perimenopause has been linked to cognitive impairment (Tilt, 1871), this is not frequently taken into account when evaluating women in this stage of life for memory and other cognitive impairments.

8.3.1. Perimenopause and Cognition

8.3.1.1. Physiologic Connections

Perimenopause may cause cognitive decline through several different mechanisms (Singh M, Toran-Allerand et al., 1999; Greendale et al., 2011; Lumsden et al., 2015). Many brain regions, including the hippocampus, striatum, and prefrontal cortex, are involved in learning, registering, and retrieving information for language and judgment. These functions are influenced by estrogen. Reduced cholinergic and serotonergic transmission, which has an immediate impact on mood and cognition, is a result of diminished cholinergic and serotonergic transmission in the hippocampus and basal forebrain, which is correlated with estrogen loss. Mood disorders exacerbate cognitive dysfunction indirectly. Hot flashes are caused by the vasovagal effects of perimenopause, which raise cortisol levels and may impair memory. Loss of estrogen may also lead to a decline in cardiovascular and cerebrovascular health, which could have an unintentional detrimental impact on brain health.

8.3.1.2. Clinical Connections

Numerous studies and reports have been published about the clinical implications of perimenopause on mental and physical health. In an open-label study, eight weeks of transdermal estradiol treatment were given to 19 early menopausal women who were randomly assigned to receive a reversible procedure called tryptophan-depletion, which lowers serotonin levels, or a control procedure. Verbal memory and mood both markedly declined in the women who underwent the tryptophan-depletion procedure, and both improved with treatment with estradiol. The positive effects of estrogen on serotonin function in relation to mood and memory were supported by this study (Amin et al., 2006). In a related study, treatment with estradiol improved psychomotor speed on Trails A and category fluency, two critical measures used in neuropsychological assessments (Kugaya et al., 2003).

The relationship between perimenopause and cognition or whether perimenopausal physical symptoms (such as flushing or night sweats) contribute to subtle deficits in cognitive function have been the main topics of longitudinal studies of perimenopause and cognitive performance.

The Kinman Women Health Investigation (KIWI) examined the cognitive function of 694 premenopausal Chinese women living in Taiwan who were 46 years old. The women were followed over an extended period of time. Measures were taken of verbal memory, verbal fluency, mental flexibility, and processing speed at baseline and after 18 months. As was to be expected given the learning effect of repeated neuropsychologic testing, all cognitive tests showed improvement. However, compared to women who did not enter the perimenopause, those who did showed less improvement in verbal memory. In the US, comparable studies monitored 800 women between the ages of 42 and 52 from all ethnic backgrounds for two years. Repeated testing, as in the KIWI study, revealed slight gains in working memory and processing speed in the premenopausal group. There were no such gains in those who had entered the perimenopause. It should be mentioned that in middle age, a lack of improvement on multiple tests could be taken as a sign of cognitive dysfunction (Lamar et al., 2003).

8.3.2. Overlap and Misdiagnosis

In studies of perimenopausal women, 35 to 62% reported memory changes across cultures. These symptoms were not associated with perimenopausal symptoms (such as hot flashes, sleep disturbances, depression, and anxiety), as evidenced by their correlation with lower performance on objective neurocognitive tests and decreases in verbal memory, verbal fluency, and executive function. While the recorded cognitive deficits seem similar to those observed in mild cognitive impairment (MCI) and some early cases of dementia, there is a suggestion that this condition be referred to as menopause-related cognitive impairment rather than MCI due to the absence of the high incidence (50%) of conversion to dementia seen in MCI. It has been observed that common hot flash symptoms and laboratory indicators of impending menopause may not manifest early, which can mislead doctors and patients to believe that another cognitive disorder is present. Likewise, a different cause needs to be taken into account if menopause-related cognitive impairment symptoms last after the shift or seriously impair functioning.

8.3.3. Menopause-Related Cognitive Impairment

In a case study, a 55-year-old woman with a 4-year history of depression and menopause at age 54, as well as a year of progressive memory loss and behavioral changes (losing objects, not caring for personal grooming), was found to have overall cognitive ability at the 98th percentile, but working memory was in the 12th percentile and verbal fluency was in the 20th percentile. Hormone therapy was prescribed for her menopause-related cognitive disorder. Repeat cognitive testing conducted after 15 months revealed that behavioral symptoms had subsided and cognitive abilities had stabilized, with working memory reaching the 88th percentile. After completing a graduate program, she held a leadership role in education for four years following her presentation (Devi, 2018).

8.3.4. Hormone Treatment and Cognition

A prospective, double-blind study compared the cognitive effects of starting estradiol six years after menopause versus starting it ten years or later. Cognitive testing took place at baseline, two, five, and seven years. Women who took estradiol within six years of menopause exhibited no different verbal memory, executive function, or global cognition than those who took it ten or more years after menopause. In this study, postmenopause was defined as absence of vaginal bleeding for at least 6 months (natural menopause) or bilateral oophorectomy (surgical menopause) and serum total estradiol of < 25 pg per mL (Henderson et al., 2016).

Regardless of the length of time since menopause, estradiol neither improved nor harmed cognitive abilities. The researchers addressed that other studies (Lethaby et al., 2008; Gleason et al., 2015; Grady et al., 2002) showed cognitive improvements, especially in verbal and episodic memory, in women treated with estrogen postmenopausally, noting that these studies had small sample sizes, smaller age range, and shorter treatment duration. However, the study's sample sizes were small, its age range was narrow, and the treatment period was short. This large trial was limited by the fact that serum levels of estradiol were higher than those linked to significant outcomes in other studies, such as the prevention of fractures and the reduction of vasomotor symptoms, and the study lacked the power to exclude small treatment effects in subgroups. Overall, the findings suggest that there is no reason for postmenopausal women who are close to or past menopause to be unduly concerned about the potential negative effects of hormone therapy on cognitive function over a five-year period.

Hormone therapy is recommended by the North American Menopause Society for the treatment of cognitive symptoms after surgical menopause, but not after an early natural menopause due to some studies showing neutral benefits. Hormone therapy is advised for indirect treatment of vasomotor symptoms and sleep disturbances, but not for the prevention or treatment of dementia or cognitive decline at any age. Positive indirect effects on memory and concentration may result from symptomatic relief.

Research indicates that estrogen is involved in healthy cognitive function. A decrease in estrogen during the perimenopause may cause flushing, mood swings, and mild cognitive changes (such as slowed psychomotor speed, verbal fluency impairment, and mild memory loss), according to certain studies. This very mild cognitive decline associated with menopause may resemble MCI, but it is not dementia. It is crucial to consider the possibility of low estrogen and mild cognitive decline, even though there is disagreement in the literature regarding the existence of cognitive decline during the perimenopause and insufficient evidence to conclude that it never happens.

Menopause should be taken into account by neurologists assessing women experiencing memory loss. As with any other cognitively impaired person, a comprehensive neuropsychologic battery of tests, a brain MRI, and standard laboratory testing are recommended for individuals with memory impairment.

Menopause usually cures mild cognitive impairments that may develop during the perimenopause. Counselling perimenopausal women who are concerned about memory issues can be aided by this information. Concomitant symptoms of depression or anxiety that can impair cognition should also be addressed. The perimenopause is a great time to assess and manage cardiovascular risk factors that can be changed to improve cardiovascular health and reduce the chance of dementia and cognitive decline brought on by blood vessel disease. A short-term (6–12 months) estrogen trial should be considered if the patient fits the recommended criteria for menopause-related cognitive impairment. During the trial, a gynecologist consultation may be necessary, and careful follow-up should be maintained.

Estrogen therapy is not a good option for women who have a high risk of stroke or clinically evident cardiovascular disease, especially if there is mild cognitive decline and MRI evidence of multiple small white matter strokes. These women often worsen clinically. The impact of perimenopause on the hypothalamic pituitary axis in relation to mood and cognition requires further research (Maki et al., 2018).

A Closer Look

Attitudes and Experiences of Society

Hormonal, menstrual, and usually vasomotor changes are all part of the process of the menopause transition. However, psychological and social factors, including past experiences, lifestyle choices, cultural and social interpretations of menopause, and a woman's social and material circumstances, greatly influence the menopause experience overall. Menopause has been defined as a biopsychosocial experience, meaning that social and cultural contexts greatly influence how menopause is felt and understood.

Women's perceptions of menopause are influenced by the paradigm they live in; those who see menopause as a medical condition tend to rate it much lower than those who see it as a life transition or an indication of aging. It's interesting to note that postmenopausal women tend to have more positive beliefs and attitudes toward menopause than do premenopausal women. There is evidence to suggest that negative attitudes and expectations held prior to the menopause predict the experience of symptoms during the menopause. More symptoms during this transition are reported by women who have more negative attitudes toward the menopause.

There are various ways to experience the menopause as a stage of life. It can be defined by changes in one's personal roles within the family and society, as well as personal challenges. Women's perspectives on the changes that come with menopause are shaped by their social, familial, and personal experiences. Women from various nations and areas also have diverse perspectives. Compared to perimenopausal or premenopausal women, postmenopausal women had more positive attitudes regarding menopause. The following additional variables may also impact attitudes regarding menopause: age, menopausal symptoms, socioeconomic and psychological status, occupation, and ethnicity (Lui et al., 2003).

Geography and ethnicity have an impact on menopause experiences. Diverse ethnic groups of American women report markedly different menopausal effects. According to a significant study, African-American women were more likely to report vasomotor symptoms, whereas Caucasian women were more likely to report what are sometimes referred to as psychosomatic symptoms.

Women from diverse ethnic backgrounds may have differing experiences with menopause and related care. Compared to non-immigrant women, immigrant women reported more vasomotor symptoms, other physical symptoms, worse mental health, and overall dissatisfaction with the care they had received. Culture also had an impact on menopausal symptom self-management techniques.

Hot flushes were not the most often reported symptoms, according to two international studies of Asian women; instead, body and joint aches, memory issues, insomnia, irritability, and migraines were. Another study comparing the menopausal experiences of White Australian women and women in Laos found that Australian women had higher rates of depression and expressed fears of cancer, weight gain, and aging, fears that Laotian women did not share, as they saw menopause as a positive experience. Japanese women differ from American women in how they experience the menopause's effects, or konenki. Hot flashes and night sweats are less common in Japanese women; there are several biological and social reasons for this. In the past, wealthy middle-class Japanese housewives were linked to konenki, i.e., women from traditional, multigenerational rural households did not report this "luxury disease." In Japan, menopause was not considered a "revolutionary transition" or a "deficiency disease" that required medical attention, but rather as a natural part of aging (Santoro et al., 2015).

According to a 2005 study, hot flashes were common in 22.1% of 140 Japanese participants, indicating that reporting of vasomotor symptoms has increased in Japanese culture. This was nearly twice as much as it was 20 years earlier. Although the precise cause of this is unknown, dietary modifications, middle-aged women becoming more medicalized, and increased media attention to the issue are all potential contributing factors. Vasomotor symptom reporting is still "significantly" lower than in North America, though.

Furthermore, studies suggest that women from some Asian cultures understand menopause in a way that emphasizes a sense of liberation and celebrates being free from the risk of pregnancy, in contrast to the majority of American women who seem to view it negatively as a period of decline or deterioration. One study seemed to indicate, in contrast to these findings, that many American women "experience this time as one of liberation and self-actualization."

Menopause can cause a sense of loss in some women because it means their fertility is ending. Furthermore, this transition frequently coincides with other stressful situations, like having to care for aging parents or handling the emotional difficulties associated with "empty nest syndrome" after children leave the family home. This condition may be made worse in societies where growing older is seen negatively.

Summary

- During the menopausal transition, which begins four to six years before cessation of menses, middle-aged women experience a progressive change in ovarian activity and a physiologic deterioration of hypothalamic-pituitary-ovarian axis function associated with fluctuating hormone levels.
- During their lifetime women experience dramatic fluctuations in the levels of the sexual hormones estradiol, progesterone and also androgens when going through the different stages of life, from menarche to menopause. These fluctuations have a significant impact on the whole body including the central nervous system (CNS) and can be responsible for modifications in behavior, cognition and mood.
- The time leading up to menopause (called perimenopause) is a physical and emotional roller coaster for some women. The so-called "change of life" comes with a host of symptoms triggered by hormonal shifts—hot flashes, insomnia, mood fluctuations and even depression.
- Changing hormone levels during menopause may affect your physical and emotional health. Also, the rapid drop in estrogen may not be the only thing affecting your mood.
- Depression during menopause is treated in much the same way it's treated at any other time in life. Your doctor may prescribe lifestyle changes, medications, therapy, or a combination of these options. Before attributing your depression to menopause, your doctor will first want to rule out any physical reasons for your symptoms, such as thyroid problems. After making a diagnosis, your doctor may suggest the following lifestyle changes to see if they provide natural relief from your depression or anxiety.
- Neurologists must consider perimenopause when evaluating women with memory decline. A detailed neuropsychologic battery of tests are indicated as in any individual with memory impairment, along with a brain MRI and standard laboratory testing as for any other cognitively impaired individual.

References

1. Amin, Z., Gueorguieva, R., Cappiello, A., et al. (2006). Estradiol and tryptophan depletion interact to modulate cognition in menopausal women. *Neuropsychopharmacology, 31*(11), 2489–2497. https://doi.org/10.1038/sj.npp.1301044.
2. Barrett-Connor, E., & Goodman-Gruen, D. (1999). Cognitive function and endogenous sex hormones in older women. *Journal of the American Geriatrics Society, 47*(10), 1289–1293. https://doi.org/10.1111/j.1532-5415.1999.tb07427.x.
3. Davis, S. R., Lambrinoudaki, I., Lumsden, M., et al. (2015). Menopause. *Nature Reviews Disease Primers, 1*, 15004. https://doi.org/10.1038/nrdp.2015.4.
4. de Kruif, M., et al. (2016). Depression during the perimenopause: A meta-analysis. *Journal of Affective Disorders, 206*, 174–180. https://doi.org/10.1016/j.jad.2016.07.040.
5. Devi, G. (2018). Menopause-related cognitive impairment. *Obstetrics & Gynecology, 132*(6), 1325–1327. https://doi.org/10.1097/AOG.0000000000002935.

6. Fuh, J. L., Wang, S. J., Lee, S. J., Lu, S. R., & Juang, K. D. (2006). A longitudinal study of cognition changes during early menopausal transition in a rural community. *Maturitas, 53*(4), 447–453. https://doi.org/10.1016/j.maturitas.2005.07.009.
7. Girdler, S. S., O'Briant, C., Steege, J., Grewen, K., & Light, K. C. (1999). A comparison of the effect of estrogen with or without progesterone on mood and physical symptoms in postmenopausal women. *Journal of Women's Health & Gender-Based Medicine, 8*(5), 637–646. https://doi.org/10.1089/jwh.1.1999.8.637.
8. Gleason, C. E., Dowling, N. M., Wharton, W., et al. (2015). Effects of hormone therapy on cognition and mood in recently postmenopausal women: Findings from the randomized controlled KEEPS-cognitive and affective study. *PLoS Medicine, 12*(3), e1001833. https://doi.org/10.1371/journal.pmed.1001833.
9. Gordon, J. L., Rubinow, D. R., Eisenlohr-Moul, T. A., Leserman, J., & Girdler, S. S. (2016). Estradiol variability, stressful life events, and the emergence of depressive symptomatology during the menopausal transition. *Menopause, 23*(3), 257–266. https://doi.org/10.1097/GME.0000000000000528.
10. Grady, D., Yaffe, K., Kristof, M., et al. (2002). Effect of postmenopausal hormone therapy on cognitive function: The Heart and Estrogen/Progestin Replacement Study. *American Journal of Medicine, 113*(7), 543–548. https://doi.org/10.1016/S0002-9343(02)01309-6.
11. Greendale, G. A., Derby, C. A., & Maki, P. M. (2011). Perimenopause and cognition. *Obstetric and Gynecologic Clinics of North America, 38*(3), 519–535. https://doi.org/10.1016/j.ogc.2011.05.008.
12. Greendale, G. A., Huang, M. H., Wight, R. G., Seeman, T., Luetters, C., Avis, N. E., Johnston, J., & Karlamangla, A. S. (2009). Effects of the menopause transition and hormone use on cognitive performance in midlife women. *Neurology, 72*(21), 1850–1857. https://doi.org/10.1212/WNL.0b013e3181a71193.
13. Henderson, V. W., & Sherwin, B. B. (2007). Surgical versus natural menopause: Cognitive issues. *Menopause, 14*(4), 572–579. https://doi.org/10.1097/gme.0b013e318032ff12.
14. Henderson, V. W., St John, J. A., Hodis, H. N., et al. (2016). Cognitive effects of estradiol after menopause. *Neurology, 87*(7), 699–707. https://doi.org/10.1212/WNL.0000000000003080.
15. Imtiaz, B., Taipale, H., Tanskanen, A., Tiihonen, M., Kivipelto, M., Heikkinen, A. M., Tiihonen, J., Soininen, H., Hartikainen, S., & Tolppanen, A. M. (2017). Risk of Alzheimer's disease among users of postmenopausal hormone therapy: A nationwide case-control study. *Maturitas, 98*, 7–13. https://doi.org/10.1016/j.maturitas.2017.01.002.
16. Khoo, S. K., Coglan, M., Battistutta, D., Tippett, V., & Raphael, B. (1998). Hormonal treatment and psychological function during the menopausal transition: An evaluation of the effects of conjugated estrogens/cyclic medroxyprogesterone acetate. *Climacteric, 1*(1), 55–62. https://doi.org/10.3109/13697139809080682.
17. Kugaya, A., Epperson, C. N., Zoghbi, S., et al. (2003). Increase in prefrontal serotonin 2A receptors following estrogen treatment in postmenopausal women. *American Journal of Psychiatry, 160*(8), 1522–1524. https://doi.org/10.1176/appi.ajp.160.8.1522.
18. Lamar, M., Resnick, S. M., & Zonderman, A. B. (2003). Longitudinal changes in verbal memory in older adults: Distinguishing the effects of age from repeat testing. *Neurology, 60*(1), 82–86. https://doi.org/10.1212/01.WNL.0000049471.84885.0F.

19. Lethaby, A., Hogervorst, E., Richards, M., Yesufu, A., & Yaffe, K. (2008). Hormone replacement therapy for cognitive function in postmenopausal women. *Cochrane Database of Systematic Reviews, 2008*(1), CD003122. https://doi.org/10.1002/14651858.CD003122.pub3.

20. Lui, L. Y., Stone, K., Cauley, J. A., Hillier, T., & Yaffe, K. (2003). Bone loss predicts subsequent cognitive decline in older women: The Study of Osteoporotic Fractures. *Journal of the American Geriatrics Society, 51*(1), 38–43. https://doi.org/10.1046/j.1601-5215.2003.51007.x.

21. Maki, P. M., et al. (2018). Guidelines for the evaluation and treatment of perimenopausal depression: Summary and recommendations. *Journal of Women's Health*. https://doi.org/10.1089/jwh.2018.27099.mensocrec.

22. Maki, P. M., Kornstein, S. G., Joffe, H., Bromberger, J. T., Freeman, E. W., Athappilly, G., Bobo, W. V., Rubin, L. H., Koleva, H. K., Cohen, L. S., et al. (2018). Guidelines for the evaluation and treatment of perimenopausal depression: Summary and recommendations. *Menopause, 25*(9), 1069–1085. https://doi.org/10.1097/GME.0000000000001174.

23. Morgan, K. N., Derby, C. A., & Gleason, C. E. (2018). Cognitive changes with reproductive aging, perimenopause, and menopause. *Obstetrics and Gynecology Clinics of North America, 45*(4), 751–763. https://doi.org/10.1016/j.ogc.2018.07.011.

24. Rentz, D. M., Weiss, B. K., Jacobs, E. G., Cherkerzian, S., Klibanski, A., Remington, A., Aizley, H., & Goldstein, J. M. (2017). Sex differences in episodic memory in early midlife: Impact of reproductive aging. *Menopause, 24*(4), 400–408. https://doi.org/10.1097/GME.0000000000000771.

25. Rocca, W. A., Mielke, M. M., Vemuri, P., & Miller, V. M. (2014). Sex and gender differences in the causes of dementia: A narrative review. *Maturitas, 79*(3), 196–201. https://doi.org/10.1016/j.maturitas.2014.05.008.

26. Santoro, N., Teal, S., Gavito, C., Cano, S., Chosich, J., & Sheeder, J. (2015). Use of a levonorgestrel-containing intrauterine system with supplemental estrogen improves symptoms in perimenopausal women: A pilot study. *Menopause, 22*(12), 1301–1307. https://doi.org/10.1097/GME.0000000000000557.

27. Savolainen-Peltonen, H., Rahkola-Soisalo, P., Hoti, F., Vattulainen, P., Gissler, M., Ylikorkala, O., & Mikkola, T. S. (2019). Use of postmenopausal hormone therapy and risk of Alzheimer's disease in Finland: Nationwide case-control study. *BMJ, 364*, l665. https://doi.org/10.1136/bmj.l665.

28. Schmidt, P. J., Ben Dor, R., Martinez, P. E., Guerrieri, G. M., Harsh, V. L., Thompson, K., Koziol, D. E., Nieman, L. K., & Rubinow, D. R. (2015). Effects of estradiol withdrawal on mood in women with past perimenopausal depression: A randomized clinical trial. *JAMA Psychiatry, 72*(7), 714–726. https://doi.org/10.1001/jamapsychiatry.2015.0111.

29. Shao, H., Breitner, J. C., Whitmer, R. A., Wang, J., Hayden, K., Wengreen, H., Corcoran, C., Tschanz, J., Norton, M., Munger, R., et al. (2012). Hormone therapy and Alzheimer disease dementia: New findings from the Cache County Study. *Neurology, 79*(18), 1846–1852. https://doi.org/10.1212/WNL.0b013e318271f823.

30. Soares, C. N., Almeida, O. P., Joffe, H., & Cohen, L. S. (2001). Efficacy of estradiol for the treatment of depressive disorders in perimenopausal women: A double-blind, randomized, placebo-controlled trial. *Archives of General Psychiatry, 58*(6), 529–534. https://doi.org/10.1001/archpsyc.58.6.529.

31. Sullivan Mitchell, E., & Fugate Woods, N. (2001). Midlife women's attributions about perceived memory changes: Observations from the Seattle Midlife Women's Health Study. *Journal of Women's Health & Gender-Based Medicine, 10*(4), 351–362. https://doi.org/10.1089/152460901750269670.

32. Tang, M. X., Jacobs, D., Stern, Y., Marder, K., Schofield, P., Gurland, B., Andrews, H., & Mayeux, R. (1996). Effect of oestrogen during menopause on risk and age at onset of Alzheimer's disease. *Lancet, 348*(9025), 429–432. https://doi.org/10.1016/S0140-6736(96)03356-9.

33. Tilt, E. (1871). *The Change of Life in Health and Disease: A Practical Treatise on the Nervous and Other Afflictions of Women at the Decline of Life.* Philadelphia, PA: Lindsey and Blakiston.

34. Toran-Allerand, C. D., Singh, M., & Sétáló, G. Jr. (1999). Novel mechanisms of estrogen action on the brain: New players in an old story. *Frontiers in Neuroendocrinology, 20*(1), 97–121. https://doi.org/10.1006/frne.1999.0175.

35. Waring, S. C., Rocca, W. A., Petersen, R. C., O'Brien, P. C., Tangalos, E. G., & Kokmen, E. (1999). Postmenopausal estrogen replacement therapy and risk of Alzheimer's disease: A population-based study. *Neurology, 52*(5), 965. https://doi.org/10.1212/WNL.52.5.965.

36. Weber, M. T., Maki, P. M., & McDermott, M. P. (2014). Cognition and mood in perimenopause: A systematic review and meta-analysis. *Journal of Steroid Biochemistry and Molecular Biology, 142*, 90–98. https://doi.org/10.1016/j.jsbmb.2013.11.007.

37. Weber, M. T., Mapstone, M., Staskiewicz, J., & Maki, P. M. (2012). Reconciling subjective memory complaints with objective memory performance in the menopausal transition. *Menopause, 19*(7), 735–741. https://doi.org/10.1097/GME.0b013e318247a535.

38. Yaffe, K., Sawaya, G., Lieberburg, I., & Grady, D. (1998). Estrogen therapy in postmenopausal women: Effects on cognitive function and dementia. *JAMA, 279*(9), 688–695. https://doi.org/10.1001/jama.279.9.688.

39. Zandi, P. P., Carlson, M. C., Plassman, B. L., Welsh-Bohmer, K. A., Mayer, L. S., Steffens, D. C., Breitner, J. C. S., & the Cache County Memory Study Investigators. (2002). Hormone replacement therapy and incidence of Alzheimer disease in older women: The Cache County Study. *JAMA, 288*(17), 2123. https://doi.org/10.1001/jama.288.17.2123.

40. Zárate, S., Stevnsner, T., & Gredilla, R. (2017). Role of estrogen and other sex hormones in brain aging: Neuroprotection and DNA repair. *Frontiers in Aging Neuroscience*. Retrieved from: http://journal.frontiersin.org/article/10.3389/fnagi.2017.00430/full (accessed on 10 September 2024).

Chapter 9

SLEEP DISTURBANCES

Contents

Introduction

Any number of problems that make it difficult to go asleep, stay asleep, or get deep, rejuvenating sleep are referred to as sleep disturbances. Since getting enough sleep is crucial for both physical and mental health, these disruptions can have a serious negative influence on general health and quality of life. Insomnia, sleep apnea, restless legs syndrome (RLS), and circadian rhythm abnormalities are common forms of sleep disturbances. Every kind has different difficulties and calls for different management techniques (Zammit et al., 1999). One of the most common sleep disorders is insomnia, which is characterized by trouble getting to sleep, remaining asleep, or waking up too early and not being able to go back to sleep. It can be chronic, continuing for months or more, or acute, lasting a few days or weeks. Insomnia has many different causes, such as stress, anxiety, depression, bad sleeping habits, and some medications. The effects of insomnia are not limited to the evening hours; they frequently result in daytime tiredness, agitation, trouble focusing, and poor performance at work or school. Another common sleep disturbance is sleep apnea, which is characterized by recurrent breathing interruptions while you're asleep. The most prevalent type of sleep apnea, known as obstructive sleep apnea (OSA), is brought on by the throat muscles' inability to maintain an open airway. Although less common, central sleep apnea is a condition in which the brain malfunctions in sending the correct signals to the muscles that regulate breathing. Loud snoring, gasping for air while you sleep, morning headaches, and excessive daytime sleepiness are all signs of sleep apnea. Severe health problems like hypertension, heart disease, and stroke can result from untreated sleep apnea.

A neurological condition known as restless legs syndrome (RLS) is typified by an insatiable desire to move the legs, usually as a result of discomfort. These feelings, which are usually felt when a person is sleeping in the evening or at night, are frequently characterized as throbbing, pulling, or creeping. Although it eases the pain, moving around can make it harder to fall asleep and stay asleep. Periodic limb movement disorder (PLMD), characterized by involuntary leg movements during sleep, is frequently linked to restless legs syndrome (RLS), which can cause severe disruptions to sleep. Disorders of the circadian rhythm refer to disturbances in the body's natural clock, which governs the cycle of sleep and wakefulness. These conditions include advanced sleep phase disorder (ASPD), in which people wake up much earlier, and delayed sleep phase disorder (DSPD), in which people fall asleep and wake up much later than desired. Circadian rhythm disruptions also include jet lag and shift work disorder. These conditions may make it difficult to fall asleep at regular times, which could result in inadequate or inadequate sleep. For sleep disturbances to be effectively managed, a multifaceted approach involving behavioral therapies, lifestyle modifications, and occasionally medication is necessary. Cognitive-behavioral therapy for insomnia (CBT-I), which focuses on altering sleep-related behaviors and misconceptions, is regarded as the gold standard treatment for insomnia. Continuous positive airway pressure (CPAP) therapy is frequently recommended for sleep apnea to maintain an open airway while you sleep. Medication that affects dopamine levels and lifestyle modifications like cutting back on alcohol and caffeine intake can help manage RLS. Treatment options for circadian rhythm disorders include melatonin supplements, light therapy, and sleep schedule modifications (Gauld et al., 2021)

Orientation and Directional Terms:

Term	Definition	Illustration
Corticosteroids	A class of steroid hormones that are produced in the adrenal cortex of vertebrates, as well as the synthetic analogs of these hormones.	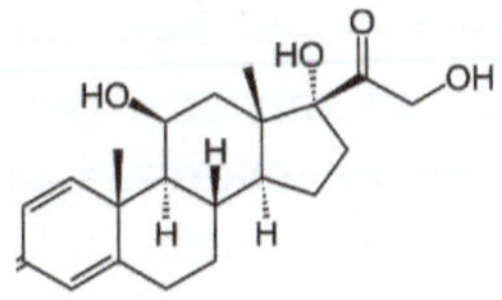
Bipolar disorder	A mental illness that causes unusual shifts in a person's mood, energy, activity levels, and concentration.	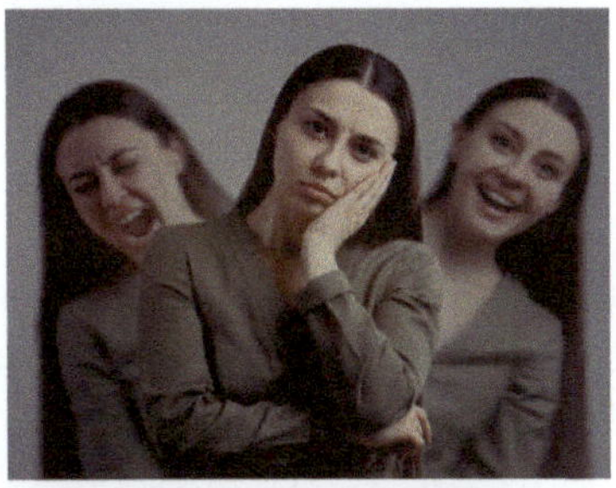
Central Nervous System	A processing center that manages everything that your body does, from your thoughts and feelings to your movements.	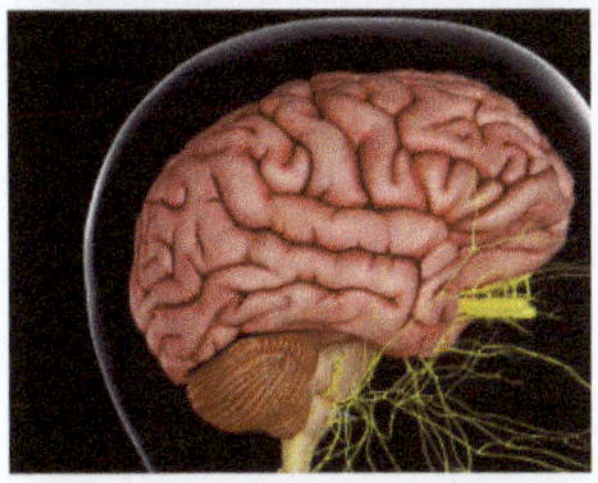
Cataplexy	A type of sudden weakness in your muscles that can make you go limp or temporarily lose your ability to move.	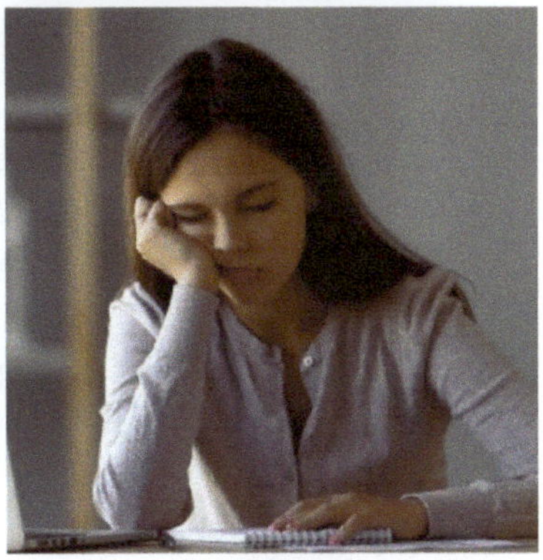
Narcolepsy	A chronic neurological disorder that affects the brain's ability to control sleep-wake cycles. People with narcolepsy may feel rested after waking, but then feel very sleepy throughout much of the day.	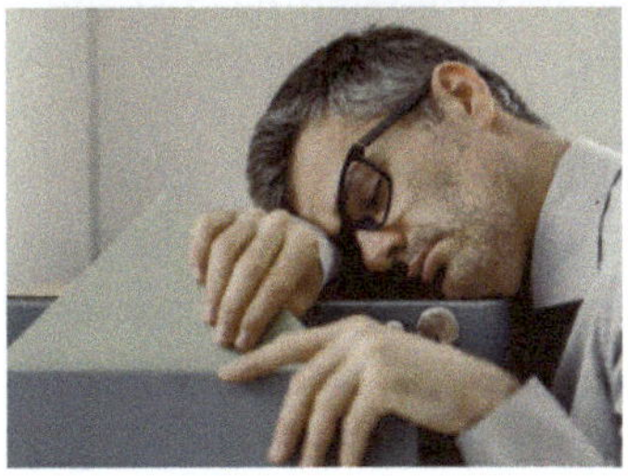

9.1. Sleep Disturbances Technique

The clinician should familiarize themselves with the broad categories of sleep disorders that the Association of Sleep Disorders Centers (1979) has detailed a diagnostic classification of sleep and arousal disorders to shed light on the patient's complaint of sleep disturbance. The fact that the diagnoses covered in the first two classification divisions were arranged in accordance with the patient's complaint of insomnia or excessive daytime sleepiness is clinically significant. The best chance of gaining meaningful information about the underlying ailment is to investigate the patient's past sleep-related complaints.

9.1.1. Ways to Manage Sleep Disturbance

There are many ways you can manage and cope with sleep disturbance:

- Daily log of sleep (including naps and the amount of time you sleep at night), sleep disturbances, and what are doing to manage the sleep disturbances using the My STORI™ app or a journal.
- Cognitive behavioral therapy.
- Good sleep hygiene
- Medication schedule. Corticosteroids and other medications may interfere with sleep if taken late in the day.
- Explore self-care activities that can help the cope with and improve the sleep, including diet, exercise, etc.

9.1.2. Disorders of Initiating and Maintaining Sleep

The most common arousal and sleep disorders that clinicians see are insomnias, or problems starting and staying asleep. When a patient complains of having trouble sleeping, what are the symptoms? Is the patient having trouble falling asleep? Can the patient stay asleep for the desired amount of time? How long does the patient sleep? How does the patient feel about the quality of the sleep? Since both the waking and the sleeping states are essential to a 24-hour continuum, the patient's waking state is just as important. Some patients wake up feeling rested and perform flawlessly even though they slept far less than anticipated. How does the patient feel when they wake up in the morning? How does he or she function during the day? Does the patient feel tired and/or involuntarily fall asleep during the day? With the exception of brevity, their sleeping seems typical. These so-called short sleepers frequently get less than 75% of the recommended amount of sleep each day for their age (Huyett et al., 2021).

Other patients who appear psychologically well but complain of insomnia do not exhibit any signs of sleep pathology, according to objective studies. These patients believe that their sleep is insufficient, even though they have slept for more than 6.5 hours and fallen asleep in less than 15 to 20 minutes (insomnia without objective findings). About 30% of patients who complain of insomnia do so in combination with short sleepers and these pseudoinsomniacs. In certain cases, some very basic components of good sleep hygiene may be involved in restless nights. Every person has a different threshold for environmental factors. Does the patient have a regular wake-up time? Does the lighting change while they sleep? Is the room's temperature appropriate for their specific sleeping needs? Is the patient's bed partner bothersome? When attempting to determine a causal relationship between an environmental factor and sleep disturbance, the clinician must take into account whether the disturbance is temporally correlated with a stimulus that is both physically measurable and disturbing. Second, rather than the stimulus's emotional significance to the patient, its physical characteristics should be the source of its upsetting aspects. Third, after the stimulus is eliminated, there ought to be a gradual return to restful sleep. Does the patient take naps during the day? Naps can help with sleep at night, but they also frequently get in the way of it. This is especially valid for senior patients. How long has any sleep disturbance lasted? This information is important for both the problem's management and the differential diagnosis of the complaint. When a disturbance arises recently, the clinician will look for contributing factors. Psychological disturbance is the most frequent cause of chronic insomnia (Kaur et al., 2023).

When considered appropriately, a sleep disturbance could provide compelling evidence supporting a unipolar depression diagnosis. How's your sleep? "No good" is a common reply. What is the bad news? Usually, the patient wakes up and finds it hard to fall back asleep. When do you wake up? 2:00 or 3:00 a.m. is a common response. m. Can you fall back asleep? Most of the time, the answer is no. Different sleep symptoms may be linked to other mental health conditions. Excessive yet restless sleep is more frequently linked to bipolar depression. Manic patients frequently appear to need little sleep. The patient who is generally anxious may experience restless sleep, trouble falling asleep, or both. Sleep disturbances are common in psychotic disorders. The degree of sleep disturbance and the severity of the mental illness appear to be directly correlated. An emotionally charged incident may be the cause of insomnia even when there is no significant mental illness. We call this insomnia situational psychophysiological. When the emotional response to the incident fades, you can anticipate that the sleep will return to normal. A disruption that lasts for less than three weeks is considered temporary. When psychophysiological insomnia is chronic, there is typically a history of mediocre to nonexistent prestress sleep. The additional weight of overstress causes sleep quality to further deteriorate, which has a detrimental impact on daytime functioning. Intense attempts to fall asleep may incite arousal in and of themselves. In the end, even going to bed on time might raise arousal levels long after the initial stressful event has subsided. These patients typically get a better night's sleep on the weekends or during vacations. A drug history is crucial in any insomnia case. Alcohol is used by some patients as a sleep aid. Due to the short-lived nature of the effect, the patient might wake up in a few hours and find it difficult to fall back asleep. On the other hand, a chronic alcoholic might have little overall sleep due to frequent sleep disruptions. A marked delay in the onset of sleep may accompany acute withdrawal, and this delay may worsen into delirium tremens (Momin et al., 2023).

Certain patients have extremely high caffeine sensitivity. Not only should coffee be the subject of inquiry, but also tea, cola, and chocolate. Smoking cigarettes can disrupt sleep, most likely by activating the catecholaminergic systems. Furthermore, the heavy smoker who quits might momentarily have trouble sleeping as a result of nicotine withdrawal. It is imperative to inquire about more conventionally prescribed sleep aids from the patient as well. Hypnotic medications generally lose their efficacy within a few weeks, which frequently prompts an increase in dosage. How long have any such medications been used? Has the dose been increased gradually? Any further sleep reaction also becomes only momentary. Chronic use of hypnotic drugs may result in recurrent awakenings during the night that last longer than five minutes each. A history of difficulty maintaining sleep in the later part of the night could indicate that a drug's effectiveness has been shortened as a result of tolerance developing. On the other hand, sudden withdrawal can result in a noticeable worsening of sleep disturbance, which is frequently connected to nightmares. Does the patient use any stimulants that target the central nervous system (e.g., amphetamines)? Steroid drugs and centrally acting adrenergic blocking agents can also cause insomnia. Sleep disturbances may result from xanthines used as bronchodilators and adrenergic agonists. Chemically speaking, the latter compounds are connected to caffeine. What is the overall health status of the patient? Pain is especially painful when trying to fall asleep. Is there nocturia, fever, pruritus, paresthesias, nocturnal dyspnea or coughing, hyperthyroidism, renal failure, or an organic brain syndrome? Does the patient have frequent headaches, angina pectoris, reflux esophagitis, peptic ulcer disease, or arthritis?

Some patients with sleep disturbances express greater complaints about the resulting problems with daytime wakefulness. This is typically the case when it comes to sleep apnea, a syndrome marked by several instances of interrupted breathing that last for at least 10 seconds and happen at least 30 times over the course of a 6-hour sleep study. Sleep apnea may be central, in which the cessation of airflow occurs simultaneously with disruption of thoracic and diaphragmatic movements, or it may be purely secondary to obstruction of the upper airway, in which case there is no airflow through the nose or mouth despite continuous respiratory efforts of the thorax and abdomen. The latter kind most likely indicates a problem with the way the brain controls breathing. The majority of cases are mixed—central at first, and obstructive later. The central form of sleep apnea is more common in patients who complain of insomnia, so a bed partner's history may not always indicate loud snoring or gasping respirations. However, a watchful bed partner might detect apnea episodes. Patients with nocturnal myoclonus may describe themselves as restless sleepers, but they usually aren't aware of the leg twitches that occur repeatedly during seemingly normal sleep intervals. The patient's bed partner may report that the patient has kicked them. The patient might disclose past experiences with leg cramps, unkempt bedding, or even bed falls. A patient may have restless legs syndrome if they complain of having trouble relaxing or even going asleep due to strange crawling sensations in their thighs and calves. With exercise, the dysesthesias frequently go away for a while. The majority of patients with sleep-related myoclonus also do not have restless legs syndrome, but nearly all of them also suffer from it.

9.1.3. Disorders of Excessive Somnolence

As with sleep apnea, the main complaint of the patient may be that he or she is too sleepy during the expected window of wakefulness. The clinician has to differentiate between the more widespread symptoms of fatigue and daytime sleepiness. The inability to stay awake during the hours that the patient would typically expect to be awake is referred to as sleepiness. The patient might not wake up fully aroused, and their cognitive and motor abilities might be compromised. The term "sleepiness" should not be used clinically to describe the fatigue that follows physical activity or the lassitude, irritability, or difficulty concentrating that are brought on by insufficient sleep. Even after the patient has had the typical full night of sleep, the clinician may conclude that the patient does in fact experience excessive daytime sleepiness. The majority of these complaints have an organic basis. Although CNS infections or brain tumors should be ruled out, the majority of these patients will have either sleep apnea syndrome or narcolepsy. Making the distinction can be aided by historical data. When did the symptoms start to appear? Any time in the teens or 20s is suggestive of narcolepsy. The patient might mention a protracted history of social challenges brought on by excessive sleepiness. When narcolepsy manifests after the age of thirty, the likelihood of it diminishes. After age 40, hypersomnolence would increase the likelihood of having sleep apnea syndrome. However, some types of apnea can affect people at any age (Maggard et al., 2023).

Patients with narcolepsy typically cannot delay an attack, while those with sleep apnea may be able to do so if necessary. Are the sleep attacks completely uncontrollable? When the narcoleptic patient wakes up from an episode, is he or she at least momentarily refreshed? The narcoleptic patient typically has the ability to function normally when performing tasks like driving and may even have developed self-management skills by taking multiple quick naps throughout the day. On the other hand, the patient with sleep apnea wakes up from extended naps feeling unchanged. How well does the patient sleep at night? While a lot of narcoleptic patients wake up a lot at night and/or have nightmares, some may sleep through the night quite peacefully. Patients with sleep apnea typically report experiencing restless nights and exhaustion when they wake up. The diagnosis of sleep apnea syndrome is strengthened when a collateral history explains periods of apnea, prominent nocturnal snoring, or both, in addition to restlessness. Many narcoleptics experience some degree of muscular helplessness in response to a wide range of emotional experiences. Does the patient experience any unusual phenomena related to emotions? This entails the paralysis of some antigravity muscles, either completely or partially. The presence of this phenomenon, cataplexy, supports the narcolepsy diagnosis. Cataplexy can occur in certain patients even when they don't experience excessive daytime sleepiness (Rana and Sankari, 2023).

The doctor needs to look for two additional narcolepsy-related symptoms. While most normal people have occasionally experienced a mild, fleeting, generalized paralysis upon awakening, narcoleptic patients exhibit a much more marked manifestation of this phenomenon, which typically occurs at the onset of sleep. Moreover, dream images, or hallucinations, can happen either when you wake up or right before you go to sleep (hypnagogic) (hypnopompic). Even though the majority of narcoleptic patients do not exhibit every one of the aforementioned symptoms, the existence of the entire tetrad alone historically confirms the diagnosis. About 50% of narcoleptic patients also exhibit automatic behavior. In the absence of sleep attacks, persistent daytime sleepiness increases the remote possibility of idiopathic CNS hypersomnolence. Raynaud's disease complaints, headaches, and syncope are frequently associated symptoms. Similar symptoms are frequently seen in other family members. Some of these patients may experience sleep drunkenness, a condition marked by a protracted awakening process that is frequently accompanied by confused thoughts and illogical conduct. To fully understand hypersomnia, a comprehensive personality profile must be obtained. Situations related to grief may be linked to heightened drowsiness, which is thought to be psycho-physiological. Usually temporary in nature, this disorder can sporadically persist as a tendency toward fatigue. A common feature of bipolar depression is excessive daytime sleepiness. In these situations, the depressed patient sleeps more during the day than usual.

A past drug and alcohol use history is especially significant. An individual may be addicted to opiates, barbiturates, or other sleep-inducing drugs and may use these agents primarily for their somnolent effects. Is the patient regularly using CNS depressants? When taking moderate to high doses of drugs meant for other therapeutic purposes, other patients may inadvertently suffer similar side effects (e.g., beta-adrenergic blocking agents, antihistamines, some antihypertensive medications, and numerous psychotropic medications). Just as elderly patients are more vulnerable to hypnotic medications that are specifically intended to combat insomnia, they are also more susceptible to the somnolent effects of these drugs. Moreover, very high doses of CNS depressants before bed may cause the alveolar hypoventilation syndrome, a sleep-related breathing impairment that is not linked to noticeable apneic pauses. This syndrome can also manifest without the use of CNS depressants. Excessive sleepiness may be brought on by CNS stimulants. Even though they are frequently taken to combat daytime fatigue, when the drug's effects wear off, sleepiness frequently follows. Moreover, the drug's duration of action shortens with tolerance, and mini withdrawals with accompanying drowsiness may occur. When CNS stimulants are deliberately stopped, excessive sleepiness may also be observed (Ghimire et al., 2024).

Patients who use caffeine-containing drugs excessively may also build up a tolerance to the drug and eventually become dependent on it. Caffeine withdrawal may be the cause of the morning need for multiple cups of coffee to wake up. Alcohol should not be ruled out as a potential cause of excessive sleepiness. The overall state of health may be a factor in hypersomnolence. Conditions to be taken into account include uremia, hepatic encephalopathy, morbid obesity, and endocrinologic disorders of the pancreas and thyroid gland. Multiple nocturnal mini-arousals may be linked to Cheyne-Stokes respirations, which can cause excessive daytime sleepiness. The restless legs syndrome and nocturnal myoclonus can both cause this. Lastly, some patients may just be at the high end of the spectrum when it comes to their needs for typical sleep, requiring more sleep than is typically recommended for a given age. As long as their sleep is not interrupted, these long-sleepers do not complain about poor sleep quality, daytime tiredness, or issues with attitude or performance during the day.

9.1.4. Disorders of Sleep–Wake Schedule

An additional cluster of disturbances, disorders of the sleep-wake schedule, may be represented by a complaint related to sleep. To understand these disorders, it is necessary to consider wakefulness and sleep as behaviors that are closely linked to social and physiological processes. Moreover, the 24-hour day-night cycle that is a natural byproduct of the earth's rotation is superimposed upon and influences this relationship. Disorders pertaining to the sleep-wake schedule are a group of syndromes that are characterized by a dyssynchrony between the wakeful and sleeping behaviors and the processes of human physiology and/or societal expectations in the context of a 24-hour day. These disorders can be either temporary or chronic. Inquire about recent long-distance air travel across different time zones if you have any transient disorders. The typical inclination of the person to adjust their sleep and wake schedule as soon as possible in accordance with the destination's local time cues causes jet lag syndrome. There is a temporary misalignment between the internal sleep-wake phases and the clock times for sleeping and waking because physiological processes other than sleep and wake may take a week or more to adjust. As a result, a syndrome develops that is typified by sleepiness and reduced physical and mental functioning during the desired wake period, and insomnia during the desired sleep period. The rapid time zone change syndrome does not occur after north-south jet travel if there is no more than a 1- or 2-hour change in time zone.

It is typically prolonged after eastward flights and often less severe after the return trip to the time zone of origin (Antoine et al., 2024).

An analogous condition is known as the shift in work schedule in traditional sleep-wake patterns. In this instance, symptoms come from establishing a sleep-wake pattern that is inconsistent with the local schedule rather than from an attempt to adjust to local time cues. The outcome is a disruption of both the waking and sleeping cycles. Frequent changes to the sleep-wake schedule may lead to a persistent disorder. The resulting clinical picture incorporates aspects of disorders of excessive somnolence as well as insomnias. Typically, sleep durations are shortened and disturbed, performance during the intended waking state is compromised, and brief attempts to return to a regular sleep schedule are fruitless. The frequency of schedule changes and the severity of symptoms may be correlated with answers to the following questions: How many hours of shifting are involved with each shift, how frequently do the shifts occur, and how long does it take between schedule changes? Scheduling changes that occur less frequently than three to four weeks apart place additional demands on physiological processes that haven't fully adapted to the previous shift. The hour the patient typically goes to bed is another important historical detail. A very early bedtime may be the cause of early morning awakenings, especially in the elderly, which the patient may interpret as disturbed sleep. Young adults, on the other hand, frequently wait until after midnight to go to bed and then stay up until about noon. In either scenario, it could be challenging to change the sleeping schedule when external factors call for more regular sleeping hours.

A patient may be diagnosed with advanced sleep phase syndrome or delayed sleep phase syndrome if the clinician finds that the patient's paired sleep onset and wake times are not only earlier or later than desired, but also significantly so. Due to an apparent uncontrollable lack of correlation between their physiologic clock and the standard time clock, these patients may complain about social or occupational conflicts (Slowik et al., 2023). When the body's natural urge to sleep is complied with, the patient in these disorders finds it easy to fall asleep, and when sleep is allowed, it is restorative and long enough. A patient may complain of periodic excessive daytime sleepiness or insomnia when they first arrive. A log of the patient's sleep and wake times over a few weeks should show the pattern of the phenomenon in this situation, and it may even show that the patient is going to bed at progressively later hours. This may suggest that the patient has non-24-hour sleep-wake syndrome, which is characterized by a circadian rhythm that is noticeably longer than the typical 24 or 25 hours. The patient's complaint is periodic, which indicates that as their internal physiological clock gradually advances through a 24-hour day, it will momentarily align with the conventional clock. But the patient will once more experience a prolonged physiological clock that is out of sync with society, which will cause them to experience excessive somnolence during the day and difficulty falling asleep at the appropriate hour.

9.1.5. Disorders Associated with Sleep, Sleep Stages, or Partial Arousals (Parasomnias)

Patients who complain of disturbing events related to sleep, stages of sleep, or partial arousals occasionally come before clinicians. Even though children are most commonly affected by these parasomnias, adults can also occasionally experience these disorders. The CNS is activated during sleep, as evidenced by the fact that most complaints are related to events in the autonomic nervous system or skeletal muscle. Sleep terrors or nightmares may be the cause of disturbing dreams. When does the disturbance happen during the night? If it happens within the first two hours of the onset of sleep, the diagnosis of sleep terror is more likely to be made. These episodes typically start with a scream and are followed by distress signals like perspiration, fast breathing and heartbeat, and seemingly erratic body movements. The patient is typically difficult to wake during these episodes, according to household members. But after a short while, regular sleep appears to return on its own. Dream anxiety attacks, or nightmares, are more common in the later hours of the night when the unsettling dreams happen. There is one exception to this timing: a relatively new kind of nightmare where the patient experiences terrifying dream imagery just as they are drifting off to sleep. These phenomena could represent an early stage of psychotic illness or be a component of posttraumatic stress disorder. Can the patient recall the content of the dreams? Patients who are able to describe their disturbing dreams in some degree of detail are more likely to be suffering from nightmares. Typically, the patient experiencing sleep terrors won't remember those episodes (Shah and Gupta, 2023).

When a patient complains of nightmares, it's a good idea to inquire about the patient's medication usage (e.g., serpine). Alcohol, CNS stimulants, hypnotics, and abrupt withdrawal can all cause nightmares. Even without drug use, sleep deprivation can occasionally result in nightmares. Another sleep disturbance that typically happens in the early stages of sleep is somnambulism, or sleepwalking. Once more, rousing a patient during an episode can be challenging, and the patient may not remember the episode afterwards. For this reason, a collateral history is crucial. In adults, frequent sleepwalking is often indicative of an emotional disorder. A medical history is crucial because alcohol and hypnotics can either cause this disorder or exacerbate it. Long stretches of purposeful wakefulness may also make the condition worse. Different types of parasomnias should be known to the physician. The most well-known of these, bedwetting (also known as sleep-related enuresis), is a rare complaint that adults first present with. The possibility of underlying diseases like a lower urinary tract infection, neurogenic bladder, seizure disorder, or stress urinary incontinence must be taken into account by the clinician in such situations. Usually, these underlying issues are the patient's main complaint, not the bedwetting itself. Numerous other complaints could be signs of additional sleep-related dysfunctions. Bruxism, or teeth grinding, may be the secondary cause of headaches. Cluster headaches are typified by a history of abrupt nocturnal awakenings with severe unilateral frontal headaches, frequently accompanied by ipsilateral lacrimation and rhinorrhea. Dreams about attacks are not uncommon in asthmatics. While you sleep, you run the risk of developing arrhythmias and your cardiovascular symptoms getting worse. Heartburn brought on by gastroesophageal reflux disease may cause some patients to wake up from sleep. A delayed clearance of acid from the esophagus during sleep may cause multiple miniarousals in certain patients, even if they do not have heartburn. These patients may not be aware of these miniarousals. These merely represent a handful of the numerous instances that highlight the influence that sleep has on the autonomic nervous system in particular as well as the central nervous system generally (Okawa et al., 2007).

9.1.6. Basic Science

9.1.6.1. Normal Sleep

Electroencephalogram (EEG) recordings of brain wave activity, electrooculogram (EOG) recordings of eye movements, and transcutaneous electromyogram (EMG) recordings of facial muscular activity have been used to characterize sleep in recent years. The fundamental methods of polysomnography are these three study approaches, which facilitate the somewhat arbitrary but practical staging of the sleep-wake cycle. The EEG's characteristics serve as the primary means of defining the stages, but the EOG and EMG's features are frequently more helpful in defining transitions between stages. Three distinct states of the basic sleep-wake cycle have been identified based on polysomnographic studies: rapid eye movement (REM) sleep, non-rapid eye movement (NREM) sleep, and wakefulness. When an individual is awake, the EEG usually shows low voltage and frequencies between 4 and 25 Hz, or cycles per second. Theta waves are clusters with frequencies between 4 and 7 Hz. Alpha rhythm, which typically manifests as relaxed but awake patients with closed eyes, is made up of sinusoidal waves in the 8–13 Hz range. Beta rhythm clusters are those whose frequency is higher than 13 Hz. The EMG recorded while awake reveals a baseline tone of the face muscles. The waking EOG shows rapid, conjugate eye movements even when the patient is at rest. Four stages make up NREM sleep, which typically occurs after wakefulness. Phase I is characterized by an EEG rhythm loss (alpha wave), a progressive, widespread decrease in EEG voltage, and the subsequent emergence of theta activity. Slow, random, circular, and occasionally disconjugate eye movements are the most consistent indicator of stage I. There is a slight relaxation of the facial muscles. The sleeping patient is most easily aroused during stage I, drowsiness. Daydreaming is possible.

An EEG showing regular, spindle-shaped clusters in the 10–16 Hz range is indicative of Stage II (also known as light sleep or spindle sleep). Slow, blunted, high voltage, biphasic waves (K-complexes), which are often linked to hypnagogic myoclonus, may accompany these. Vertex (or V) waves may signal nonspecific arousal during stage II sleep. During this phase, the electrical activity of the face muscles continues to decrease, and eye movements are typically quiet. Slow wave sleep refers to stages III and IV of sleep. When delta waves (1 to 3 Hz) account for at least 20% of an EEG epoch and have an amplitude of 75 μV or higher, Stage III is typically considered to be present. As a result, delta sleep is another term for this stage of sleep as well as stage IV. Stage IV is defined as the presence of 50% or more delta waves within an epoch. This distinction should be considered biologically insignificant because it is somewhat arbitrary. Muscle tone is comparable to stage II sleep and eye movements are typically absent during slow wave sleep. One clinical characteristic of slow wave sleep—hence the synonym deep sleep—is marked resistance to arousal.

A random, mixed-frequency spectrum in the 4–25 Hz range and a relatively low voltage are two characteristics of the EEG readings associated with REM sleep. Typically, there are groups of quick, conjugate eye movements. When paired with a loss of postural tone and resistance to arousal, these bursts of eye movements and phasic body movements are referred to as paradoxical sleep. Dream sleep also fits in here because the most vivid dreams happen during REM sleep. Normal sleep is defined as the sequential progression of NREM sleep from stages I through IV, usually preceded, if only momentarily, by a return to stage II sleep, which sets up the first and subsequent periods of REM sleep. The interval between one REM period and the next, known as a REM cycle, lasts roughly ninety minutes. Since most REM periods get longer as the night goes on, the majority of REM sleep happens in the second half of the night, with slow wave sleep predominating in the first half. The latter type of sleep is primarily characterized by extended periods of immobility of the body, which is thought to be the source of the relaxed sensations commonly associated with sleep. 30 to 35% of the total amount of sleep time is spent in REM sleep at all ages, with the remaining portion being split between the different stages of NREM sleep. But as people age, their percentage of sleep falls into different NREM stages. Between the ages of 20 and 60, nocturnal sleep duration is generally maintained. Elderly individuals sleep for a smaller percentage of the night. Despite this, the total average amount of time spent sleeping over the course of a typical 24-hour period is comparable for adults over 60 and younger adults. The elderly supplement the reduced amount of nocturnal sleep with daytime naps and/or microsleeps, which last from 1 to 10 seconds and are linked to a lowering of the eyelids, to reach that average of 7:45 hours (Basit et al., 2023).

9.1.6.2. Abnormal Sleep

When younger people experience increasing sleep deprivation, they too develop the microsleeps that are so characteristic of the elderly. Shorter daytime sleep onset latencies are observed as a lack of nocturnal sleep becomes more pronounced, even prior to the emergence of microsleeps. Additionally, research involving the deprivation of a specific sleep stage has shown that an excess of that stage will occur when sleep is later allowed freely. This is especially true for REM sleep, when there will be a rebound in the quantity of REM sleep afterward and it will get harder to suppress that sleep state. When pharmacological REM sleep suppressants are used, the aforementioned phenomenon—known as REM pressure—may also come into play. These substances (e.g., amphetamines, tricyclic antidepressants, and some hypnotics) suppress the onset and length of REM sleep at first. Even if the drug is used continuously, the normal quantity of REM sleep will eventually return due to REM pressure. But stopping the substance doesn't stop REM pressure from happening right away. REM rebound, which is frequently manifested as nightmares and generally disrupted sleep, is the outcome. It is an increase in the frequency, duration, and intensity of REM periods.

This is also the case when alcohol is abruptly stopped after long-term use. Exaggerated levels of REM sleep occur after alcohol is stopped because REM deprivation occurs during alcohol consumption. Delirium tremens is preceded by this REM rebound. Beyond the discussion of drug use, knowledge of the different phases of sleep promotes a better comprehension of enuresis associated with sleep, sleepwalking, sleep terrors, and nightmares. The first three disorders happen during slow wave sleep and most likely represent partial arousals. The correlation with this stage of sleep is in line with the fact that these events typically occur in the first part of the night, when slow wave sleep predominates. The fact that the person resists arousal during each of the first three disorders and typically does not remember the episodes is consistent with the deep sleep synonym for this stage. In contrast, nightmares usually entail waking up from REM sleep. The higher percentage of REM sleep that occurs in the second half of the night is consistent with their more frequent occurrence in the mid-to-late segment of nocturnal sleep. Furthermore, the vivid dream imagery of REM sleep is consistent with the memory of nightmares. One of the purposes of REM sleep and dreaming might be the integration of emotionally significant information. It's possible that a nightmare signifies the integration process' failure.

The basic polysomnographic findings have particular clinical significance for a few other disorders. Short REM sleep latency, or the interval between the start of stage II and the onset of REM sleep, is now recognized as a biologic marker for non-bipolar depression. In narcolepsy, REM sleep latency is even shorter, which could indicate an imbalance between the REM, NREM, and wake states. The wake state is continuously invaded by the REM system. As a result, rather than focusing mostly on nighttime sleep, polysomnographic documentation of narcolepsy usually includes the demonstration of abnormalities of daytime sleep. The emergence of REM sleep within 10 minutes of the onset of sleep is a hallmark of narcolepsy. REM sleep-onset periods do not occur in idiopathic CNS hypersomnolence, on the other hand. In relation to narcolepsy's auxiliary symptoms, hypnagogic hallucinations most likely correspond to REM dreaming that precedes unconsciousness. Sleep-onset paralysis is a reflection of REM sleep's inhibitory mechanisms. When a patient experiences cataplexy, they are fully conscious and experience the paralysis of their muscles during REM sleep in response to an emotional stimulus. Sometimes cataplexy develops into a full-blown REM sleep episode. Many narcoleptics exhibit automatic behavior that resembles sleepwalking during the day when they have recurrent microsleep episodes.

9.1.7. Clinical Significance

Sleep disruptions should be considered symptoms rather than sleep and arousal disorders in and of themselves. They are made up of a wide range of clinical presentations involving various physiological, psychological, and behavioral abnormalities. In keeping with the 24-hour day-night cycle, these anomalies frequently manifest primarily during the waking hours and do not limit themselves to the sleep period. Thus, in addition to taking into account many of the patient's daytime complaints, the clinician needs to be alert for the potential of sleep and arousal disorders. Proficiency in taking historical accounts is necessary to investigate such issues. Only a small percentage of patients will benefit from polysomnography, and even in those situations, the studies' primary purpose is typically to confirm the clinician's preexisting suspicions based on the patient's medical history (Hublin and Kaprio, 2003).

9.2. Prevalence and Types of Sleep Disorders

Sleep disorders are a broad category of clinical issues that arise in outpatient settings. Standardized definitions and classifications are crucial because sleep disorders have a wide differential diagnosis. The various kinds of sleep disorders are numerous. A standardized classification and definition of sleep disorders can be obtained by using the International Classification of Sleep Disorders (ICSD). Sleep disturbances are prevalent in both juveniles and adults. On the other hand, compared to adults, children with sleep disorders may exhibit distinct symptoms. A collection of illnesses known as sleep disorders interfere with regular sleep cycles. One of the most prevalent clinical issues that are encountered is sleep disorders. It is possible for normal physical, mental, social, and emotional functioning to be hampered by inadequate or non-restorative sleep. Sleep problems can impact one's general well-being, safety, and standard of living. A study revealed that patients with insomnia had a markedly reduced quality of life. The various kinds of sleep disorders are numerous. A standardized classification and definitions for sleep disorders are provided by the International Classification of Sleep Disorders (ICSD).

Specifically, the third edition of the ICSD (ICSD-3) includes the following categories of sleep disorders:

- Insomnia
- Sleep-disordered breathing
- Central disorders of hypersomnolence
- Circadian rhythm sleep-wake disorders
- Parasomnias
- Sleep-related movement disorders

9.2.1. Etiology

A medical condition that affects a person's sleep patterns is called somnipathy, or sleep disorder. Certain sleep disorders can affect a person's ability to function normally on a physical, mental, social, and emotional level. Sleep disturbances are common and can negatively impact a patient's quality of life and overall health. Tests like actigraphy and polysomnography are frequently requested to diagnose sleep disorders. The general categories of sleep disorders include parasomnias, dyssomnias, circadian rhythm sleep disorders, which affect when people sleep, and other disorders, such as those brought on by physical or mental health issues. The most common type of sleep disorder is insomnia, which is defined as difficulty falling or staying asleep without a clear cause. The others include night terrors, sleep apnea, narcolepsy, and hypersomnia (excessive sleepiness at inappropriate times). Sleeping sickness is caused by an infection that disrupts the sleep cycle. Several problems, such as night terrors and teeth grinding (bruxism), can interfere with sleep. When treating sleep disturbances resulting from mental, physical, or substance abuse disorders, the primary focus should be on treating the underlying conditions.

Adolescents and adults alike frequently experience primary insomnia. Because most cases of childhood sleep disorders go undiagnosed, there is, however, a marked lack of awareness about them. Stress, age-related changes in circadian rhythms, environmental changes, changes in lifestyle, pre-diagnosed physiological issues, and increased medication use are some of the common factors that contribute to the onset of a sleep disorder. Elderly people are particularly susceptible to sleep disorders such as breathing problems during sleep, REM sleep behavior disorders, periodic limb movements, restless legs syndrome, insomnia, and circadian rhythm disturbances (Acquavella et al., 2020).

There are different causes for different sleep disorders. For each sleep disorder listed below, more details are discussed in the pertinent section referenced below.

- **Insomnia:** The exact causes of insomnia are unknown. Some contributing factors include environmental, genetic, psychological, and behavioral, leading to hyperarousal.
- **Sleep-Disordered Breathing (SDB):** Breathing control issues, as well as problems with upper airway and chest wall mechanics that impair ventilatory and resistive loading, are among the causes of SDB. SDB is a group of conditions that includes central sleep apnea (CSA), OSA, and syndrome. Obesity is a major factor in the obstructive type of SDB; further details are covered in the sections on OSA, CSA, and obesity hypoventilation syndrome.

- **Central Disorders of Hypersomnolence:** The central nervous system's intrinsic abnormalities in regulating sleep-wake are frequently the cause of central causes of hypersomnolence. The three primary subtypes of central hypersomnia that are typically identified are idiopathic hypersomnia (IH), narcolepsy type 2, and narcolepsy type 1. These subtypes are covered in more detail in their own sections. Furthermore, Kleine-Levin syndrome, hypersomnia brought on by a medical condition, drug or substance abuse, psychiatric condition, and sleep insufficiency syndrome are additional causes of central hypersomnolence.
- **Circadian Rhythm Sleep-Wake Disorders (CRSD):** The two main categories of causative factors for CRSD are as follows: (1) the environment is not in harmony with the body's natural circadian rhythm (2) those that arise when the circadian timing system is changed in relation to the external environment (e.g., shift work, jet lag), irregular sleep-wake rhythm, advanced sleep phase syndrome, non-24, delayed sleep phase syndrome).
- **Parasomnias:** Parasomnias have various causes, including environmental factors, genetic predisposition, and interactions between genes and the environment, all of which play a significant role in the development of parasomnias. There are three main categories of parasomnia: Non-rapid eye movement (NREM)-related parasomnias, rapid eye movement (REM)-related parasomnias, and other parasomnias. NREM-related parasomnia encompasses confusional arousal, sleepwalking, sleep terrors, and sleep-related eating disorder. REM-related parasomnias include REM sleep behavior disorder (RBD) and nightmare disorder (Fariba et al., 2023).
- **Sleep-Related Movement Disorders:** Disorders of motor control excitation or disinhibition that are frequently linked to sleep disturbances are abnormal movements during sleep. Depending on the kind of disorder, different sleep-related movements have different etiologies. For instance, the etiology of restless legs syndrome (RLS) may be secondary to iron deficiency or primarily attributed to familial and genetic predisposition.

9.2.2. Causes

A published review of research has shown that childhood trauma, such as family conflicts or sexual abuse, can significantly increase the likelihood of developing various sleep disorders in adulthood, including sleep apnea, narcolepsy, and insomnia. Additionally, evidence suggests that idiopathic REM sleep behavior disorder (iRBD) may have a genetic component. In a study involving 632 participants, half with iRBD and half without, it was found that those with iRBD were more likely to have a first-degree relative with the same disorder compared to those without it. Further research is needed to fully understand the genetic factors involved in sleep disorders. Individuals who have suffered a traumatic brain injury (TBI) are also at a higher risk for developing sleep disorders. A systematic review of existing studies found that those who have experienced a TBI are particularly vulnerable to narcolepsy, obstructive sleep apnea, excessive daytime sleepiness, and insomnia. Researchers emphasize the importance of continued investigation into the relationship between TBIs and sleep disorders (Bargiotas et al., 2017).

9.2.3. Epidemiology

Depending on the condition, there are differences in the prevalence of sleep disorders. Recent reports have suggested a connection between SDB, short sleep duration, and non-restorative sleep. According to a recent study, there is a connection between sleep disorders and other sleep problems. For instance, in a group of diabetes patients, 61% reported having trouble sleeping, 47% tested positive for RLS, and 51% were at higher risk of developing OSA. The prevalence of each major sleep disorder as defined by the ICSD-3 will be briefly listed here.

9.2.3.1. Children and Young Adults

Confusional arousals and sleepwalking are the two most prevalent sleep disorders in children, per a meta-analysis of pediatric sleep disorders. It is estimated that 17:3% of children aged 3 to 13 have confusional arousals. The disorder affects roughly 17% of kids, with boys experiencing it more frequently than girls. Sleepwalking peaks between the ages of 8 and 12. A different systematic review provides a wide range of child sleep bruxism prevalence rates. The initial phase of an individual's sleep cycle, known as the first slow wave of sleep, is when insomnias such as sleepwalking and talking usually happen. During this phase, the body and mind slow down, making one feel relaxed and sleepy. Since this is the easiest time to wake up, many kids don't remember what happened during this period. Children who experience nightmares are also thought to suffer from parasomnia, as they usually recall the events of the nightmare. But nightmares only come during Rapid Eye Movement (REM), the final stage of sleep. The deepest stage of sleep, known as REM, gets its name from the variety of awake-like neurological and physiological reactions people can exhibit at this time of the sleep cycle.

Preschoolers who grind their teeth at least one night a week range from 15:29 to 38:6%. In every study that was included, the prevalence of bruxists decreased with age, with the exception of one, and the prevalence was higher in boys than in girls. 7–16% of young adults have delayed sleep phase disorder, according to another systematic review. People in their 20s experience the highest prevalence of this disorder. 20 to 26% of teenagers say they sleep onset later than thirty minutes. Additionally, 7–36% report having trouble falling asleep. All of these negative sleep outcomes are more common in Asian teens than in their North American and European counterparts. Due to a person's growth, parasomnias usually go away by adulthood; however, 4% of people experience recurrent symptoms (Mansur et al., 2023).

9.2.3.2. Effects of Untreated Sleep Disorders

Due to sleep disorders, children and young adults who don't get enough sleep also face a host of other health issues, including obesity and physical issues that can interfere with daily living. Children and young adults should follow the CDC's recommended sleep guidelines as it promotes better mental and physical health, among other benefits.

9.2.3.3. Insomnia

One common result of sleep deprivation is insomnia. People who suffer from insomnia may experience hyposomnia, or difficulty staying asleep, or a combination of the two inadequate sleep in terms of both quantity and quality. A pooled prevalence of 15.0% is reported for China based on the combination of data from 17 studies on the subject. This result is comparable to those of other East Asian nations, but it is significantly lower than those of several Western nations (Poland: 50.5%, France and Italy: 37.2%, USA: 27.1%). In China, the prevalence of insomnia is similar in men and women. According to a different meta-analysis on this sleeping disorder in the elderly, people who have more than one physical or mental illness are 60% more likely to experience it than people who only have one or fewer conditions. Additionally, it mentions that compared to men, women over 50 are more likely to experience insomnia (Pham et al., 2022).

An algorithm to identify patients with sleep disorders using electronic medical records was developed, according to a study that came about as a result of a collaboration between Massachusetts General Hospital and Merck. More than 36,000 people with physician-documented insomnia were found using an algorithm that combined structured and unstructured variables. Basic cases of insomnia are not uncommon, but approximately 40% of sufferers experience more severe symptoms. Cognitive behavioral therapy (Espie, 2009.), medication, sleep schedule planning, and self-imposed caffeine limits are among the treatments for insomnia that can be helpful.

9.2.3.4. Obstructive Sleep Apnea

In the United States, 2% of women and 4% of men suffer from obstructive sleep apnea (OSA). This disorder is generally more common in men. With age, though, this difference tends to disappear. Pregnant women are most at risk for obstructive sleep apnea (OSA), and they also frequently report co-occurring depression and insomnia. China and India have the highest rates of the disorder in a meta-analysis of the different Asian nations. In particular, it is estimated that 7% of people in Hong Kong and 13.7% of people in India suffer from OSA. Similar rates of daytime OSA symptoms, such as difficulty concentrating, mood swings, or elevated blood pressure, are experienced by the two study groups (prevalence of 3 percent and 3.57 percent, respectively).

9.2.3.5. Obesity and Sleep Apnea

The increasing prevalence of obesity in society is a major contributing factor to the rising incidence of obstructive sleep apnea (OSA) worldwide. Obesity-related upper respiratory tract fat deposits can cause breathing problems while you sleep, which can result in OSA. Since there is a clear link between obesity and OSA, screening obese people for OSA and related conditions is crucial. Furthermore, patients with OSA and obesity have an increased risk of developing metabolic syndrome. Introducing dietary control in obese people can improve their sleep quality and lessen related conditions like anxiety, depression, and insomnia. Obesity may have an impact on the sleep pattern disruption that leads to OSA. Because obesity can impair the upper respiratory system by causing fat to accumulate around the muscles that surround the lungs, it is a risk factor for OSA. Furthermore, OSA can exacerbate obesity by extending drowsiness throughout the day, which lowers physical activity and promotes an inactive lifestyle (Matsumoto et al., 2019).

9.2.3.6. Sleep Paralysis

According to a systematic review, 7 percent of people in general will at some point in their lives experience sleep paralysis. Men are 15.9% likely to experience it, compared to 18.9% of women. Regarding particular demographics, 31.9% of mental health patients and 28.3% of students have encountered this phenomenon at least once in their lives. 36% of those in mental health have panic disorder. Students of Asian descent are slightly more likely to experience sleep paralysis (39.9%) than students of other ethnicities (Hispanics: 34.5%, African Americans: 31.4%, and Caucasians: 30.8%).

9.2.3.7. Restless Leg Syndrome

The average prevalence rate for Western Europe and North America is estimated to be 14.5±8.0 percent, based on one meta-analysis. Using strict diagnostic criteria, the prevalence of restless leg syndrome is estimated to be between 5 and 15% in the United States. Compared to men, American women experience restless leg syndrome (RLS) at a rate that is more than 35% higher. A sensorimotor disorder called RLS is characterized by lower limb discomfort. Usually, symptoms get worse at night, get better when you move, and get worse when you're sleeping.

9.2.4. History and Physical

The way that sleep disorders manifest clinically varies depending on the ailment. In general, sleep disturbances can manifest in a variety of clinical ways, with insomnia, hypersomnia, and unusual sleep-related behaviors being the most common presentations. To avoid complications and negative health effects, early detection of the underlying sleep disorder is crucial. The evaluation depends heavily on the patient's medical history, sleep patterns, and work schedule. When evaluating patients who experience sleep disturbances, it is crucial to obtain a comprehensive list of all prescribed and over-the-counter medications. Evaluating a patient's complete social and family history is also crucial, as is learning about any substance use that may have affected their ability to breathe or sleep.

9.2.4.1. Insomnia

Difficulties getting to sleep and/or remaining asleep are common symptoms of insomnia. Patients with sleep initiation difficulties report taking thirty minutes or longer to fall asleep, and those with sleep maintenance difficulties report staying awake for thirty minutes or longer during the night. Compromised daytime function, comprising one or more of the following symptoms: weariness, daytime sleepiness, inattentiveness, increased accidents, aggression, decreased motivation, or energy, is another prerequisite for diagnosing insomnia. Many times, insomnia is a chronic or recurrent illness, with medical, psychological, and psychosocial stressors being linked to its exacerbations. Insomnia was recently divided into two categories: chronic and short-term.

The three conditions listed below are included in the ICSD-3 criteria for the diagnosis of chronic insomnia disorder: (1) difficulty initiating or maintaining sleep; (2) adequate opportunity to sleep; and (3) presence of daytime consequences resulting from difficulty sleeping. These circumstances ought to persist for a minimum of three months, thrice a week. It's important to diagnose insomnia as soon as possible, and suspicion must be low. It is important to determine from history the clinical characteristics that predispose, precipitate, and perpetuate symptoms of insomnia (Demirtaş and Dolu, 2023).

9.2.4.2. Hypersomnia

Individuals who suffer from hypersomnia lament their incapacity to sleep during the day. They struggle to stay awake for long stretches of time during the day, and they frequently fall asleep accidentally or at inappropriate times that disrupt their regular schedule. Numerous patients refer to a significant impairment in their cognitive abilities as "brain fog." Furthermore, there has been a correlation found in idiopathic hypersomnia between excessive sleepiness, depressive symptoms, and a reduced quality of life. A wide range of sleep disorders can manifest as fatigue, which is sometimes mistaken for sleepiness. Measures of hypersomnia and fatigue severity, such as the Epworth sleepiness scale and the fatigue severity scale, are frequently used in research. Other characteristics of sleepiness, like idiopathic hypersomnia (IH) or particular neurological disorders like narcolepsy, are connected to the length of sleep. In addition to the severity of hypersomnia, IH has unique clinical characteristics like sleep inertia and extended nighttime sleep (more than 10 hours). On the other hand, narcolepsy is a persistent neurological condition because the brain cannot regulate wakefulness and sleep. It is linked to a low level of orexin-A/hypocretin-1 in the cerebrospinal fluid.

Individuals suffering from narcolepsy typically report symptoms such as excessive, chronic daytime sleepiness, sleep paralysis (inability to move immediately after awakening), hallucinations while falling asleep (hypnagogic hallucinations) or while waking (hypnopompic hallucinations), and cataplexy (type I or type II)—a temporary loss of muscle tone in response to intense emotion, such as laughter. 30% of cases of cataplexy involve partial cataplexy, which affects the jaw and face, and more than 50% of cases involve nontypical presentations, such as spontaneous cataplectic attacks or cataplexy brought on by non-humorous triggers like anger. Among the most prevalent clinical manifestations of sleep-disordered breathing (SDB), which typically affects up to 50% of patients, are excessive daytime sleepiness, loud snoring, and gasping or apnea that is witnessed by a bed partner. Nonetheless, a large number of SDB patients do not exhibit any symptoms, especially in specific populations with heart failure, stroke, and other neurological conditions.

9.2.4.3. Unusual Sleep-Related Behaviors

Certain behaviors that occur before, during, or after sleep can give important hints about specific sleep disorders, such as eating disorders, movement disorders, or parasomnia. To confirm the diagnosis, more information is required. For instance, reporting movement disorders related to sleep, such as the urge to move legs at a specific time of night, may indicate periodic or restless leg movements. One common symptom of hypersomnolence disorder is confusional arousal or sleep drunkenness during arousal or awakening from sleep. This condition is known as idiopathic hypersomnia or, less frequently, sleep-related sex (sexsomnia). Unusual sexual behaviors, such as masturbating, vocalizing during sex, or having sex with a bed partner while unconscious, are known as sexsomnia. Patients may have REM sleep behavior disorder (RBD) if they report engaging in violent dreams that cause them to kick, punch, flail their arms, or jump out of bed. If the patient wakes up during the episode, he can remember the dream. Other illnesses like Parkinson's disease, multiple system atrophy, or Lewy body dementia may be linked to this disorder. Other sleep-related symptoms that need a thorough medical history to be diagnosed include sleepwalking, sleep talking, and night terrors, which are common in kids between the ages of two and twelve and usually go away on their own as the child gets older. They mostly happen during non-REM sleep, when there is no recall of the incident. Conversely, nightmares happen during REM sleep, usually in the wee hours of the morning. The person may cry out and scream during a nightmare (Morin et al., 2020).

One distinguishing feature between night terrors and nightmares is that the former can cause a person to become completely conscious upon awakening. In addition, there is a nightmare memory of the incident, i.e., one can remember having a nightmare. To distinguish sleep-eating disorders from other uncommon sleep-related behaviors, comprehensive medical histories are necessary. The hallmark of sleep-related eating disorders (SRED) is recurrent episodes of compulsive eating during the first third of unconscious sleep. But night eating syndrome (NES) is characterized by binge eating right before bedtime or right after fully waking up from sleep. Complex sleep behaviors are those associated with nonrapid eye movement (NREM) that, when present in middle-aged and older patients with chronic insomnia, can result in major injuries or even death. Examples of these behaviors include sleepwalking. Lack of sleep, physical or emotional stress, traumatic experiences, and the use or abuse of drugs or alcohol are all known to aggravate the symptoms of sleep disorders. Several medications have been associated with atypical sleep-related behaviors, including antipsychotics and psychotropic drugs (e.g., anticholinergics), hypnotics, and sedatives, especially those in the Z drug class, also known as nonbenzodiazepine benzodiazepine receptor agonists (e.g., the US Food and Drug Administration (FDA) has issued a black box warning for two medications (zolpidem and eszopiclone) due to an increased risk of complex sleep behaviors.

9.2.5. Evaluation

A multitude of data points are needed to assess sleep issues. Several clinical and investigative tools may be able to assist in reducing the differential diagnosis and determining the specific type of sleep disorder following a thorough medical history, medication history, and physical examination. A selection of these tests and questionnaires is provided here.

- **Epworth Sleepiness Scale (ESS):** ESS is an eight-item self-administered questionnaire that measures the presence and severity of sleepiness.
- **Fatigue Severity Scale (FSS):** FSS is a nine-item instrument that can help distinguish sleepiness from fatigue and estimate fatigue severity.
- **Insomnia Severity Index (ISI):** ISI is the most widely accepted clinical assessment tool that helps identify and monitor insomnia severity in addition to a sleep diary.
- **Sleep Diary:** The sleep diary, or sleep log, is a personal paper record of sleep and wakefulness over weeks to months. Patients should record a detailed description of sleep, such as bedtime, duration until sleep onset, the number of awakenings, duration of awakenings, and nap times.
- **Sleep Studies:** Sleep studies, such as polysomnography (PSG) or home sleep apnea testing (HSAT), can yield objective measures of sleep. The most reliable method for identifying OSA and other sleep disorders is PSG. The patient is connected to multiple monitoring devices during PSG, which enables the patient to sleep. Numerous physiological parameters are evaluated, including electrical heart rate, respiratory effort, sleep stages, airflow, body posture, and limb movements. The data gathered from these parameters is useful in diagnosing a range of REM and NREM sleep disorders as well as identifying the root causes of sleep disruption. Follow-up PSG can be used to reevaluate patients and make sure they are receiving enough PAP in cases

where OSA has been diagnosed and there is still hypersomnia after PAP therapy with appropriate adherence. Nonetheless, it is not advised to perform a routine follow-up sleep study (PSG or HSAT) on asymptomatic patients (Rodriguez et al., 2015).

- **Laboratory Studies:** Some of the lab studies appropriate for those with sleep disorders include:
  - Arterial blood gases (ABG)
  - Thyroid function tests
  - Drug and alcohol toxicity screening
  - Iron studies and ferritin level
  - Cerebrospinal fluid (CSF) hypocretin-1 deficiency (<110 pg/ml).
- **Actigraphy:** An actigraph device, similar to a watch, is worn on the wrist during this test. Movement triggers the signals, and periods of inactivity or sleep record very few or no signals at all. This tool can diagnose advanced or delayed sleep phase syndrome by measuring sleep-wake cycles or circadian rhythm over an extended period of time.
- **Multiple Sleep Latency Testing (MSLT):** The degree of sleepiness is ascertained by this objective test. Many refer to this test as a nap study. The patient is instructed to sleep for eight to ten hours the day after an overnight PSG study, taking four or five naps. Every nap lasts roughly twenty minutes. These examinations aid in determining the reasons behind excessive daytime sleepiness, which can be found in several conditions, including narcolepsy, hypersomnia, and sleep apnea.

9.2.6. Treatment/Management

Treatments for sleep disorders depend on the type of sleep disorder.

Treatment of insomnia can be broadly categorized into non-pharmacological and pharmacological treatments.

Non-Pharmacological

- A variety of behavioral and psychological strategies are used in cognitive-behavioral therapy for insomnia (CBT-I), which is designed specifically to treat insomnia. Based on individual or group therapy techniques and, more recently, digital CBT-I formats, studies show that CBT-I is the preferred psychological treatment. In addition to significantly increasing sleep parameters like sleep efficiency and total sleep time, CBT-I also significantly reduces sleep onset latency, wake after sleep onset, and the severity of insomnia, according to a meta-analysis of 61 randomized controlled trials with 11,571 participants. The trials evaluated various CBT-I delivery formats (individual, group, guided self-help, digital assisted, and unguided self-help) with control conditions. Because of the higher risk of side effects, addiction, and tolerance to using Z drugs, CBT-I therapy is especially important for patient groups like older patients who may not be able to tolerate pharmaceutical treatment. Other interventions are not proven to have a clinical effect if used alone. These interventions include:

- **Sleep Restriction Therapy (SRT):** SRT limits the total time allowed in bed to increase the drive to sleep.

Patients who receive stimulus control therapy can alter their sleeping patterns and no longer experience difficulty falling asleep. Patients ought to wait until they are tired before going to bed. Additionally, the bed should only be used for sleeping—it shouldn't be used for reading or watching TV.

- **Relaxation Therapy:** Relaxation techniques may be implemented before sleep. Meditation and breathing exercises are some of the relaxation techniques.
- **Sleep Hygiene:** A series of instruction concerning environmental and lifestyle factors (e.g., factors that could impede sleep, such as temperature, light, and noise). Education about healthy sleep patterns, abstaining from drugs, exercising frequently, maintaining a comfortable bedroom environment, observing wake and sleep schedules, and avoiding midday naps are all examples of good sleep hygiene. However, CBT-I is more effective than sleep hygiene education alone in treating insomnia or poor sleep.

Pharmacologic

- **Inhibitors of the Histamine Type 1 Receptor:** Because of their sedative properties, diphenhydramine, and chlorpheniramine, are frequently used for sleep problems. But these medications ought to be avoided because of their anticholinergic effect.
- **Benzodiazepines (BZD):** Insomnia is frequently treated with these medications. The medications increase the activity of neurotransmitters by attaching to a specific benzodiazepine site on the gamma-aminobutyric acid (GABA) receptor complex. These medications increase stage 2 sleep while suppressing REM sleep and decreasing stage 3 sleep. Temazepam and flurazepam are two examples.
- **Non-Benzodiazepine Hypnotics or z-Drugs:** these agents are used to treat acute and short-term insomnia. These drugs have non-BZD-like chemical structures but interact with the GABA-BZD receptor, causing sedation. Examples include zolpidem and zaleplon.
- **Melatonin Receptor Agonists:** The regulation of sleepiness and the sleep-wake cycle is associated with the melatonin receptors MT1 and MT2. Melatonin receptor agonists work by binding to these receptors and enhancing sleep via the body's own regulatory mechanism. These medications are used to treat delayed sleep-wake phase disorder (insomnia with difficulty in initiating sleep), jet lag, and circadian rhythm sleep disorders. Ramelteon serves as one illustration.
- **Orexin Receptor Antagonists:** orexin promotes wakefulness. Thus, the antagonism of this receptor helps in sleep. An example includes suvorexant, which improved ISI through improvement in sleep onset and maintenance.

The mainstays of treatment for OSA are lifestyle modifications, oral appliances, and, in some cases, surgical procedures. Mechanical positive airway therapy (PAP) is also used. In certain patients, medication therapy such as solriamfetol, stimulants (like amphetamines or modafinil), and norepinephrine reuptake inhibitors may be used to treat daytime symptoms of OSA and persistent hypersomnia that persists despite appropriate PAP adherence and respiratory event elimination. Long-term safety and effectiveness of solriamfetol under open-label, double-blind, placebo-controlled conditions was demonstrated in a long-term study. Side effects, including headache, nausea, nasopharyngitis, insomnia, dry mouth, anxiety, decreased appetite, and upper respiratory tract infection, were reported in less than 5 percent of patients with narcolepsy or OSA. Treatment options for narcolepsy include a variety of medications. Since it lessens daytime sleepiness, is well tolerated, and has less potential for abuse than traditional stimulants (methylphenidate and amphetamines), modafinil—a non-amphetamine stimulant that promotes wakefulness—is thought to be the first-line therapy for narcolepsy. They are second-line drugs, these conventional medications. REM-suppressing drugs like sodium oxybate and antidepressants may help patients who exhibit severe cataplexy (Slowik et al., 2022).

Treatment for sleep disturbances linked to irregular circadian rhythms involves light-phase shift therapy. Bright light exposure may be used to help patients return to a regular sleep schedule. A prodrug formulation of gabapentin called gabapentin enacarbil has been shown to significantly improve restless leg syndrome, which in turn can help reduce sleep disturbance.

9.2.7. Differential Diagnosis

The differential diagnosis of sleep disorders is as follows:

- Post-traumatic stress disorder (PTSD)
- Depression
- Anxiety disorder
- Bipolar disorder
- Opioid abuse
- Alcoholism
- Stimulant abuse (amphetamine)
- Chronic obstructive pulmonary disease (COPD)
- Hyperthyroidism

9.2.8. Prognosis

Reduced productivity at work, impaired cognitive function, and industrial or auto accidents can all be caused by sleep deprivation. The cause of a sleep disorder has a significant impact on the prognosis of the condition. Patients with chronic insomnia are more likely to experience depression, anxiety, and a lower quality of life. In contrast, insomnia brought on by open airway breathing (OSA) usually goes away with treatment (Yazaki et al., 1999).

9.2.9. Complications

Sleep disorders that go untreated can raise the risk of accidents and cause several serious side effects. Anxiety and mood disorders could emerge. Lack of sleep can impair cognitive function and cause false memories. Individuals with sleep disorders related to periodic limb movement may be more susceptible to cerebrovascular accidents. Untreated OSA can result in several cardiovascular conditions, particularly if it is severe and accompanied by hypersomnia.

9.2.10. Deterrence and Patient Education

All patients should be educated well and encouraged to practice good sleep hygiene. "Sleep hygiene" is a term used to describe good sleep habits.

The following advice should be given to the patients to practice good sleep hygiene:

- Maintain a regular schedule, i.e., go to bed and wake up at the same time every day
- Use the bed for sleep and sex only. Avoid watching television, looking at phones, or reading in the bed
- Exercise almost every day, but not right before bedtime
- Avoid caffeine or smoking, mainly during the evening
- Maintain a dark, calm, and quiet environment in the bedroom
- Avoid struggling to fall asleep in bed. If you can't sleep, get up and try again later or change the bed.

Also, if the patient takes sedative-hypnotic medications, this should be documented in the medical record. Patients should be counseled to avoid driving and operating machines when under these medications.

9.2.11. Enhancing Healthcare Team Outcomes

An interdisciplinary healthcare team comprising (physicians, dentists, nurse practitioners, pharmacists, social workers, counselors, and other mental health professionals is needed to properly manage sleep disorders), as well as a dietician and sleep clinic in certain situations. Certain underlying causes of insomnia necessitate surgical consultations; for example, OSA patients may require palate surgery. For patients with sleep disorders to have positive outcomes, interprofessional collaboration is crucial (Schrader et al., 1993).

In addition to counseling patients and responding to inquiries, nurses can serve as a liaison between the case's other medical specialists and managing clinicians. The pharmacist will confirm the dosage of medications, look for drug interactions, and give patients advice on how to take them. When necessary, sleep clinics will investigate the case further, possibly involving sleep studies. Psychologists will address any concerns that might be linked to sleep disorders and provide updates to the other members of the interdisciplinary team. When choosing their therapy plan, clinicians would be well to take into account the opinions of all team members, including the patient and potentially the family (e.g., parents, and spouses) are additional team members providing care. Every interaction or intervention made by the interprofessional team members is accountable for keeping accurate and current records about the patient's case. When there are worries about the patient's state or advancement, they must also be able to freely discuss them with every other member of the team. This interprofessional approach will support patients with sleep disorders of any kind in achieving the best possible results.

9.3. Impact on Quality of Life

9.3.1. Sleep Disorders and Neurodegenerative Diseases

Sleep disturbances are frequently linked to neurodegenerative diseases, particularly those that exhibit aberrant alpha-synuclein accumulation, such as multiple system atrophy (MSA), Parkinson's disease (PD), and Lewy body disease (LBD). For example, individuals with Parkinson's disease (PD) have frequently presented with various sleep-related issues. These issues are typically related to insomnia (affecting approximately 70% of the PD population), hypersomnia (affecting over 50% of the PD population), and REM sleep behavior disorder (RBD), which affects approximately 40% of the PD population and is linked to increased motor symptoms. Moreover, RBD has been shown over the past few years to be a potent predictor of the development of those neurodegenerative diseases, which presents a wonderful chance to advance the disease's therapies. Neurodegenerative diseases are frequently associated with structural brain impairment, which can interfere with circadian rhythm, motor or non-motor functioning, and the states of wakefulness and sleep. However, poorer quality of life, emotional state, and cognitive functioning are often linked to sleep disturbances in patients. Furthermore, their relatives and caregivers are negatively impacted by these abnormal behavioral symptoms. A more thorough understanding of the connection between sleep disorders and neurodegenerative disease is necessary, given the paucity of existing research on the subject and the rising average lifespan.

9.3.2.1. Sleep Disturbances and Alzheimer's Disease

About 45% of people with Alzheimer's disease (AD) also experience sleep disturbances. This percentage rises to roughly 70% when caregiver reports are taken into account. Insomnia and hypersomnia are commonly identified in AD patients, as well as in the PD population. These conditions have been linked to beta-amyloid accumulation, circadian rhythm sleep disorders (CRSD), and melatonin alteration. Moreover, AD is associated with modifications in the architecture of sleep. Even though the architecture of sleep seems to naturally alter with age, AD patients appear to have more pronounced changes in this area. Spindles, the amount of time spent in REM sleep, and SWS may all decrease (or occasionally disappear entirely) as its latency rises. Poor sleep onset in AD has been linked to sundowning, a common chronobiological phenomenon seen in the disease, as well as dream-related hallucinations, increased restlessness, wandering, and agitation (Takaesu et al., 2016).

Alzheimer's disease is associated with altered sleep architecture, significant sleep disturbances, and cognitive decline as well as memory impairment. The latter may include insomnia, sleep fragmentation, shorter sleep duration, increased naps during the day, fewer stages of sleep overall, and an increasing similarity between certain stages (N1 and N2). This kind of insomnia affects over 65% of those who have Alzheimer's disease. A shift in the circadian rhythm, which controls sleep, is one element that might account for this alteration in the architecture of sleep. Disturbances in the circadian rhythm would result in insomnia. According to certain research, individuals with AD exhibit a delayed circadian rhythm, while those who normally exhibit an advanced circadian rhythm. There are two primary neurological symptoms of Alzheimer's disease in addition to these psychological ones. The first is the build-up of waste beta-amyloid, which results in aggregate plaques. An accumulation of tau protein is the second.

Research has demonstrated that the beta-amyloid burden, a key factor in AD, is influenced by the sleep-wake cycle. The production of beta-amyloid protein during sleep is not as regular as it is during wakefulness. There are two phenomena that explain this. The first is that when you're awake, your metabolism will be more active, which will lead to more beta-amyloid protein being secreted. The second is that more oxidative stress will result in increased production of AB. On the other hand, beta-amyloid residues are broken down to stop plaque from forming while you sleep. This is caused by the glymphatic system and the phenomenon known as glymphatic clearance. Because of this, the AB burden is higher during wakefulness due to increased metabolic activity, oxidative stress, and lack of glymphatic clearance-mediated protein degradation. The burden is lessened while we sleep because there is less oxidative stress and metabolic activity (along with the glymphatic clearance that takes place). Sleeping in the NREM SWS allows for the clearance of lymph. As we age, this sleep stage diminishes, leading to a decrease in glymphatic clearance and an increase in AB burden, which ultimately forms AB plaques. Consequently, sleep disturbances in AD patients will make this phenomenon more pronounced (Liu et al., 2022).

Hence, an increase in AB plaques will result from a reduction in both the quantity and quality of NREM SWS as well as sleep disruptions. This starts in the hippocampus, a region of the brain essential to the formation of long-term memory. There is a decrease in memory function and cognitive deterioration associated with AD, which is partly caused by hippocampal cell death. There is a correlation between the emergence of prominent sleep disorders and AD, albeit the exact cause of the relationship remains unclear. Similarly, there is a positive feedback relationship between sleep disorders and the advancement of the disease. Consequently, sleep disruptions are now more than just an indication of AD; rather, there is a reciprocal relationship between sleep disruptions and AD. At the same time, it has been demonstrated that NREM sleep is when long-term memory consolidation—which is dependent on the hippocampus—occurs. According to this, a reduction in NREM sleep will lead to less consolidation, which will impair hippocampal-dependent long-term memory function. One of the main signs of AD is this decline in performance. Neurogenesis, AD, and sleep disturbances have all been related in recent studies. In adult brains, new neurons were still being produced in the subgranular and subventricular zones. Following that, these new cells are integrated into the hippocampus's subgranular zone and neural circuits. These new cells are important for hippocampal-dependent memory and have a role in both learning and memory.

Nonetheless, recent research has demonstrated that several variables, such as stress and extended sleep deprivation (more than one day), can impede neurogenesis. Thus, sleep disturbances associated with AD may inhibit neurogenesis, thereby compromising hippocampal functions. This would exacerbate sleep disturbances and accelerate the development of AD, which would also lead to decreased memory performance. AD preclinical phase is characterized by changes in sleep architecture in patients. These alterations may be used to identify people who are most vulnerable to AD. This is still merely theoretical, though. Even though the precise processes and the causal link between sleep disorders and AD are still unknown, these findings already improve our understanding of the condition and present opportunities for better targeting at-risk populations and developing treatments to slow the cognitive decline of AD patients.

9.3.2. Sleep Disorder Symptoms in Psychiatric Illnesses

9.3.2.1. Schizophrenia

A wide range of clinical symptoms, such as excessive daytime sleepiness, trouble falling or staying asleep, nightmares, sleep talking, sleepwalking, and poor sleep quality, can be present in people with psychiatric illnesses who suffer from sleep disorders. Insomnia, hypersomnia, and delayed sleep-phase disorder are three common sleep disturbances associated with severe mental illnesses, including psychotic disorders. Sleep issues are a contributing factor to cognitive deficits in learning and memory in individuals with schizophrenia. Sleep problems frequently arise before the onset of psychosis. Delusions, depression, and hallucinations can also result from sleep deprivation. In a 2019 study, 617 people with schizophrenia-spectrum (SCZ), 440 people with bipolar (BP) disorder, and 173 healthy controls (HC) were examined for the three sleep disturbances previously mentioned with these conditions. The Inventory for Depressive Symptoms – clinician rated scale (IDS-C) was used to identify sleep disturbances (Lundetræ et al., 2018). According to the findings, 78% of SCZ people, 69% of BD patients, and 39% of healthy controls had experienced at least one type of sleep disturbance. In comparison to the BD and HC groups, the SCZ group reported the highest frequency of sleep disturbances; in particular, hypersomnia was more common in those with SCZ, and delayed sleep phase disorder was three times more common in the SCZ group than in the BD group. Among the three groups, insomnias were the most commonly reported sleep disturbance.

9.3.2.2. Bipolar Disorder

Sleep abnormalities are a primary behavioral symptom of bipolar disorder. Research indicates that between 23 and 78% of people with bipolar disorders frequently report symptoms of hypersomnia, or sleeping for an extended period of time. Sleep disturbances are a good predictor of mood swings, and bipolar disorder may have a circadian rhythm variability component to its pathogenesis, which includes an increased risk of suicidal ideation. In addition to hypersomnia, nightmares, poor sleep quality, OSA, excessive daytime sleepiness, and other sleep-related symptoms, insomnia is the most prevalent sleep-related symptom of bipolar disorder. Furthermore, sleep debt has been demonstrated in animal models to cause bipolar mania episodes in lab mice; however, the capacity of these models to fully explain human bipolar illness and all of its complex symptoms, including sleep disturbances, is still limited (Gulia and Kumar, 2018).

9.3.2.3. Major Depressive Disorder (MDD)

Although not a mandatory diagnostic criterion, sleep disturbances, such as insomnia or hypersomnia, are common symptoms of major depressive disorder (MDD). Insomnia and hypersomnia are estimated to be prevalent in 88% and 27% of MDD patients, respectively, while the likelihood of developing MDD is tripled in those who experience insomnia. Although sleep regulation issues may come before depressive episodes, depressive episodes themselves can also lead to sleep deprivation. Depressed mood and sleep efficiency are highly correlated. Depression symptoms and fatigue, including sleep disturbances like excessive and irregular sleepiness, are related. Even weariness and sleep issues have been implicated in recent research as possible mediators between the symptoms of MDD and co-occurring generalized anxiety disorder.

9.4. Insomnia: Treatment and Management Strategies

One common sleep ailment that can make it difficult to get to sleep or stay asleep is insomnia. It may also result in excessive waking and difficulty falling back asleep. Long-term sleep issues such as insomnia can be successfully treated with cognitive behavioral therapy, also known as CBT (Vgontzas et al., 2010). It is typically the first course of treatment advised. CBT assists you in identifying the ideas and actions that either exacerbate or cause sleep issues. You discover how to swap out these ideas and actions for routines that promote restful sleep. CBT aids in resolving the root causes of your sleep issues, as opposed to pharmaceutical sleeping aids. Your sleep specialist may ask you to keep a thorough sleep diary for one to two weeks to determine the best course of treatment for your insomnia (Vgontzas et al., 2010).

9.4.1. How Does CBT Work?

Cognitive behavioral therapy (CBT) teaches you to identify and modify beliefs that interfere with your ability to fall asleep. This kind of therapy can assist you in managing or eliminating unfavorable ideas and anxieties that keep you up at night. The behavioral component of CBT aids in the development of healthy sleeping habits and the avoidance of bad sleep-inducing behaviors. Depending on your needs, your sleep specialist may recommend that you:

- **Change Your Routine:** This can help you sleep better. Set a consistent bedtime and wake time. Avoid naps. Use the bed only for sleep and sex.
- **Set Sleep Limits:** Poor sleep can result from making it a habit to lie in bed when you're awake. Get out of bed and wait to go back to bed until you are tired if, after twenty minutes, you are unable to fall asleep. However, do not alter your wake-up time. This prolongs your fatigue the following evening. But you gradually increase the amount of time you spend in bed as your sleep improves.
- **Change Certain Lifestyle Habits:** Give up bad sleeping habits like smoking, consuming large amounts of caffeine late in the day, and excessive alcohol consumption. Insufficient physical activity can also contribute to restless nights. You might pick up tricks to improve your quality of sleep, like how to unwind an hour or two before bed.
- **Improve Your Sleep Area:** Create a comfortable sleep area. Keep your bedroom quiet, dark and cool. Don't have a TV in the bedroom. Hide the clock from view.
- **Learn Relaxation Techniques:** These techniques help you calm your mind and body. Approaches include meditation, imagery and muscle relaxation.
- **Remain Passively Awake:** With this method, once you're in bed, you try not to think about falling asleep. That's because worrying that you can't sleep can keep you awake. Letting go of this worry can help you relax and make it easier to fall asleep.
- **Use Biofeedback:** Using a device that displays indicators like your heart rate and muscle tension is part of this technique. Next, you discover how to assist in their management. Your sleep specialist might ask you to record your

daily patterns with a biofeedback device at home. These data may reveal trends that influence sleep.

The most effective treatment approach may combine several of these methods.

9.4.2. CBT Versus Pills

Before getting treatment for insomnia, many people attempt over-the-counter sleeping pills. Certain prescription sleep aids may work well as a temporary remedy. For instance, they can offer instant comfort when you're experiencing extreme stress or grief. Certain more recent sleep aids are authorized for extended usage. However, for many people, sleeping pills are not the most effective long-term treatment for insomnia. It's unlikely that taking medication by itself will cure all of your insomnia symptoms. Furthermore, there is a chance that some medications will cause major side effects, such as addiction, withdrawal symptoms, amnesia, and suicidal thoughts. These medications typically cause fatigue when you need to be alert, like when driving or at work. If you have persistent sleep issues or are concerned about developing a drug dependency on sleep aids, cognitive behavioral therapy (CBT) might be a good option for your care. It may also be a wise decision in cases where medications are ineffective or have unpleasant side effects. CBT targets the root cause of your insomnia rather than just treating the symptoms, in contrast to sleep aids (Vgontzas et al., 2010). However, to make it work, it requires time and effort. Sometimes the best treatment is a combination of CBT and sleep aids. If cognitive behavioral therapy (CBT) is not offered where you live, ask your medical professional for CBT-based sleep advice.

9.4.3. Insomnia and Other Disorders

A lot of illnesses can make it difficult to sleep. Heart disease, asthma, arthritis, and chronic obstructive pulmonary disease (COPD) are a few of these. Disorders of the mind can also cause sleep disturbances. Anxiety, depression, bipolar disorder, and post-traumatic stress disorder are a few examples. Chronic sleep deprivation raises the risk of heart disease, diabetes, high blood pressure, anxiety, depression, and chronic pain. Certain medications, including over-the-counter ones, can also make you sleepy. Speak with your healthcare provider about the best ways to handle sleep issues if your insomnia is caused by a medical condition or a medication you're taking. If treatment is not received, insomnia is unlikely to improve.

9.4.4. Finding Help

A wide range of healthcare professionals, such as primary care physicians and behavioral sleep medicine specialists, can offer CBT guidance for insomnia. The number of certified specialists in behavioral sleep medicine is restricted. It might be necessary for you to look for a qualified professional and a treatment plan that works for you. To find a sleep center in the United States, do an online search at sleepeducation.org/sleep-center, such as the Mayo Clinic Center for Sleep Medicine, are accredited by the American Academy of Sleep Medicine. Alternatively, you can look up a list of behavioral sleep medicine providers by visiting the website of the Society of Behavioral Sleep Medicine at behavioral sleep. org. There may be variations in the kind of treatment, duration, and frequency of sessions. One session might be all you need, or you might need eight or more. It is contingent upon your progress, the program, and your sleep expert. Most patients require six to eight sessions. Make sure to inquire about the treatment plan and what to anticipate when scheduling an appointment. Additionally, confirm ahead of time if the necessary treatments will be covered by your health insurance. If possible, schedule in-person consultations with a sleep medicine specialist in your area. However, a phone conversation or video conference could also be beneficial. For advice on CBT methods for insomnia, you can also search for self-help books and internet resources.

9.4.5. Evaluation and Diagnosis

- **Acute Insomnia:** To distinguish between insomnia and sleep disturbance, a complete medical history is crucial. Even though trouble falling asleep and staying asleep is a common complaint, many people manage to function normally all day. On the other hand, insomnia affects how one functions during the day. Sleep disturbances in presentations are more often the result of the perception that sleep is not meeting expectations than actual negative outcomes (Vgontzas et al., 2010). The emphasis placed by society on the necessity of getting the ideal sleep to maintain good health and wellbeing frequently serves to reinforce this belief.
- **Chronic Insomnia:** A sleep disturbance that causes significant distress or interferes with daytime functioning and occurs three or more nights a week for a duration of three months is referred to as chronic insomnia or insomnia disorder. A prior history of insomnia is a strong indicator of the development of insomnia disorder in the future due to the high recurrence rate. In a long-term study involving 388 individuals suffering from chronic insomnia, 46% of patients still experienced symptoms after three years, and 14% experienced a relapse after experiencing remission.
- **Comorbidities:** It is common for comorbid disorders like depression and anxiety to coexist with long-term medical conditions. Given the potential for mutual effects, a thorough evaluation and treatment of all comorbidities and insomnia are crucial. A concomitant sleep disorder may also manifest as insomnia. It is possible for up to 50% of individuals with obstructive sleep apnea to experience symptoms of insomnia and struggle to comply with continuous positive airway pressure (CPAP) therapy. Although weariness and lethargy are typical signs of insomnia, excessive daytime sleepiness is rare and needs to be ruled out in favor of sleep disordered breathing. Insomnia can also be a symptom of other sleep disorders, such as circadian rhythm disorders and restless legs syndrome.

9.4.6. Initial Management

It is appropriate to use a short-term strategy to improve sleep quality in patients with acute insomnia. This could entail techniques to lessen acute discomfort as well as perhaps a brief hypnotic medication course. To improve outcomes, longer term management strategies are needed for chronic insomnia, given its worse prognosis. The main goals of treating insomnia are to address comorbidities and precipitating factors, as well as to lessen anxiety associated with sleep and maladaptive sleep-related behaviors. Educating people about sleep is crucial because it addresses erroneous or unrealistic expectations about sleep, which frequently exacerbate the symptoms of insomnia. The high prevalence of insomnia and the dearth of practitioners of specialized sleep medicine and sleep psychology may warrant a stepped-care approach to insomnia in primary care (Hillman et al., 2018).

9.4.6.1. Cognitive Behavioral Therapy

Cognitive behavioral therapy for insomnia is recommended as first-line therapy. It has five components (See Table 9.1):

Table 9.1. Components of Cognitive Behavioral Therapy for Insomnia

Components	Rationale	Directions
Sleep hygiene	Promotes healthy bedtime behaviors and an ideal environment for sleep	Behaviors: • Avoid caffeine and nicotine before bedtime • Maintain a regular bed and wake time • Take regular daytime exercise Environment: • Maintain bedroom as a place to sleep • Reduce noise and light • Control temperature • Avoid bedroom clutter
Sleep/time in bed restriction	Aims to balance estimated total sleep time with opportunity to sleep. This reduces the unnecessary amount of time spent in bed awake and increases sleep drive and sleep debt to consolidate sleep on subsequent nights	Assess patient's natural time of feeling sleepy and estimated total sleep time overnight (a sleep diary is often helpful in this setting). Schedule a fixed bed and wake time based on estimated total sleep time, with at least six hours of opportunity for sleep, aiming for no longer than 30 minutes of wakefulness. Maintain a consistent sleep–wake schedule regardless of how much sleep is obtained overnight. Lengthen sleep window in 30-minute increments on subsequent reviews depending on progress
Stimulus control	Promotes a consistent sleep–wake schedule and reduces conditioned response around sleep	Avoid naps during the day to increase natural homeostatic sleep drive Only go to bed when sleepy If unable to fall asleep or waking for prolonged periods during the night, engage in another activity Only return to sleeping position or bed when sleepy
Relaxation strategies	Aim to reduce hyperarousal that often underpins insomnia and to improve stress management	Meditation Breathing exercises Progressive muscle relaxation Guided visualization practices Implement short relaxation periods at various times during the day

Cognitive therapy	Encourages thought restructuring around sleep and promotes mindfulness	Challenge unhelpful beliefs and attitudes around sleep including the requirement for a certain number of hours of sleep, the health impacts of insomnia and attributional biases attached to inadequate sleep (Hillman et al., 2018)

Source: https://www.ncbi.nlm.nih.gov/pmc/articles/PMC8377300/.

The goal of good sleep hygiene is to create an environment that is conducive to healthy behavior and better sleep. Patients run the risk of acquiring maladaptive sleep-related behaviors, and there is little evidence to support sleep hygiene as the only behavioral strategy. By matching the total amount of time spent in bed with the estimated duration of sleep, sleep restriction is a behavioral strategy designed to reduce the amount of time spent awake in bed. In a randomized trial with 45 patients suffering from chronic insomnia, 73% of the patients who received both sleep restriction therapy and good sleep hygiene reported better symptom outcomes than the 35% of patients in the control group who only received good sleep hygiene. By building cues that encourage sleep and adhering to a regular sleep-wake schedule, stimulus control techniques seek to enhance the quality of sleep. One strategy is to tell patients to go to bed only when they are tired and to leave the bedroom to do something else if they can't sleep or wake up during the night. These techniques aim to lessen anxiety associated with sleep as well as a conditioned reaction related to sleep (Hillman et al., 2018).

Strategies for both sleep restriction and stimulus control are combined in brief behavioral therapy for insomnia. After six months of follow-up, 36% of the 82 patients in a randomized controlled trial experienced remission, and 60% of them showed improvement. Two in-person sessions make up the therapy: a 45–60 minute assessment and intervention session and a 30-minute follow-up session held after two weeks. GPs and practice nurses are encouraged to use it by the Royal Australian College of General Practitioners because it can be administered effectively and doesn't require specialized training. Patients may need cognitive therapies for insomnia if they don't improve with brief behavioral therapy. A sleep psychologist referral ought to be taken into consideration. According to a meta-analysis, cognitive behavioral therapy is a successful long-term intervention that significantly improves sleep onset latency and sleep efficiency up to a 12-month period. It is often given by a psychologist or other qualified health professional once a week for two to eight sessions. However, due to the lack of specialists in sleep medicine and sleep psychology, access to primary care may be severely hampered.

9.4.7. Drug Management

Despite receiving cognitive behavioral therapy, up to 40% of insomnia patients will still experience symptoms. When considering medication therapy, it's critical to assess the underlying cause of the patient's insomnia as well as the intended result of the prescription.

9.4.7.1. Acute Insomnia

To stop acute insomnia from becoming chronic, short-term medication therapy may be suitable if there is a clear stressor, illness, or other circumstances that preceded the insomnia. This would typically last no more than four weeks, during which time the acute precipitating circumstances would be addressed concurrently.

9.4.7.2. Chronic Insomnia

When used in conjunction with cognitive behavioral therapy, medication can help patients with chronic insomnia and high levels of distress by establishing sleep patterns and preventing the exacerbation of anxiety related to sleep. During the first six weeks of a trial involving 160 adults with chronic insomnia, patients were randomly assigned to receive cognitive behavioral therapy alone or in combination with zolpidem. With remission rates of 68% at six months, the group that received combined therapy for six weeks and then cognitive behavioral therapy alone during six months of extended therapy had the best results. This study showed how important it is to address insomnia-related distress during the first six weeks of treatment, as individuals are working through cognitive behavioral therapy and developing their abilities and self-assurance in the cognitive and behavioral strategies. Nonetheless, it is important to explain to patients that any medication prescribed for chronic insomnia is only meant to be used temporarily because the effects usually wear off over time. Over the course of three weeks, adults over the age of 55 can effectively treat their insomnia with melatonin (2 mg extended-release formulation). Additionally, it might help patients whose circadian rhythm is disrupted and they experience insomnia or wakefulness in the early morning. But aside from melatonin's approved indication of insomnia in adults over 55, there isn't much data to support the design, dosage, or length of therapy (Hillman et al., 2018).

A dual orexin receptor antagonist called suvorexant has been shown to be a useful treatment for hyperarousal-induced insomnia. When compared to a placebo, it can enhance sleep latency, maintenance, and overall sleep duration. For insomnia that affects both the onset and maintenance of sleep, benzodiazepines and their receptor agonists, such as zolpidem and zopiclone, are useful short-term treatments. There are few data on long-term effectiveness. Although there is a chance of drug abuse, tolerance, and dependency, these risks should be reduced with frequent monitoring and dose escalation restrictions. A harm-benefit analysis should be done before prescribing these medications for insomnia, especially for elderly patients. It is important to use caution when using sleep-promoting medications in combination with other sedatives, such as alcohol. Drugs that induce hypnosis may raise the chance of falls, but so does sleep deprivation. Despite having serious potential side effects, antidepressants, sedating antipsychotics, and antihistamines are frequently prescribed for the treatment of insomnia despite the lack of supporting data. These medications' side effects and the scant evidence supporting them make them unrecommended.

9.4.7.3. Stopping Drugs

It is only advised to use benzodiazepines and benzodiazepine receptor agonists for a maximum of four weeks at a time, so a safe withdrawal plan is necessary. A systematic review and meta-analysis found that cognitive behavioral therapy plus gradual drug tapering over three months was a more successful combination for drug cessation than gradual tapering on its own. The combination was linked to a temporary reduction in insomnia symptoms (Espie, 2009).

A Closer Look

Early Symptoms Obstructive Sleep Apnea (OSA) of Menopause

Obstructive sleep apnea (OSA) is a common yet potentially serious sleep disorder characterized by repeated episodes of complete or partial obstruction of the upper airway during sleep. These obstructions result in disruptions to normal breathing patterns, leading to brief pauses in breathing known as apneas. These apneic episodes can occur numerous times throughout the night, often accompanied by loud snoring, gasping, or choking sounds as the individual struggles to resume breathing. OSA can significantly impact sleep quality and overall health, as it disrupts the normal sleep cycle, preventing individuals from achieving restorative, deep sleep stages.

The primary cause of obstructive sleep apnea is the relaxation of the muscles in the throat and tongue during sleep, which causes the airway to become narrowed or completely blocked. This narrowing or obstruction restricts airflow, leading to breathing difficulties. Certain factors can increase the risk of developing OSA, including obesity, anatomical abnormalities in the upper airway, such as enlarged tonsils or a narrow throat, aging, male gender, family history of OSA, and certain medical conditions like hypertension, diabetes, or hormonal disorders.

One of the hallmark symptoms of obstructive sleep apnea is excessive daytime sleepiness, as individuals with OSA often experience fragmented sleep due to repeated awakenings throughout the night to resume breathing. Consequently, they may struggle to stay awake or alert during the day, leading to impaired cognitive function, decreased concentration, memory problems, irritability, and mood changes.

Summary

- Sleep disturbances refer to a range of issues that interfere with the ability to fall asleep, stay asleep, or achieve restful and restorative sleep. These disturbances can significantly impact overall health and quality of life, as adequate sleep is essential for physical and mental well-being.
- Sleep apnea is another common sleep disturbance, marked by repeated interruptions in breathing during sleep. Obstructive sleep apnea (OSA), the most common form, occurs when the muscles at the back of the throat fail to keep the airway open.
- Restless legs syndrome (RLS) is a neurological disorder characterized by an uncontrollable urge to move the legs, usually due to uncomfortable sensations.
- Circadian rhythm disorders involve disruptions in the body's internal clock, which regulates the sleep-wake cycle.
- The sleep and arousal disorders most frequently encountered by the clinician are disorders of initiating and maintaining sleep, the insomnias.
- A few patients awaken refreshed and function perfectly well, despite sleeping much less than expected. Except for brevity, their sleeping appears to be normal. These so-called short sleepers regularly have a daily sleep total that is less than 75% of that usually expected for their age.
- Patients who excessively use caffeine-containing substances may similarly develop tolerance and become progressively dependent on caffeine. The need for several cups of coffee to wake up in the morning may reflect caffeine withdrawal. Alcohol should not be overlooked as a possible etiologic agent in excessive somnolence.
- A sleep-related complaint may represent another cluster of disturbances: disorders of the sleep–wake schedule. To conceptualize these disorders, one must view sleep and wake as behaviors that are intimately related to physiological and societal processes.
- Clinicians occasionally encounter patients whose complaints deal with disturbing events associated with sleep, sleep stages, or partial arousals. Although these parasomnias constitute perhaps the most common group of sleep disorders found in children, occasionally adults present with these disorders.
- The microsleeps so typical of the elderly also appear in younger individuals when they are progressively deprived of sleep. Even before the appearance of microsleeps, shorter daytime sleep onset latencies are noted as a lack of nocturnal sleep becomes progressive.
- Sleep disorders encompass several clinical problems encountered in outpatient settings. Sleep disorders have a broad differential diagnosis; therefore, standardized definitions and classifications are essential. There are many different types of sleep disorders.
- A sleep disorder, or somnipathy, is a medical disorder of an individual's sleep patterns. Some sleep disorders are severe enough to interfere with normal physical, mental, social and emotional functioning.
- Insomnia is a prevalent form of sleep deprivation. Individuals with insomnia may have problems falling asleep, staying asleep, or a combination of both resulting in hyposomnia – i.e., insufficient quantity and poor quality of sleep.

References

1. Zammit, G. K., Weiner, J., Damato, N., Sillup, G. P., & McMillan, C. A. (1999). Quality of life in people with insomnia. *Sleep, 22*(Suppl 2), S379–S385.
2. Gauld, C., Lopez, R., Geoffroy, P. A., Morin, C. M., Guichard, K., Giroux, É., Dauvilliers, Y., Dumas, G., Philip, P., & Micoulaud-Franchi, J. A. (2021). A systematic analysis of ICSD-3 diagnostic criteria and proposal for further structured iteration. *Sleep Medicine Reviews, 58*, 101439. https://doi.org/10.1016/j.smrv.2021.101439.
3. Huyett, P., Siegel, N., & Bhattacharyya, N. (2021). Prevalence of sleep disorders and association with mortality: Results from the NHANES 2009–2010. *Laryngoscope, 131*(3), 686–689. https://doi.org/10.1002/lary.29196.
4. Kaur, H., Spurling, B. C., & Bollu, P. C. (2023). Chronic insomnia. In *StatPearls*. StatPearls Publishing. Retrieved from: https://www.statpearls.com (accessed on 10 September 2024).
5. Momin, R. R., & Ketvertis, K. (2023). Short-term insomnia. In *StatPearls*. StatPearls Publishing. Retrieved from: https://www.statpearls.com (accessed on 10 September 2024).
6. Maggard, M. D., Sankari, A., & Cascella, M. (2023). Upper airway resistance syndrome. In *StatPearls*. StatPearls Publishing. Retrieved from: https://www.statpearls.com (accessed on 10 September 2024).
7. Rana, A. M., & Sankari, A. (2023). Central sleep apnea. In *StatPearls*. StatPearls Publishing. Retrieved from: https://www.statpearls.com (accessed on 10 September 2024).
8. Ghimire, P., Sankari, A., & Kaul, P. (2024). Pickwickian syndrome. In *StatPearls*. StatPearls Publishing. Retrieved from: https://www.statpearls.com (accessed on 10 September 2024).
9. Antoine, M. H., Sankari, A., & Bollu, P. C. (2024). Obesity-hypoventilation syndrome. In *StatPearls*. StatPearls Publishing. Retrieved from: https://www.statpearls.com (accessed on 10 September 2024).
10. Slowik, J. M., Collen, J. F., & Yow, A. G. (2023). Narcolepsy. In *StatPearls*. StatPearls Publishing. Retrieved from: https://www.statpearls.com (accessed on 10 September 2024).
11. Shah, F., & Gupta, V. (2023). Kleine-Levin syndrome (KLS). In *StatPearls*. StatPearls Publishing. Retrieved from: https://www.statpearls.com (accessed on 10 September 2024).
12. Okawa, M., & Uchiyama, M. (2007). Circadian rhythm sleep disorders: Characteristics and entrainment pathology in delayed sleep phase and non-24-h sleep-wake syndrome. *Sleep Medicine Reviews, 11*(6), 485–496. https://doi.org/10.1016/j.smrv.2007.05.001.
13. Basit, H., Damhoff, T. C., & Huecker, M. R. (2023). Sleeplessness and circadian disorder. In *StatPearls*. StatPearls Publishing. Retrieved from: https://www.statpearls.com (accessed on 10 September 2024).
14. Hublin, C., & Kaprio, J. (2003). Genetic aspects and genetic epidemiology of parasomnias. *Sleep Medicine Reviews, 7*(5), 413–421. https://doi.org/10.1016/S1087-0792(03)00040-5.
15. Acquavella, J., Mehra, R., Bron, M., Suomi, J. M., & Hess, G. P. (2020). Prevalence of narcolepsy and other sleep disorders and frequency of diagnostic tests from 2013-2016 in insured patients actively seeking care. *Journal of Clinical Sleep Medicine, 16*(8), 1255–1263. https://doi.org/10.5664/jcsm.8448.

16. Fariba, K. A., & Tadi, P. (2023). Parasomnias. In *StatPearls*. StatPearls Publishing. Retrieved from: https://www.statpearls.com (accessed on 10 September 2024).

17. Bargiotas, P., & Bassetti, C. L. (2017). Sleep-related movement disorders and disturbances of motor control. *Current Opinion in Neurology, 30*(4), 405–415. https://doi.org/10.1097/WCO.0000000000000475.

18. Mansur, A., Castillo, P. R., Rocha Cabrero, F., & Bokhari, S. R. A. (2023). Restless legs syndrome. In *StatPearls*. StatPearls Publishing. Retrieved from: https://www.statpearls.com (accessed on 10 September 2024).

19. Pham, C. K., Sankari, A., & Slowik, J. M. (2022). Rapid eye movement sleep behavior disorder. In *StatPearls*. StatPearls Publishing. Retrieved from: https://www.statpearls.com (accessed on 10 September 2024).

20. Matsumoto, T., & Chin, K. (2019). Prevalence of sleep disturbances: Sleep disordered breathing, short sleep duration, and non-restorative sleep. *Respiratory Investigation, 57*(3), 227–237. https://doi.org/10.1016/j.resinv.2019.01.007.

21. Demirtaş, H., & Dolu, İ. (2023). The prevalence of poor sleep quality and its association with the risk of obstructive sleep apnea and restless legs syndrome in diabetic patients treated with cyanoacrylate glue for varicose veins. *Sleep and Breath, 27*(2), 745–755. https://doi.org/10.1007/s11325-022-02791-8.

22. Morin, C. M., Jarrin, D. C., Ivers, H., Mérette, C., LeBlanc, M., & Savard, J. (2020). Incidence, persistence, and remission rates of insomnia over 5 years. *JAMA Network Open, 3*(11), e2018782. https://doi.org/10.1001/jamanetworkopen.2020.18782.

23. Rodriguez, J. C., Dzierzewski, J. M., & Alessi, C. A. (2015). Sleep problems in the elderly. *Medical Clinics of North America, 99*(2), 431–439. https://doi.org/10.1016/j.mcna.2014.12.005.

24. Slowik, J. M., Sankari, A., & Collen, J. F. (2022). Obstructive sleep apnea. In *StatPearls*. StatPearls Publishing. Retrieved from: https://www.statpearls.com (accessed on 10 September 2024).

25. Yazaki, M., Shirakawa, S., Okawa, M., & Takahashi, K. (1999). Demography of sleep disturbances associated with circadian rhythm disorders in Japan. *Psychiatry and Clinical Neurosciences, 53*(2), 267–268. https://doi.org/10.1046/j.1440-1819.1999.00535.x.

26. Schrader, H., Bovim, G., & Sand, T. (1993). The prevalence of delayed and advanced sleep phase syndromes. *Journal of Sleep Research, 2*(1), 51–55. https://doi.org/10.1111/j.1365-2869.1993.tb00040.x.

27. Takaesu, Y., Inoue, Y., Murakoshi, A., Komada, Y., Otsuka, A., Futenma, K., & Inoue, T. (2016). Prevalence of circadian rhythm sleep-wake disorders and associated factors in euthymic patients with bipolar disorder. *PLoS One, 11*(7), e0159578. https://doi.org/10.1371/journal.pone.0159578.

28. Liu, C., Tang, X., Gong, Z., Zeng, W., Hou, Q., & Lu, R. (2022). Circadian rhythm sleep disorders: Genetics, mechanisms, and adverse effects on health. *Frontiers in Genetics, 13*, 875342. https://doi.org/10.3389/fgene.2022.875342.

29. Lundetræ, R. S., Saxvig, I. W., Pallesen, S., Aurlien, H., Lehmann, S., & Bjorvatn, B. (2018). Prevalence of parasomnias in patients with obstructive sleep apnea: A registry-based cross-sectional study. *Frontiers in Psychology, 9*, 1140. https://doi.org/10.3389/fpsyg.2018.01140.

30. Gulia, K. K., & Kumar, V. M. (2018). Sleep disorders in the elderly: A growing challenge. *Psychogeriatrics, 18*(3), 155–165. https://doi.org/10.1111/psyg.12337.

31. Vgontzas, A. N., Liao, D., Pejovic, S., Calhoun, S., Karataraki, M., Basta, M., & Bixler, E. O. (2010). Insomnia with short sleep duration and mortality: The Penn State cohort. *Sleep, 33*(9), 1159–1164. https://doi.org/10.1093/sleep/33.9.1159.

32. Hillman, D., Mitchell, S., Streatfeild, J., Burns, C., Bruck, D., & Pezzullo, L. (2018). The economic cost of inadequate sleep. *Sleep (Basel), 41*(zsy083). https://doi.org/10.1093/sleep/zsy083.

33. Espie, C. A. (2009). "Stepped care": A health technology solution for delivering cognitive behavioral therapy as a first-line insomnia treatment. *Sleep, 32*(12), 1549–1558. https://doi.org/10.1093/sleep/32.12.1549.

Chapter 10

WEIGHT MANAGEMENT AND METABOLIC CHANGES

Contents

Introduction

Managing weight is a complex process linked to changes in the body's metabolism. It all starts with the basic idea of caloric balance, which states that the energy expenditure from physical activity, basal metabolic rate (BMR), and the thermic effect of food (TEF) must equal the energy intake from food. The state of this delicate equilibrium determines whether weight is maintained, gained, or lost (Allison et al., 2012).

The complex network of biochemical reactions that support life, metabolism, controls these energy dynamics (Anderson et al., 2011). While the thermic effect of food (TEF) includes the energy used in the digestion and metabolism of food, basal metabolic rate (BMR) measures the amount of energy needed for fundamental body processes while at rest. Exercise also alters metabolism, increasing energy expenditure and impacting weight control in general (Apovian et al., 2015).

The way we eat has a major impact on how our metabolism functions. The macronutrient makeup—proteins, lipids, and carbohydrates—affects energy utilization, metabolic rate, and satiety. Similarly, micronutrients have a significant impact on metabolic processes because they are necessary for enzymatic reactions and cellular function. Consuming enough fiber, which comes from whole grains, fruits, and vegetables, promotes satiety, controls blood sugar, and aids in weight management (Aronne et al., 2013).

Physical exercise plays a key role in achieving metabolic health and managing weight. Both cardio and resistance workouts have positive effects on metabolism, increasing calorie burn, building muscle, and improving metabolic flexibility (Astrup et al., 2005). Consistent exercise not only helps burn calories but also creates a healthy metabolic environment that supports maintaining a healthy weight in the long term.

Beyond nutrition and physical activity, metabolic regulation and weight management are intricately entwined with factors like sleep, stress management, hormone balance, and underlying medical conditions. Comprehensive approaches to metabolic health include addressing hormonal imbalances, adopting stress coping mechanisms, and placing a high priority on getting enough sleep. Effective weight management involves more than just counting calories; it involves a comprehensive approach that incorporates physical activity, diet, lifestyle modifications, and metabolic control. Building a symbiotic relationship with metabolism enables people to effectively and resiliently manage their weight while maintaining long-lasting metabolic vitality (Avery et al., 2016).

Orientation and Directional Terms:

Terms	Definition	Illustration
Basal metabolic rate	Basal metabolic rate is the rate of energy expenditure per unit time by endothermic animals at rest.	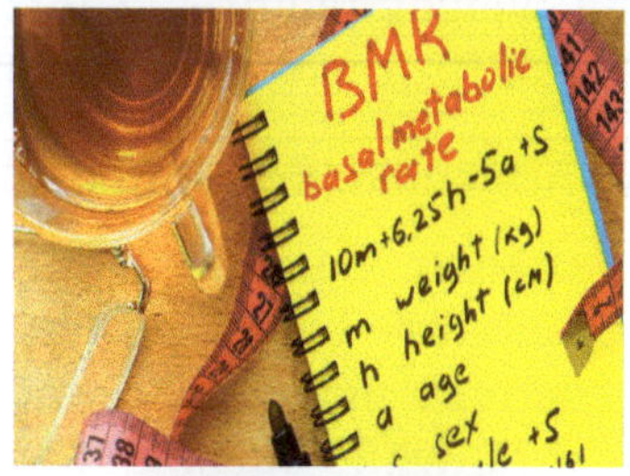
Homeostasis	Homeostasis is any self-regulating process by which an organism tends to maintain stability while adjusting to conditions that are best for its survival.	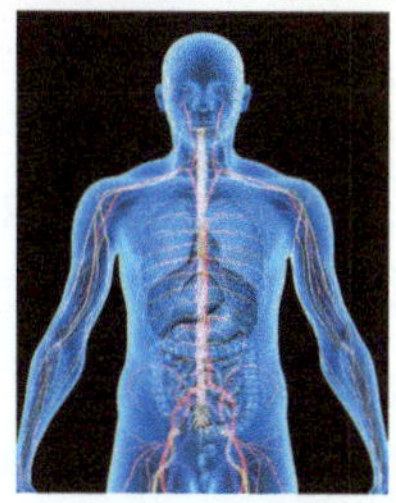
Anaerobic glycolysis	Anaerobic glycolysis is the transformation of glucose to lactate when limited amounts of oxygen are available.	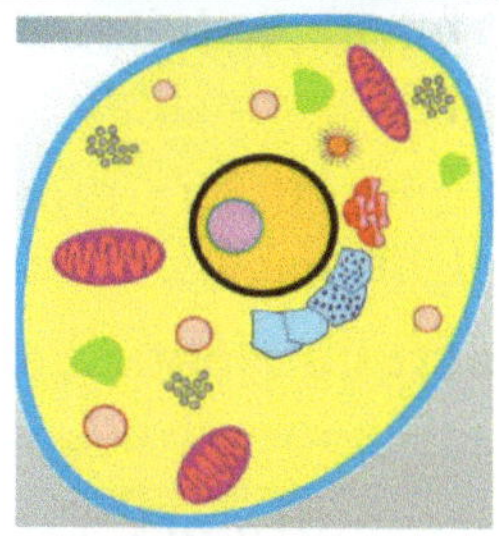
Gastrectomy	Gastrectomy is surgery to remove part or all of the stomach. If only part of the stomach is removed, it is called partial gastrectomy.	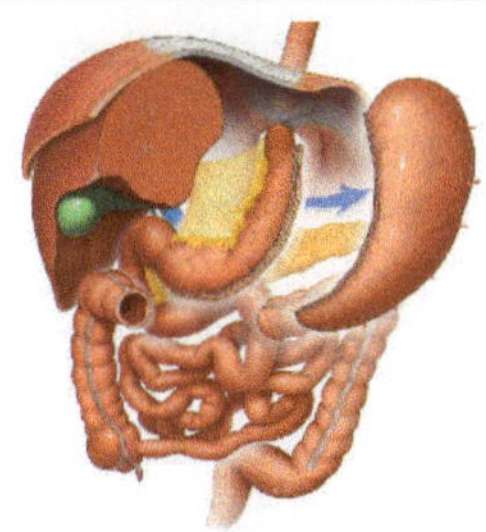
Pathophysiologies	Pathophysiology is a branch of study, at the intersection of pathology and physiology, concerning disordered physiological processes that cause, result from, or are otherwise associated with a disease or injury.	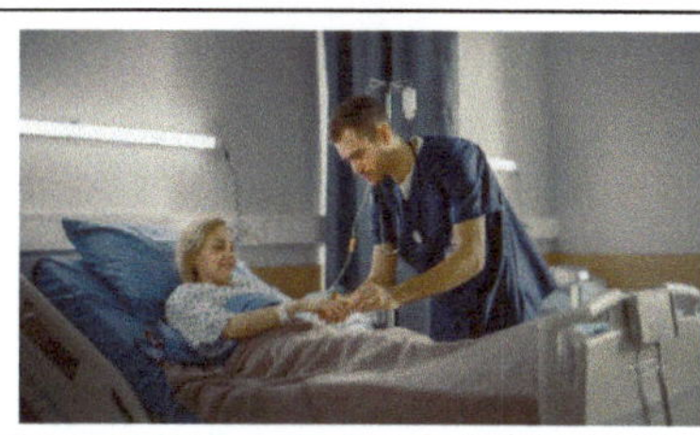

10.1. Overview of Weight Management and Metabolic Changes

Managing weight requires a mix of diet, exercise, and lifestyle adjustments. When addressing metabolic shifts, there are multiple factors to take into account (Bellicha et al., 2021).

Here are some key points:

1. **Caloric Balance**: Weight management often revolves around the concept of caloric balance—balancing the calories you consume with those you expend through physical activity and bodily functions. Consuming more calories than you burn leads to weight gain, while burning more calories than you consume leads to weight loss.
2. **Metabolism**: Metabolism refers to the chemical processes that occur within the body to maintain life. It's commonly divided into two main components:

- **Basal Metabolic Rate (BMR)**: This is the number of calories your body needs to perform basic functions at rest, such as breathing and circulating blood.
- **Thermic Effect of Food (TEF)**: This is the energy expenditure associated with digesting, absorbing, and processing nutrients from food.
- **Physical Activity**: This includes any movement you do, from walking to intense exercise, which also contributes to your overall energy expenditure.

3. **Nutrition**: The types of foods you eat can significantly impact your metabolism and weight management. For example:

- **Macronutrients**: Balancing intake of carbohydrates, fats, and proteins is crucial. Each macronutrient has a different effect on satiety, metabolism, and energy levels.
- **Micronutrients**: Essential vitamins and minerals play key roles in metabolism and overall health. Deficiencies can impair metabolic processes.
- **Fiber**: High-fiber foods can help with weight management by promoting feelings of fullness and regulating blood sugar levels.

4. **Physical Activity**: Exercise is a crucial component of weight management and can also influence metabolic health. Both aerobic exercise (such as walking, running, or cycling) and strength training (lifting weights or bodyweight exercises) can boost metabolism and help burn calories.
5. **Hormonal Factors**: Hormones such as insulin, cortisol, and thyroid hormones play important roles in metabolism and weight regulation. Imbalances in these hormones can contribute to weight gain or difficulty losing weight.
6. **Sleep**: Poor sleep habits can disrupt hormonal balance, leading to increased hunger, cravings for unhealthy foods, and weight gain. Adequate sleep is essential for metabolic health and overall well-being.
7. **Stress Management**: Chronic stress can lead to overeating or unhealthy food choices, which can contribute to weight gain. Finding healthy ways to manage stress, such as exercise, meditation, or hobbies, is important for both weight management and metabolic health.

8. **Medical Conditions**: Certain medical conditions, such as thyroid disorders or insulin resistance, can affect metabolism and make weight management more challenging. It's important to address any underlying health issues with the help of a healthcare professional.

A comprehensive strategy that takes into account diet, exercise, sleep, stress management, and any underlying medical conditions is necessary for both successful weight management and maintaining metabolic health. The comparison of calories in vs. calories out; it's also important to consider the type of calories you consume and how they affect your body's metabolism (Ben Slama et al., 2002).

10.1.1. Changes in Body Composition and Metabolism

Over the course of a person's life, their body composition and metabolism change dynamically in response to a variety of factors, including age, genetics, nutrition, physical activity, and hormonal fluctuations. It's essential to comprehend these changes if you want to manage your weight, prevent metabolic disorders, and maximize your health (Brehm et al., 2003).

Age-related changes in bone density, muscle mass, and fat mass are the hallmarks of changes in body composition. Sarcopenia is characterized by a progressive loss of lean muscle mass and an increase in adiposity. Numerous factors, including reduced physical activity, hormonal changes, and impaired protein metabolism, are responsible for this age-related decline in muscle mass. Changes in bone mineral density could occur concurrently, raising the risk of osteoporosis and fractures (Bueno et al., 2013). As we age, the body experiences changes in metabolism, which is the collection of all biochemical processes. The basal metabolic rate (BMR), or the energy used at rest to sustain essential functions, typically decreases with age. This is mainly because of declines in lean body mass and metabolic function of organs like the liver and kidneys. Despite this general trend, there are variations in metabolic rate among individuals, influenced by genetic makeup, body composition, and lifestyle choices (Caprio et al., 2019).

Body composition and metabolism can change in response to lifestyle factors like diet and physical activity, in addition to age-related changes. Unhealthy eating patterns that involve consuming large amounts of calories, consuming a lot of processed foods, and consuming little nutrient-dense food are the main causes of weight gain, obesity, and metabolic dysfunction. On the other hand, maintaining a healthy body composition and metabolic process is supported by eating a balanced diet high in fruits, vegetables, lean proteins, and whole grains.

An essential part of controlling body composition and metabolism is physical activity. Frequent exercise, which includes resistance and aerobic training, increases metabolic rate, aids in weight management, and supports the maintenance of lean muscle mass. Walking, running, or swimming are examples of aerobic exercise that raises heart rate and strengthens the heart, whereas resistance training increases muscular growth, strength, and metabolic efficiency (Carraca et al., 2021).

Throughout life, hormonal fluctuations also affect metabolism and body composition. Hormonal changes accompanying puberty lead to modifications in body composition, such as the emergence of secondary sexual traits and gains in lean body mass. In adulthood, changes in fat distribution, loss of muscle mass, and changes in metabolic rate can result from hormonal changes linked to menopause in women andropause in men (Castellana et al., 2020).

Additionally, conditions like obesity, insulin resistance, and metabolic syndrome have a significant effect on body composition and metabolism. The accumulation of excess visceral fat is linked to insulin resistance, dyslipidemia, and inflammation, increasing the risk of type 2 diabetes and cardiovascular disease. Metabolic syndrome, with its combination of central obesity, hypertension, dyslipidemia, and impaired glucose metabolism, further elevates the likelihood of cardiometabolic issues.

Age, genetics, lifestyle choices, and hormonal changes all play a role in the complex and multifaceted processes that alter body composition and metabolism. It is crucial to comprehend these changes to manage weight and maintain metabolic health, as well as to promote optimal health and prevent metabolic disorders. Healthy lifestyle choices can support a healthy body composition, preserve metabolic function, and improve general well-being throughout life. These choices include a balanced diet, frequent exercise, and stress management (Castelnuovo et al., 2017).

10.1.1.1. Metabolism

Metabolism is a complex system of biochemical processes that support life by converting nutrients into energy, creating biomolecules, and controlling cellular functions. This system is constantly adjusting to new physiological needs, environmental signals, and nutritional conditions to keep metabolism balanced.

The process of energy metabolism, which involves converting macronutrients like proteins, fats, and carbohydrates into adenosine triphosphate (ATP), the universal energy unit of cells, is at the center of metabolism. The two main processes that produce this energy are anaerobic glycolysis, which happens in the cytoplasm and doesn't require oxygen, and aerobic respiration, which happens in the mitochondria and requires oxygen (Chiu et al., 2017).

Carbohydrates are the main fuel source for the body, supplying energy for cellular processes. Once consumed, carbohydrates are converted into glucose, which is used by cells for energy production through glycolysis. Any extra glucose can be stored in the liver and muscles as glycogen for later use.

Triglycerides, which are fats that are stored in adipose tissue, are essential for hormone synthesis, cellular structure, and insulation. They are also a concentrated source of energy. In reaction to an energy demand, triglycerides are broken down into fatty acids and glycerol, a process known as lipolysis. This releases the fatty acids into the mitochondria for oxidation, which produces ATP.

Additionally, during times of fasting or low carbohydrate intake, ketogenesis—the process of converting fatty acids into ketone bodies—offers an alternate fuel source. Amino acid-based proteins function as the building blocks of tissues and as enzymes in metabolic processes. Although proteins are not usually used as the main source of energy, they can be used during extended fasting or energy deprivation to produce energy by breaking down into amino acids through a process called proteolysis (Corica et al., 2018).

A complex web of hormones, enzymes, and signaling pathways coordinate metabolic processes and preserve energy balance through intricate regulation of metabolism. In response to nutritional cues and metabolic demands, hormones like insulin, glucagon, leptin, and ghrelin are important in controlling the uptake, storage, and utilization of nutrients. When blood glucose levels rise, the pancreas releases insulin, which encourages cells to absorb glucose and increases the production of glycogen and lipogenesis. On the other hand, glucagon, which is released in reaction to low blood glucose, increases blood glucose levels by promoting gluconeogenesis and glycogenolysis. Adipose tissue secretes the hormone leptin, which signals fullness and encourages energy expenditure to control appetite and energy expenditure. In reaction to fasting and energy deficiency, the stomach secretes the hormone ghrelin, which increases appetite and food intake.

Moreover, a person's age, sex, body composition, genetics, and degree of physical activity all affect their metabolic rate—the speed at which their body uses energy. The majority of total energy expenditure is made up of basal metabolic rate (BMR), which varies from person to person depending on various factors. BMR is the amount of energy used at rest to maintain vital functions. The total energy expenditure also includes the energy used for physical activity, thermic effect of food (TEF), and the energy required for nutrient digestion, absorption, and metabolism (Dalle et al., 2013).

In general, metabolism is a sophisticated and highly controlled system that manages the synthesis of energy, the use of nutrients, and the maintenance of metabolic homeostasis. Maintaining metabolic health, controlling weight, and avoiding metabolic disorders all depend on an understanding of the complexities of metabolism. A balanced diet, frequent exercise, and stress reduction are just a few of the healthy lifestyle choices people can make to support optimal metabolic function and improve general well-being (de Lannoy et al., 2021).

10.2. Strategies for Weight Management

A healthy body weight can be attained and maintained through a variety of strategies that are part of the multifaceted endeavor that is weight management. These tactics usually include dietary changes, upping physical activity, altering behavior, and changing one's way of living. People can effectively manage their weight and promote overall health and well-being by putting into practice a comprehensive approach.

A key component of weight management is dietary changes. Consuming whole, nutrient-dense foods and limiting processed and high-calorie foods is one important tactic. In addition to providing necessary nutrients, placing an emphasis on fruits, vegetables, lean proteins, whole grains, and healthy fats also helps control calorie intake and encourages satiety. Another crucial component of diet management is portion control, which promotes better calorie regulation and helps avoid overeating. Meal schedule and frequency, in addition to food selections, can affect weight control. Some people find success with methods like intermittent fasting, which alternates between eating and fasting periods. Spreading their meals throughout the day might help others avoid being overly hungry and encourage a better energy balance. The secret to long-term success is ultimately determining a dietary strategy that suits personal preferences and lifestyle while also being sustainable (Ditschuneit et al., 1999).

Exercise is still another essential part of managing weight. Frequent exercise increases metabolism and promotes weight loss and maintenance by burning calories and assisting in the development and maintenance of lean muscle mass. For best effects, combine aerobic exercises like walking, running, or cycling with strength training exercises like bodyweight exercises or weightlifting. Finding sustainable and enjoyable activities is also crucial for maintaining a regular exercise schedule.

Making behavioral adjustments is crucial for successful long-term weight management. This may entail techniques like goal-setting that is grounded in reality, monitoring food consumption and exercise, engaging in mindful eating, and creating constructive coping strategies for stress and emotional regulation. Enhancing motivation and accountability can also be accomplished by creating a supportive environment, looking for social support, and obtaining the assistance of a weight loss coach or medical professional (Donnelly et al., 2009).

A change in lifestyle that includes less sedentary behavior, stress management, and better sleep quality can help with weight management. The hormones that control appetite and metabolism depend on getting enough sleep, and stress-reduction methods like yoga, meditation, or deep breathing exercises can help stop emotional eating and improve general wellbeing. Reduced screen time and increased movement in daily activities, like walking after meals or using the stairs instead of the elevator, can also help boost calorie expenditure and assist weight loss objectives. A multifaceted strategy involving dietary adjustments, increased physical activity, behavioral modifications, and lifestyle adjustments is necessary for effective weight management. People can improve their metabolic health, attain and maintain a healthy weight, and generally improve their quality of life by combining these strategies with the adoption of healthy habits (Donnelly et al., 2013).

10.2.1. Medical Weight Management: A Multidisciplinary Approach

Under the supervision of medical professionals, medical weight management is a multidisciplinary approach to addressing obesity and related health concerns. Evidence-based interventions such as dietary changes, physical activity guidelines, behavioral counseling, and, in certain situations, medication or surgical interventions are all integrated into this all-encompassing approach (Donnelly et al., 2000).

The evaluation of a patient's unique metabolic health, medical history, and lifestyle factors is essential to medical weight management to customize interventions to meet their specific needs. To support long-term weight loss and metabolic health, healthcare professionals work in tandem with patients to set reasonable goals, create customized diet plans, and put into practice long-lasting behavioral changes (Donnelly et al., 2005).

To attain energy balance and promote weight loss, nutritional interventions concentrate on calorie restriction, portion control, and the makeup of macronutrients. Health care providers stress the value of eating a diet high in nutrients and minimizing processed foods, sugar-filled drinks, and high-calorie snacks. Furthermore, depending on personal preferences and metabolic profiles, dietary approaches like meal replacements, low-carb diets, and intermittent fasting may be advised (Driscoll et al., 2021).

Beyond just burning calories, physical activity provides several metabolic advantages that make it a crucial component of medical weight management. To improve muscle strength, metabolic rate, and cardiovascular fitness, doctors prescribe customized exercise programs that include resistance, flexibility, and aerobic exercises. In addition to helping people lose weight, regular exercise enhances their lipid profiles, insulin sensitivity, and general metabolic health. When it comes to addressing psychological issues, emotional eating patterns, and lifestyle choices that lead to weight gain, behavioral counseling is essential. Healthcare providers empower patients to make long-lasting lifestyle changes and get past obstacles by using cognitive-behavioral techniques, motivational interviewing, and goal-setting strategies.

Pharmacotherapy or bariatric surgery may be considered when lifestyle changes alone are not enough to achieve weight loss goals or to mitigate comorbidities related to obesity. Prescription drugs, like appetite suppressants or anti-obesity agents, are only sometimes given in addition to diet and exercise regimens. Individuals with severe obesity or significant metabolic dysfunction can achieve long-lasting and effective weight loss outcomes through bariatric surgery, which includes procedures like gastric bypass or sleeve gastrectomy (Duffey et al., 2007; Fabricatore, 2007).

Over the past few years, there has been a notable rise in obesity. The excessive buildup of fat that negatively impacts health and is brought on by consuming more energy than one needs to expend is known as obesity. Obesity has a complex etiology that involves interactions between genetic, physiological, environmental, lifestyle, psychological, social, economic, and political factors (Table 10.1). Obesity is diagnosed using body mass index (BMI, kg/m^2), weight in kilogram divided by the height in meters squared. Obesity is defined as BMI $\geq 30\ kg/m^2$ while having a BMI 25.0–29.9 kg/m^2 is considered as overweight (Forgione et al., 2018).

Table 10.1. Factors Contributing to Obesity

Factors	
Individual	
Genetic predisposition	Monogenic single gene mutation: deficiency of melanocortin-4 receptor (MC4R), leptin, or proopiomelanocortin (POMC). Polygenic obesity: contribution of many genes. Syndromic obesity: Prader-Willi syndrome
Epigenetic modifications	DNA methylation: metabolic status of mother can influence DNA methylation of leptin at birth causing obesity. Adiponectin epigenetic status related to obesity
Prenatal	Maternal obesity, high weight gain during gestation, gestational diabetes
Neonatal	Prematurity
Post-natal	Formula versus breast feeding, infant overfeeding
Family history	Parental obesity: 3 fold increase risk in offspring if 1 parent is obese and 10 fold increase if 2 parents.
Excessive energy intake	High calorie diet rich in processed fat and carbohydrates
Physical inactivity	Sedentary lifestyle: prolonged screen time, sitting at home or work
Sleep deprivation associated with obesity	Due to imbalance of hormones, impaired glucose tolerance, increased nocturnal cortisol
Psychological	Depression, anxiety, stress
Drug-induced	Steroids, insulin, antidepressants (amitriptyline), antipsychotics (clozapine, quetiapine)
Gut microbiomes	Alteration causes changes in host weight and metabolism leading to obesity

Environmental	
Obesogenic environment	Easily accessible fast food/ high calorie diets, affordability of food
Built environment	Few sidewalks/green spaces, low access to recreational resources
Transport/technology	Utilization of cars for transport, less manual jobs
Socioeconomic	
Demographic	Age, ethnicity (black, Hispanic), menopause
Socioeconomic	Low income and educational level

Source: https://www.intechopen.com/chapters/82257.

Obesity raises the risk of many illnesses, which also lowers quality of life and increases morbidity and mortality. It is connected to numerous health issues and consequences. g. obstructive sleep apnea, metabolic syndrome, hypertension, type 2 diabetes (T2DM), hyperlipidemia, cardiovascular disorders, chronic kidney disease (CKD), nonalcoholic fatty liver disease (NAFLD), osteoarthritis, depression, and certain cancers. These primarily stem from the increased body fat, which causes metabolic and endocrine disruptions in addition to increasing the mechanical pressure on different organs (Foster et al., 2010).

Given its complex pathophysiologies and multifaceted etiology, obesity is a chronic disease. It causes complications and exhibits distinctive signs and symptoms that are in line with anatomical changes in several organs, including the immune system, cardiovascular system, and endocrine system. Because of this, treatment is required for life. Additionally, due to the heterogeneous nature of the condition, management, risk assessment, and individual assessment are required. Current weight loss (WL) therapies may not be able to stop the obesity epidemic on a societal scale, but they may be helpful in lowering the morbidity and mortality linked to obesity on an individual basis. In addition to two weight-related comorbidities, the current treatment guidelines for overweight and obesity call for diet, exercise, and behavior modification for people with BMIs of 30 or higher and those with BMIs of 27 or higher (Franz et al., 2015).

10.2.2. Goals of Treatment

Management objectives ought to be reasonable and tailored to each individual based on their background, aptitude, and level of risk. This is particularly crucial because the patient's commitment to altering their daily routine and implementing the recommended changes is what determines the effectiveness of the long-term treatment. While studies have shown that even 2–3 percent weight loss (WL) can improve cardiovascular (CV) risk factors, current guidelines recommend ≥5–10% (clinically significant WL) over a 6-month period to achieve a greater reduction in CV risk. Thus, achieving WL targets of >5% of baseline weight for BMIs of 25–35 kg/m^2 and >10% of baseline weight for BMIs of >35 kg/m^2 is the goal of long-term weight reduction. Other objectives include lowering the risk of early mortality, preventing work disability and early retirement, improving quality of life, and improving obesity-associated risk factors (Gaesser et al., 2021).

10.2.3. Weight Loss Strategies

10.2.3.1. Lifestyle Modification

A comprehensive approach is needed for lifestyle modification programs, and a multidisciplinary team of interventionists—including doctors, dietitians, psychologists, exercise physiologists, and other health care professionals—should be involved in the treatment plan. Patients in this program are to be checked on every week (30–90 minutes) for 16–26 weeks to guarantee compliance, and then every other week for 6–12 months to maintain weight. Individuals receiving treatment will receive counseling on long-term weight control techniques, appropriate physical activity, and a healthy, balanced diet (Gardner et al., 2018).

There are various settings where lifestyle modification programs can be implemented, such as specialized obesity clinics, primary care, commercial weight loss centers, private dietetics practices, or academic medical centers. These programs typically lead to moderate weight loss, which in turn improves health conditions commonly associated with obesity, including sleep apnea, Type 2 diabetes, hypertension, and high cholesterol. They also have positive effects on mental well-being, quality of life, and body image. Numerous studies have shown the effectiveness of lifestyle modification in promoting weight loss and addressing obesity-related health issues. You discuss two examples of lifestyle modification interventions that demonstrate the potential for weight loss and long-term health benefits through lifestyle changes (Garvey et al., 2016).

In an effort to achieve 7% WL, the Diabetes Prevention Program (DPP) randomized over 3200 individuals who were overweight or obese and had impaired glucose tolerance to metformin, a placebo, or an intensive lifestyle intervention. Throughout the first twenty-four weeks of the study, dietitians provided individual counseling to the group receiving the lifestyle intervention. After that, for the remaining eight weeks, they met once every two months. The participants were instructed to follow a low-fat diet, cut back on calories, and engage in 150 minutes of physical activity each week. After an average of 2.8 years, the mean weight loss in the lifestyle intervention group was 5.6 kg vs. 0.1 and 2.1 kg in the placebo and metformin groups, respectively. This 5.6 kg WL was equivalent to 58% relative decrease in the likelihood of developing T2DM. Ten years after the start of the study, the lifestyle intervention group had regained most of the weight they lost, although their T2DM incidence stayed 34% below that of the placebo group (Garvey et al., 2012).

The Look AHEAD Study (Action for Health in Diabetes) enrolled >5100 overweight/obese persons with T2DM. Participants were randomized to diabetes support and education group (3 group-education meetings per year for the first 4 years) or an intensive lifestyle intervention group (weekly group treatment sessions, monthly individual visit, meal replacement with liquid supplement and 1200–1800 kcal/day dietary plan individualized by weight). After 1 year, the lifestyle intervention group lost 8.6% of their weight vs. 0.6% for the diabetes support and education group; at the fourth year, average WL was 4.7% vs. 1.1%, respectively. The WL was maintained at 8 years (4.7%) for the lifestyle intervention group vs. 2.1% for the diabetes support and education participants. In addition, the lifestyle intervention participants exhibited significantly lower HbA1C (glycated hemoglobin) and showed improvements in CV risk factors including reduced systolic, diastolic pressure and triglycerides. Moreover, the lifestyle intervention group consumed less diabetes, hypertension, and lipid-lowering medications and had remissions or decreased in the severity of obstructive sleep apnea as well as improved depression symptoms (Ghachem et al., 2017).

10.2.3.2. Dietary Therapy

Adults who are overweight or obese can achieve WL through a variety of dietary strategies (Table 10.2). To achieve a sustainable and healthy weight, individuals with obesity should receive individualized nutritional plans based on their risk factors and therapeutic goals. To help with adherence to the dietary plans, the diet selection should take their preferences into consideration. Nutritional counseling on an individual or group basis is part of dietary therapy. Sessions in groups are typically more productive (Goldstein et al., 2019). Healthy eating guidelines for managing weight emphasize cutting back on energy-dense foods, controlling portion sizes, and enhancing diet quality to create an energy deficit that causes long-term weight loss (WL) without compromising health. For example, a 500–600 kcal/day energy deficit allows for approximately 0.5 kg/week WL over 12 weeks, with a maximum of 24 weeks. Different nutrition strategies are used to achieve WL, and the selection process can be influenced by the need to control comorbidities like type 2 diabetes and hypertension (HTN), as all of the diets evaluated below have nearly equivalent short- and long-term safety (Grant et al., 2014).

Table 10.2. Summary of Weight Loss Strategies

Weight Loss Strategies	Summary
Lifestyle modification	
Dietary therapy	
Low carbohydrate diet	Restrict carbohydrates to 20–120 g per day
Low fat diet	10–30% total calorie intake from fat
High protein diet	25% of total calories from protein
Mediterranean diet	35–40% fat, rich in omega-3, whole grains, fruits, vegetables, legumes, nuts, fish
Low calorie diet	Energy deficit of 500–800 kcal/day
Ketogenic diet	Reduced carbohydrates (<50 g/day), rich in protein
Very low-calorie ketogenic Diet	Energy intake < 800 calories, protein 1.2–1.5 g/kg of ideal body weight, fat 15–30 g/day, carbohydrates < 30 g/day
Meal replacements	Liquid formula or bars
Exercise	
Aerobic	Important during weight loss phase
Resistance	Increase muscle mass, for weight maintenance
Behavioral modifications	

Behavioral skills	
Self-monitoring	Weight, food record, exercise minutes
Goal-setting	Weight, calorie intake, exercise
Stimulus control	Keep tempting foods out of sight
Behavioral substitution	Relaxation techniques
Cognitive skills	
Problem-solving	Tactics to deal with weight-related health behaviors (social eating)
Cognitive restructuring	Identify/modify maladaptive thoughts contributing to overeating/physical inactivity
Relapse prevention	Learn to get back on track, maintain long-term motivation, stress management
Pharmacotherapy	Single/combination anti-obesity medications

Source: https://www.intechopen.com/chapters/82257.

10.2.3.2.1. Low Carbohydrate Diet (LCD)

With good short- and medium-term WL as well as cardiometabolic control, LCD is used to treat obesity, T2DM, and other obesity-related conditions. It provides 20–120 g of carbohydrates per day. At one year and two years, the reported WL with LCD was 11% and 7%, respectively. During the first six months of use, LCD improves high density lipoprotein cholesterol and, to a lesser extent, low density lipoprotein cholesterol (LDL), as well as diastolic blood pressure (DBP), triglycerides (TG), and very-low-density lipoprotein cholesterol (VLDL) (Greenway et al., 2010).

10.2.3.2.2. Low Fat Diet

Comprises 10–30% of total calorie intake from fat. At 2 years, mean weight and BMI changes were −3.3 ± 4.1 kg and −1.0 ± 1.4 kg/m^2 respectively. Low fat diet also results in significant improvement in the CV risk including reduction in waist circumference (−2.8 ± 4.3 cm), systolic blood pressure (SBP), total cholesterol (TC), LDL, fasting glucose and insulin levels (Gudzune et al., 2015).

10.2.3.2.3. Low-Carbohydrate Versus Low-Fat Diets

Low-carbohydrate and low-fat diets were compared in several studies. According to a study, individuals on an LCD regimen lost noticeably more weight at six months than those following a low-calorie, low-fat diet. But at 12 months, the WL did not change (−5.1 vs. −3.11 kg). In a different study, participants were randomized to either a low-fat diet or an LCD in addition to lifestyle modification; at one and two years, respectively, both groups lost 11% and 7% of their TW, with no discernible difference between the two groups. Therefore, LCD or a low-fat diet combined with behavioral therapy can result in successful WL. Moreover, lifestyle modification that makes it possible to follow the suggested calorie targets is more important for WL than the macronutrient components in and of themselves (Harvey-Berino et al., 2010).

10.2.3.2.4. High Protein Diet

This diet consists of foods that create an energy deficit and provides protein, fat, and carbohydrates in proportions of 25%, 30%, and 45% of total calories, respectively. Predicted weight loss (WL) is approximately -3.5% at six months and may reach 15% TWL at a year. A high-protein diet may lead to a notable improvement in the lipid profile, which includes LDL, TC, TG, and HDL, as well as a significant decrease in blood pressure, fasting glucose, and insulin levels (Hayes et al., 2008).

10.2.3.2.5. Mediterranean Diet

It has moderate amount of fat (35–40%) and is rich in Omega-3, where the primary fat source is extra virgin olive oil. Mediterranean diet has more whole grains, fruits, vegetables, legumes, nuts, fish and seafood, with limited poultry, dairy, red meat and usually prescribed with energy restriction to achieve WL. Reported WL at 2 years is −3.4 kg (−5.1 to −3.0). In addition, it decreases waist circumference, improves SBP, HDL and glucose levels (Ho et al., 2012).

10.2.3.2.6. Low-Calorie Diet

A balanced diet comprising 45–55% carbohydrates, 15–25% proteins, and 25–30% fat is the foundation of a low-calorie diet. It needs to be customized for each person's unique energy needs, sex, age, and level of physical activity. To reduce comorbidities, the diet's composition should be changed. g. hyperlipidemia, T2DM, and HTN. The goal of this diet should be to produce an energy deficit of 500–800 kcal/day. Consequently, 1,200–1,500 kcal/d for women and 1,500–1,800 kcal/d for men can be prescribed. Because diet-induced thermogenesis and the preservation of lean muscle mass lead to increased satiety and energy expenditure, a low-calorie, relatively high-protein diet promotes weight loss and helps people avoid gaining weight again. At 26 weeks, studies showed an 11 kg weight loss. Additionally, this diet was shown to significantly improve lipid profiles (TC, TG), glucose, insulin level, waist circumference, blood pressure, and insulin levels (Hollander et al., 2013).

10.2.3.2.7. Ketogenic Diet

Since the 1920s, this diet has been used to treat epilepsy, and it has been demonstrated in certain cases to lessen or completely eliminate the need for epilepsy medications. It has been a widely used approach to treating obesity since the 1960s. Numerous diseases linked to obesity may benefit from this diet, including e. g. polycystic ovarian syndrome, acne, type 2 diabetes, and cancer. Ketogenic diets include more fat and protein and fewer carbohydrates (<50 g/day) (Jacob et al., 2009).

10.2.3.2.8. Very Low-Calorie Ketogenic Diet (VLCKD)

This gives the energy intake in grams. <800 calories/day, protein 1.2–1.5 g/kg of ideal body weight, carbohydrates of <30 g/day and 15–30 g of fat/day. The low carbohydrate stimulates lipolysis of stored fat and synthesis of ketone bodies utilized as fuel by extrahepatic tissues (Jensen et al., 2013). Ketosis associated with VLCKD is always moderate (ketonemia never > It differs from diabetic ketoacidosis (3 mmol/L). WL (0.5–2.0 kg/week) is attained by the satiety effect of proteins on hunger hormones, the appetite-suppressive properties of ketone bodies, and the combination of increased lipolysis and decreased lipogenesis.

To increase patient compliance, VLCKD is administered using a combination of natural foods and meal replacements that include protein (milk, peas, whey, and soy). There are also daily vitamins and minerals available. For a maximum of 12 weeks, BMI ≥30 kg/m^2 is advised to undergo VLCKD. Due to the increased risk of side effects like dehydration, nausea, diarrhea, constipation, hyperuricemia, gallstones, and vitamin/microelement deficiencies, this diet should be followed under medical supervision. Research demonstrates that at 4 weeks, VLCKD improved BMI (−5.3 kg/m^2), lipids (TG, TC, HDL), insulin resistance (HOMA-IR), and WL (6–37% TWL percent). Similar results were also observed in obese diabetic patients with VLCKD, who showed improvements in blood glucose and significant WL at 3 months (8.5%) and 12 months (11.5%). Furthermore, of the patients who finished the trial, 26% were able to stop taking any antidiabetic drugs, whereas 73% only took metformin (Juchacz et al., 2021).

10.2.3.2.9. Meal Replacements

Meal placements is produced in different forms such as drink, bars or soup to substitute solid food. They have controlled calories and nutrient contents and are commonly used in energy restricted diet to facilitate WL. It also contains the necessary vitamins and minerals. Many studies reported the effectiveness of utilizing meal replacements as dietary intervention for weight management.

Participants who replaced two meals and two snacks per day with liquid shakes and meal bars lost 7.1 kg in 3 months compared to 1.3 kg for individuals on conventional foods with the same calories (1200–1500 kcal/d). Moreover, those who substitute 1 meal and 1 snack a day during follow-up maintained a WL of 10.4 kg at 27 months. Similarly, the use of meal replacement in patients with T2DM resulted in significant WL at 12 months compared to conventional diet (−4.4 vs. −2.4 kg, P = 0.07), with significant glycemic (HbA1c) improvement and reduced medications (Kannan et al., 2014).

10.2.4. Behavioral Modifications

A diet, exercise, and behavior therapy program comprised of lifestyle modification is the cornerstone of treatment for obesity. Psychotherapists utilize either individual or group behavior therapy to teach clients how to change their eating and exercise habits and to help them reach their energy intake and expenditure objectives. When overweight/obesity is accompanied by serious symptoms (e. g. depression, eating disorders, and a lack of drive), then patients' care should involve psychiatrists. It is important to modify different tactics based on the needs of the patient and the specific circumstances.

To prevent weight regain, typical behavioral WL programs involve 60–90 minute weekly sittings for six months, followed by maintenance meetings every other week for an additional twelve months (Kelley et al., 2016).

10.2.4.1. Behavioral Skills

10.2.4.1.1. Self-Monitoring

Teaching individuals how to track and monitor their eating, physical activity, and progress is a technique in behavioral therapy known as self-monitoring. This method is essential in treating obesity as it helps individuals become more aware of their behaviors and make healthier choices. While self-monitoring food and energy intake is crucial in behavioral therapy, it can be challenging to implement. For example, some individuals may underestimate their food consumption by 50% when trying to lose weight. Therefore, patients need to be educated on using tools like measurement devices, nutrition labels, and calorie guides. They should also be encouraged to keep track of details such as the time, amount, preparation, and calorie content of their meals and beverages, and bring this information to group sessions for feedback (Knowler et al., 2002).

In behavior therapy, PA monitoring is also crucial. It is required of participants to document the kind and quantity of their PA. Pedometers offer instantaneous feedback, motivating users to progressively increase their energy expenditure and step count to meet the daily goal of 10,000 steps. Daily self-monitoring is recommended for the first six months, followed by sporadic self-monitoring during maintenance (Kuna et al., 2021). It is required of participants to bring their books to individual or group meetings and to record their intake and PA on a daily basis. Strong correlations between self-monitoring of food intake, self-weighing, and PA and WL were found in the research; higher frequency and more days of self-monitoring were associated with higher monthly WL (Kushner et al., 2020).

10.2.4.1.2. Goal-Setting

Establishing personal targets is crucial in weight management. To change behavior, individuals should set specific, measurable goals for physical activity and diet. It is more effective to link weight management goals to health benefits, like improving blood pressure or lipid levels, to increase motivation and commitment. Short-term goals are more successful than long-term ones, and goals should be challenging yet attainable. Starting with easier goals and gradually increasing them can improve adherence and provide a sense of achievement. Patients often think they need to lose a large amount of weight to succeed, but setting a realistic weight loss goal, such as 5%, can enhance adherence. Research shows that individuals who set targets are significantly more likely to achieve weight loss of 10% or more in one year compared to those who do not. Setting goals for diet and exercise has been shown to be a better predictor of adherence to healthy habits than setting goals solely for weight loss (Kushner, 2014).

10.2.4.1.3. Stimulus Control

Stimulus control strategies involve altering an individual's surroundings to support healthy behaviors. Behavioral treatment helps individuals rearrange their environment to reduce triggers for unhealthy eating habits and increase opportunities for making better dietary choices and engaging in physical activity. For example, if someone tends to snack while sitting on the couch or while watching TV, these actions become associated with snacking in the future. To combat this, individuals can limit their meal activities to the dining room to decrease the urge to snack. Additionally, they can put away tempting foods or remove them from the home to prevent overconsumption. It is also helpful to store fruits and vegetables in plain sight and make healthy reminders visible on the refrigerator or bathroom mirror. By making these changes, individuals can transform their home environment in a way that promotes healthier habits (Larsen et al., 2004).

10.2.4.1.4. Behavioral substitution

A lot of people eat in response to emotional stimuli (e.g., boredom, stress, anxiety, and frustration), which have significant effects on one's weight and overall health. Self-monitoring helps clients in behavior therapy identify cues other than hunger to snack and substitute other activities for eating. People and their loved ones must find alternative ways to cope with their bad emotions. If an individual overeats due to anxiety, it may be more beneficial to practice relaxation techniques or find other coping mechanisms, such as writing, knitting, housework, or exercise, as these activities prevent overeating (Li et al., 2005).

10.2.4.2. Cognitive Skills

Cognitive approaches to behavior change are also utilized in the behavioral treatment of obesity. The two most commonly taught skills are problem-solving and cognitive restructuring (Li et al., 2005).

10.2.4.2.1. Problem-Solving

When attempting to make changes to their lifestyle, people may encounter difficulties. It is crucial to provide participants with problem-solving skills training to support them throughout this process. Patients can examine their weight-related health behaviors with the aid of these problem-solving techniques. They identify a problem that impedes their WL, consider the possible outcomes of various options, select the healthiest option, carry out a predetermined plan, evaluate the efficacy of the chosen solution, and repeat the problem-solving process as needed by employing a multistep interactive behavioral strategy (Lichtman et al., 1992). Group visits help assist participants in solving problems related to a particular health issue, learning from the solutions of others who have faced similar issues, and developing solutions unique to their circumstances. An 8.8 percent reduction in body weight was achieved with a 6-month problem-solving-based lifestyle intervention for obesity. A shift in weight was linked to improved problem-solving abilities and better treatment compliance. Furthermore, participants with WL > 10% were better at solving problems than those with <5% reduction (Lin and Li, 2021).

10.2.4.2.2. Cognitive Restructuring

Through behavior therapy, clients learn to identify and replace illogical thoughts with more sensible ones, as well as to watch the thoughts that interfere with their ability to meet behavioral goals. Overeating and inactivity are encouraged by maladaptive thoughts, which cognitive restructuring helps to identify and modify. Such thoughts can include rationalizations like "I had a stressful day, this justifies a portion of cake" and dichotomous thinking like "As I am unable to exercise for 30 minutes, I might then not exercise at all." Participants are not aware of how these thoughts affect their actions. Through cognitive restructuring, individuals can create a positive self-statement that will support changes in behavior (Mansoor et al., 2016).

10.2.4.3. Cognitive Behavioral Therapy

Cognitive techniques are used in behavior therapy to change eating and activity habits. It focuses on modifying the behavioral and cognitive processes that give rise to the problematic behavior and applying behavioral and cognitive techniques to transform the behavior for the better. Anthropometric profile, eating habits, quality of life in the physical, psychological, social, and environmental domains, as well as a decrease in depression, all significantly improved as a result of cognitive behavioral therapy (Mb et al., 2000).

10.2.4.3.1. Relapse Prevention

Helping people get ready and make plans for preventing relapses involves teaching them how to anticipate difficult circumstances that may lead to overeating and how to use coping mechanisms to get through such times. People are driven to make plans to prevent a single overindulgence from turning into a major relapse. Following a telephone-based WL maintenance program that focused on social support, self-monitoring, relapse prevention planning, and outcome satisfaction, it was discovered that, at 56 weeks, the intervention group (0.75 kg) experienced statistically significantly less weight regain than the group receiving usual care (Min et al., 2021).

Regarding the use of technology for lifestyle modification, behavioral treatment increases adherence to lifestyle intervention; however, in-person delivery requires a significant investment of time and resources, as well as expensive and inconvenient travel. Many people can receive cost-effective lifestyle interventions by using the phone or internet. To reach 10% WL, a study comparing the effectiveness of phone and in-person clinic approaches discovered that, at 12 weeks, WL was 10.4% for phone calls and 13.7% for in-person visits, both of which were significantly higher than the control group (0.24 percent). In rural communities, individual telephone counseling reduced weight regain and raised the percentage of participants who maintained clinically significant weight loss. This type of extended care for obesity management was implemented. Evidence also suggests that while Internet-based interventions are less effective than in-person treatment, they are still superior to no or minimal intervention. An online behavioral weight-control program produced WL results of 8 kg, 5 kg, and 6 kg for in-person, online, and hybrid treatment, respectively ($p < 0.01$), indicating that the internet can be a good alternative for delivering and disseminating behavioral weight-control interventions. Although there has been a recent surge in the use of smartphone applications for weight management, their long-term efficacy has not been established. According to a randomized controlled trial conducted on young adults who were overweight or obese, those who got personalized coaching enhanced by smartphone self-monitoring lost significantly more weight than the controls at six months, but not at twelve or twenty-four months. Furthermore, the group that solely received an interactive smartphone application for lifestyle intervention did not experience WL loss outcomes that were better than control in WL (Moraes et al., 2021).

10.3. Pharmacotherapy

Pharmacotherapy can improve adherence to lifestyle modifications by reducing appetite and energy expenditure, which occur as an adaptive mechanism for weight loss. If a patient has a BMI of 30 or higher and conditions linked to obesity, pharmacotherapy may be indicated. To attain sufficient WL, it is recommended in conjunction with a well-rounded diet, exercise, and behavioral therapy (Moriconi et al., 2021). The goal is to produce clinically significant WL (≥5% mean TWL percent). Anti-obesity drugs are prescribed based on the type of obesity-related comorbidities, as well as the medication's safety and efficacy. Several drugs are authorized for the treatment of obesity (Table 10.3).

Table 10.3. Pharmacotherapy: Anti-Obesity Medications

	Mode of Action	**Dose**	**Side Effects**	**Contraindications**
Single Drug				
Phentermine * Schedule IV controlled substance	Sympathomimetic amine Adrenergic agonist	8 mg, 15 mg capsule, 37.5 mg tablet	Dry mouth, insomnia, agitation, constipation, tachycardia	G, severe HTN, CV disease, history of drug/alcohol abuse, pregnancy, MOI, selective serotonin reuptake inhibitor use
Orlistat	Pancreatic and gastric lipase inhibitor	60 mg OTC, 120 mg TID	Steatorrhea, oily spotting, flatulence/ discharge, fecal incontinence, fat-soluble vitamins deficiencies, malabsorption	P, malabsorption syndromes/ GI conditions that predispose to GI upset/diarrhea
Liraglutide	GLP-1 agonist	3.0 mg daily	Nausea, vomiting, diarrhea, constipation. Rarely pancreatitis, cholecystitis	Severe renal/hepatic insufficiency, pregnancy, Personal/family history of MTC or MEN2 and major depression/psychiatric disorder
Semaglutide	GLP-1 agonist	2.4 mg weekly	Nausea, vomiting, diarrhea, constipation, headache rarely pancreatitis, cholecystitis	Severe renal/hepatic insufficiency, pregnancy, personal/family history of MTC or MEN2. Past history of P + major depression or psychiatric disorder
Combination				
Phentermine-Topiramate. Schedule IV controlled substance	Sympatho-mimetic amine, anorectic, extended-release anti-epileptic drug	3.75/23 mg, 7.5/46 mg, 11.25/69 mg, 15/92 mg	Paraesthesia, dry mouth, constipation, insomnia, dizziness, altered taste sensation, cognitive effects Rare: closed angle glaucoma, depression, suicidal ideation	G, renal stones, pregnancy (when utilized for WL)

Naltrexone-Bupropion	Opioid receptor antagonist, inhibits dopamine/ norepinephrine reuptake	8/90 mg daily to 16/180 mg BID Tablet	Nausea, vomiting, constipation, dizziness, insomnia, headache, dry mouth	Pregnancy, uncontrolled HTN, uncontrolled pain, recent MOI use, history of seizures/ conditions that predispose to seizure e.g., anorexia/ BN, abrupt discontinuation of alcohol, benzodiazepines, barbiturates or antiepileptic drugs

Approved for short-term use; MEN2multiple endocrine neoplasia syndrome type 2; MTC, medullary thyroid carcinoma, BN bulimia nervosa, CV cardiovascular, HTN hypertension, MOI monoamine oxidase inhibitors

Source: https://www.intechopen.com/chapters/82257.

10.3.1. Single Medication

10.3.1.1. Phentermine

Phentermine, a sympathomimetic amine approved in 1959, works by increasing hypothalamic catecholamine secretion and resting energy expenditure to suppress appetite. It is the most commonly used obesity medication in the USA, typically prescribed for short-term use of >3 months due to a lack of long-term safety research (Murawski et al., 2009). However, it has been approved for long-term therapy when used in combination with topiramate extended-release (ER).

Despite the recommended short-term use, many obesity physicians prescribe Phentermine for longer periods as an off-label therapy for weight management (Muscogiuri et al., 2021). It comes in doses of 8, 15, 30, and 37.5 mg, with a single dose early in the day to prevent insomnia.

Side effects are generally mild and include dry mouth, insomnia, agitation, constipation, and tachycardia, all due to its sympathomimetic effects. Lowering the dose can help reduce these side effects. Phentermine is classified as a schedule IV-controlled substance and should not be used in patients with a history of cardiovascular disease, anxiety, hyperthyroidism, or drug/alcohol abuse/ dependence. Other contraindications include concurrent use of monoamine oxidase inhibitors, pregnancy, and breastfeeding (Nicoll et al., 2018). Expected WL with phentermine is 3.6 kg at 6 months. After 6 months, phentermine 15 mg induced a WL of 4.5 kg over placebo. 46% of participants on phentermine lost ≥5% of their weight, while 20.8% lost ≥10%.

10.3.1.2. Liraglutide

An injectable GLP-1 agonist with FDA approval is ligarglutide 3 mg. This incretin hormone, which is derived from the gut, increases the delivery of insulin, decreases the secretion of glucagon, and stimulates the GLP-1 receptor in the pancreatic islets. It suppresses gastric emptying, increases satiety, lessens hunger, and mediates WL via peripheral and central nervous system pathways, all of which lead to a decrease in food intake. The most typical liraglutide side effects include vomiting, nausea, diarrhea, constipation, and dyspepsia. These symptoms are typically not too severe and get better in a few days or weeks if the treatment is continued and the dosage is gradually increased.

In rare circumstances, WL combined with liraglutide may result in pancreatitis and raise the risk of symptomatic gallstones. When a patient has a serious mental illness, a history of pancreatitis, severe renal or hepatic insufficiency, or is pregnant, ligarglutide should not be used. Liraglutide caused a 5% weight loss at a year's end in a large randomized controlled trial (Nothwehr et al., 2007).

A total 63.2% of the participants in the liraglutide group lost at least 5% of their weight compared with 27.1% in the placebo group (P<0.001). Likewise, 33.1% of liraglutide group lost more than 10% of their body weight versus 10.6% in the control group(P<0.001). Moreover, cardiometabolic risk, inflammatory markers, glycemic parameters, blood pressure and lipids also improved. For weight maintenance, the SCALE study found that among individuals who lost 5% of their initial body weight on a low-calorie diet, liraglutide added another 6.2% TWL% vs. 0.2% in the placebo group (Paoli et al., 2013).

10.3.1.3. Semaglutide

Approved in 2019, semaglutide is a long-acting GLP-1 analog that mimics the effects of native GLP-1, stimulating WL by decreasing the energy intake and hunger, increasing satiety, and enhancing glycemic control. It is approved for treatment of T2D using ≤1.0 mg once weekly subcutaneously or as tablets at a dosage of up to 14 mg. Side effects and contraindications are similar to liraglutide (Table 10.3). In STEP 1 trail, semaglutide 2.4 mg resulted in significant TWL% at 68 weeks compared to placebo (−14.9% vs. − 2.4%). More participants on semaglutide than placebo achieved ≥5% TWL% (86.4% vs. 31.5%), ≥10% (69.1% vs. 12.0%), and ≥ 15% (50.5% vs. 4.9%). Moreover, semaglutide led to more improvement in cardiometabolic risk and physical functioning than placebo (Perri et al., 2020). In the STEP 4 trial, individuals completing a 20-week run-in period with semaglutide 2.4 mg once per week, maintenance with semaglutide resulted in continuous WL over the next 48 weeks compared to switching to placebo (−7.9% vs. +6.9%).

10.3.1.4. Orlistat

Approved in 1999, orlistat is the single anti-obesity medication that does not function via the CNS pathway. Instead, it inhibits pancreatic and gastric lipases, reducing absorption of 25–30% of ingested fat. The recommended dose is 120 mg three times per day up to 1 hour after food intake. Side effects are related to fat malabsorption and include steatorrhea, oily spotting, flatulence, and fecal incontinence. The gastrointestinal symptoms can be reduced by a low-fat diet and increasing intake the dietary fiber. Multivitamin supplementation is essential, as orlistat decreases absorption of fat-soluble vitamins (A, D, E, K). Orlistat resulted in a mean 2.9–3.4% weight loss at one year. Long term WL (4 years) can reach 5.8 kg, where 53% of participants lost ≥5% of their weight, and 26.2% lost ≥10% of their weight. Orlistat also reduces the serum glucose levels and increases insulin sensitivity. Individuals with T2DM prescribed orlistat 120 mg exhibited significantly more reduction in fasting blood glucose and HbA1c compared to placebo (Pi-Sunyer et al., 2015).

10.3.2. Combination Medications

10.3.2.1. Phentermine-Topiramate ER

In 2012, this long-acting combination received approval. Topiramate is a migraine and antiepileptic drug; phentermine is a short-term appetite suppressant. Uncertainty surrounds the mechanisms underlying appetite suppression; one possibility is gamma-aminobutyric acid receptor modulation. It is used off-label for obesity and binge eating, either by itself or in conjunction with phentermine, due to its anorexigenic qualities. The maximum daily dose of phentermine/topiramate ER is 15/92 mg. It is available in four doses per day (Table 10.2), to be taken in the morning, titrated every two weeks, and discontinued if 5 percent WL is not achieved in 12 weeks. A controlled substance listed in schedule IV is phentermine/topiramate ER. The Food and Drug Administration (FDA) mandates the development of a Risk Evaluation and Mitigation Strategy to notify medical professionals and women who are capable of bearing children about the possibility of a higher risk of orofacial clefts in children exposed to phentermine/topiramate ER in the first trimester of pregnancy. The adverse effects resemble those of topiramate and phentermine (Ross et al., 2019). Cognitive side effects such as psychomotor slowing, decreased concentration, memory impairment, and language difficulties are among the dose-dependent side effects of topiramate (Table 10.3). Because topiramate inhibits carbonic anhydrase activity, it can cause several side effects, including anhidrosis, hypokalemia, renal stones, myopia, angle-closure glaucoma, and metabolic acidosis. As a result, it is not recommended to take topiramate with other drugs that block carbonic anhydrase. Increased suicidal thoughts or ideations are another uncommon side effect that should be immediately reported and the medication discontinued (Ross et al., 2004).

Phentermine/topiramate ER resulted in significantly greater WL compared to placebo where participants in the 3.75/23, and 15/92 groups lost 5.1%, and 10.9% of their baseline weight, respectively compared with 1.6% in the placebo group. Moreover, 44.9% of 3.75/23 group, and 66.7% of 15/92 group, lost ≥5% of their weight after 56 weeks of treatment compared to 17.3% of the placebo group ($p<0.0001$). Phentermine/topiramate ER for 52 weeks also resulted in 76% reduction in the progression to diabetes in participants receiving 15/92 mg and a 54% reduction in participants receiving 7.5/46 mg compared with placebo (Rubino et al., 2021).

10.3.2.2. Naltrexone-Bupropion Sustained Release (SR)

Naltrexone is an opioid antagonist, and bupropion, a dopamine and norepinephrine reuptake inhibitor, is used as part of a combination that was approved in 2014 to treat depression and help people stop smoking. Their combined application suppresses appetite in a synergistic way. By boosting the neuropeptide pro-opiomelanocortin (POMC) and enhancing dopamine activation—which is lower in obese people—bupropion reduces food intake and raises energy expenditure. Treatment for alcohol and opioid dependence involves the use of naltrexone. It prevents beta-endorphin from stimulating cannabinoid-1 receptors, which increases appetite (Ruggenenti et al., 2017).

To reach a therapeutic dosage of two tablets twice daily (32/360 mg), the dosage is increased by one tablet every week, starting with one tablet (8 mg ER naltrexone and 90 mg ER bupropion) daily. If at 16 weeks WL ≥ 5 percent is not achieved, the medication should be stopped. In Table 10.3, the most prevalent adverse effects are indicated. When combined with chronic opioids and monoamine oxidase inhibitors, the medication should not be used. Additionally, individuals with uncontrolled hypertension and a history of seizures should not use it. Patients under 24 years old who take bupropion have a higher risk of suicidality; as such, they should be closely monitored for any changes in mood (Sacks et al., 2009).

10.4. Impact of Diet and Exercise

It is impossible to overestimate the effects of nutrition and exercise on general health, happiness, and longevity. These two lifestyle pillars are essential for avoiding chronic illnesses, keeping a healthy weight, and maximizing metabolic efficiency. As the cornerstone of health, diet is a powerful predictor of metabolic outcomes and physical fitness. The kind and quantity of food consumed has a significant impact on energy balance, metabolic processes, and physiological homeostasis (Sadeghirad et al., 2016).

Essential micronutrients, antioxidants, and dietary fibers are provided by a diet high in whole, nutrient-dense foods, such as fruits, vegetables, lean proteins, whole grains, and healthy fats. These foods also support optimal metabolic function. The macronutrients that make up the diet—carbohydrates, fats, and proteins—have different but related functions in the control of metabolism. The body uses carbohydrates as its main energy source to power cellular functions and physical activity. The kind and quality of carbohydrates, however, are very important. While processed foods and refined sugars can cause energy swings and dysregulation of the metabolism, whole grains, fruits, and vegetables provide a steady release of energy and a high fiber content, which promotes satiety and metabolic health (Samaha et al., 2003).

Although they are frequently demonized in popular culture, fats are necessary for hormone synthesis, cellular structure, and nutrient absorption. The benefits of monounsaturated and polyunsaturated fats on the cardiometabolic system include decreased inflammation and enhanced lipid profiles. These fats can be found in foods like nuts, seeds, avocados, and fatty fish (Saunders et al., 2018).

On the other hand, consuming too much saturated and trans fat—found in processed foods and fried foods—raises the risk of cardiovascular disease and metabolic dysfunction. The building blocks of tissues and enzymes, proteins are essential for maintaining muscle mass, controlling hunger, and carrying out metabolic functions. Lean protein sources, which include fish, poultry, legumes, and dairy products, improve satiety, aid in weight management, and maintain metabolic rate when calorie-restricting. They also promote muscle synthesis (Schwingshackl et al., 2013).

Unlike diet, exercise is the dynamic counterpart of lifestyle modification that has a significant impact on physical fitness, metabolic health, and general well-being. Frequent physical activity reduces the risk of obesity, type 2 diabetes, and cardiovascular disease by increasing insulin sensitivity, improving metabolic flexibility, and increasing energy expenditure. Aerobic exercise improves endurance, strengthens the heart, and encourages the burning of fat. It is defined by prolonged, rhythmic movements that raise heart rate and oxygen consumption. Exercises like jogging, cycling, swimming, and brisk walking promote mitochondrial biogenesis, which improves cellular energy production and metabolic efficiency (Shai et al., 2008).

Resistance training offers special metabolic advantages when combined with aerobic exercise, increasing muscular strength, hypertrophy, and metabolic rate. Resistance training improves basal metabolic rate and lean muscle mass, which helps with weight management and metabolic health. Resistance training also offers protective benefits against metabolic syndrome and type 2 diabetes by enhancing insulin sensitivity, glucose metabolism, and lipid profiles. A comprehensive training program that incorporates both resistance and aerobic exercise modalities maximizes metabolic outcomes, promoting cardiovascular resilience, physical performance, and metabolic flexibility. Furthermore, combining functional movements, flexibility, and balance improves overall movement proficiency and lowers the risk of musculoskeletal injuries (Sigal et al., 2006).

Exercise and nutrition work together to enhance long-term health outcomes and increase metabolic benefits beyond their individual merits. A well-rounded dietary regimen combined with consistent exercise creates a healthy metabolic environment that is enhanced in terms of energy balance, nutrient utilization, and physiological robustness. In addition, combining dietary changes with exercise regimens encourages people to take up sustainable lifestyle habits that support long-term metabolic health and overall wellbeing (Singh et al., 2017).

10.4.1. The Importance of a Healthy Diet and Exercise

There are many positive changes that can be made to one's health. Each person has different lifestyle choices, which vary depending on their habits, culture, and preferences. These choices include diet, exercise, and whether or not to smoke or drink. Daily food choices and level of physical activity have an impact on overall health and the likelihood of developing, recovering from, and surviving prostate cancer (Smethers & Rolls, 2018).

Physical activity can improve physical and mental well-being. It is critical for weight management, preserving muscle mass, reducing the risk of heart disease, and maintaining strong bones. Staying active can help maintain balance, improve sleep quality, and reduce anxiety and exhaustion. Exercise can also help reduce the chance of side effects from prostate cancer treatment (Son & Kim, 2020).

10.4.2. Diet and Exercise Recommendations

Guidelines provided by the American Institute for Cancer Research (AICR) are a good starting point for patients determined to make changes in diet and exercise (Stern et al., 2004).

To prevent cancer and improve long-term survival for cancer survivors, AICR recommends that people:

- Be as lean as possible without becoming underweight.
- Be physically active for at least 30 minutes every day, including activities such as walking, dancing, or participating in sports.
- Avoid sugary drinks. Limit consumption of high-energy foods, particularly processed foods that are high in added sugar, low in fiber, or high in fat.
- Eat a greater variety of vegetables, fruits, whole grains, and legumes.
- Limit red meat (such as beef, pork, and lamb) and avoid processed meats (such as ham, bacon, sausage, hot dogs, and salami).
- Limit alcoholic beverages, if consumed, to two per day for men (and one per day for women).
- Limit salty foods.
- Do not rely on supplements to prevent or protect against cancer.

10.4.3. Exercises

Exercise enhances CV health and body composition without regard to weight loss. Aerobic exercise improves lipids, visceral fat, and blood pressure (BP) in the absence of significant

WL. In non-diabetic people, decreased visceral fat enhances insulin sensitivity and glucose tolerance, while in diabetic patients, it improves glycemic control. Positive changes in vitality, mental health, and quality of life are also brought about by exercise. Therefore, rather than focusing just on weight loss, obese people should be encouraged to exercise to improve their cardiovascular health (Sukkar et al., 2021). Guidelines for care of patients with obesity include recommendations for "aerobic training of ≥150 min/week of moderate intensity, with better outcomes with increasing amounts and intensity of exercise." However, PA alone induces limited WL, unless it is accompanied by energy restriction. For instance, losing 0.45 kg/week, requires high PA is (e.g., walking 35 miles/week), but is feasible to be accomplished by decreasing food intake by 500 kcal/day. Hence, effective WL requires exercise >150 min/week with 1200–1800 kcal/week energy consumption. Exercise combined with decrease caloric intake produces greater WL than exercise or caloric restriction alone. Hence, PA should be paired with adjusted caloric intake to achieve optimal WL and body composition. Physical activity should be prescribed according to patient's ability, preference. It is also important to ascertain that there are no contraindications to physical activity particularly in individuals with BMI of 35 kg/m^2 or higher (Svetkey et al., 2015).

10.4.3.1. Aerobic Exercise

Aerobic exercise is essential for weight management. It facilitates weight loss and improves body composition by inducing fat and visceral fat loss. One study found that supervised exercise with 400 or 600 kcal/session five days/week for 10 months resulted in 3.9 ± 4.9 and 5.2 ± 5.6 kg among overweight or obese individuals respectively compared with weight gain (0.5 ± 3.5 kg) for controls. Aerobic exercise intensity also influences WL. Among sedentary college students with obesity, 12 weeks of high and moderate intensity training led to significant reduction in body weight, BMI, waist circumference, and body fat percentage than light intensity training. Likewise, the time of the session is essential for body weight outcomes, where early-exercise (50% of sessions between 7 and 11.59 am) led to significantly more weight loss compared to late-exercise (>50% of sessions between 3 and 7 pm). In contrast, there is no significant difference in terms of weight loss between continuous and intermittent exercise. For example a study compared the effect of 18 months of continuous (3 times/wk, 30 min/session) versus intermittent (5 times/wk, 15 min/session) aerobic exercise in overweight and obese individuals and found small reductions in weight (2.0%) in the continuous training group with no significant change in intermittent groups (Swift et al., 2018).

10.4.3.2. Resistance Exercise

When compared to aerobic exercises, this kind of exercise does not produce enough negative energy balance to produce clinically meaningful weight loss, so doing it alone may not cause WL. When comparing resistance exercises to aerobic exercises, the total energy expenditure of aerobic exercises is higher. Compared to aerobic or resistance exercise alone, combinations of the two offer greater benefits for WL, fat loss, and cardio-respiratory fitness. By increasing lean mass, resting metabolic rate, and fat oxidation, resistance training may promote negative energy balance and help with weight maintenance (Swinburn et al., 2011).

A Closer Look

Metabolism

Metabolism is the sum of all biochemical processes that occur within the body to maintain life. It encompasses the conversion of nutrients into energy, the synthesis of molecules essential for cellular function, and the elimination of waste products. At its core, metabolism revolves around energy metabolism, which involves the breakdown of macronutrients—carbohydrates, fats, and proteins—into adenosine triphosphate (ATP), the energy currency of cells. Carbohydrates are converted into glucose, fats into fatty acids, and proteins into amino acids, all of which can be oxidized to produce ATP through various metabolic pathways, including aerobic respiration and anaerobic glycolysis.

Metabolism is intricately regulated by a complex network of hormones, enzymes, and signaling molecules that coordinate metabolic activities in response to physiological cues and environmental factors. Hormones such as insulin, glucagon, leptin, and ghrelin play key roles in regulating nutrient uptake, storage, and utilization. Insulin, for example, promotes glucose uptake and storage in cells, while glucagon stimulates glycogenolysis and gluconeogenesis to increase blood glucose levels during fasting. Leptin, produced by adipose tissue, regulates appetite and energy expenditure, while ghrelin stimulates hunger and food intake (Wadden et al., 2005).

Basal metabolic rate (BMR), the energy expended at rest to maintain vital functions, is a key determinant of overall metabolic rate. Factors such as age, sex, body composition, genetics, and physical activity level influence BMR and contribute to individual variations in metabolic rate. Additionally, the thermic effect of food (TEF), the energy expended during digestion, absorption, and metabolism of nutrients, and physical activity further influence total energy expenditure and metabolic rate. Metabolism is essential for promoting metabolic health, managing weight, and preventing metabolic disorders such as obesity, type 2 diabetes, and cardiovascular disease. By adopting healthy lifestyle habits, including a balanced diet, regular physical activity, and stress management, individuals can support optimal metabolic function and enhance overall well-being.

Summary

- Weight management is a multifaceted journey intertwined with metabolic changes within the body. At its core lies the fundamental principle of caloric balance, where the energy consumed through food intake must align with the energy expended through basal metabolic rate (BMR), physical activity, and the thermic effect of food (TEF).
- Body composition and metabolism undergo dynamic changes throughout life, influenced by factors such as age, genetics, diet, physical activity, and hormonal fluctuations.
- Metabolism, the intricate network of biochemical processes that sustain life, governs the conversion of nutrients into energy, the synthesis of biomolecules, and the regulation of cellular activities.
- Weight management is a multifaceted endeavor that encompasses a variety of strategies aimed at achieving and maintaining a healthy body weight.
- The cornerstone treatment of obesity is a lifestyle modification program that consist of diet, exercise, and behavior therapy.
- The impact of diet and exercise on overall health, well-being, and longevity cannot be overstated. These two pillars of lifestyle play crucial roles in preventing chronic diseases, maintaining healthy body weight, and optimizing metabolic function.
- A good starting point if you are contemplating diet and exercise changes is the American Institute for Cancer Research (AICR) recommendations.

References

1. Allison, D. B., Gadde, K. M., Garvey, W. T., et al. (2012). Controlled-release phentermine/topiramate in severely obese adults: A randomized controlled trial (EQUIP). *Obesity*, *20*(2), 330–342. https://doi.org/10.1038/oby.2011.147.
2. Anderson, J. W., Reynolds, L. R., Bush, H. M., Rinsky, J. L., & Washnock, C. (2011). Effect of a behavioral/nutritional intervention program on weight loss in obese adults: A randomized controlled trial. *Postgraduate Medicine*, *123*(6), 205–213. https://doi.org/10.3810/pgm.2011.11.2462.
3. Apovian, C. M., Aronne, L. J., Bessesen, D. H., et al. (2015). Pharmacological management of obesity: An Endocrine Society clinical practice guideline. *The Journal of Clinical Endocrinology and Metabolism*, *100*(2), 342–362. https://doi.org/10.1210/jc.2014-3415.
4. Aronne, L. J., Wadden, T. A., Peterson, C., Winslow, D., Odeh, S., & Gadde, K. M. (2013). Evaluation of phentermine and topiramate versus phentermine/topiramate extended-release in obese adults. *Obesity*, *21*(11), 2163–2171. https://doi.org/10.1002/oby.20506.
5. Astrup, A., Carraro, R., Finer, N., et al. (2012). Safety, tolerability and sustained weight loss over 2 years with the once-daily human GLP-1 analog, liraglutide. *International Journal of Obesity*, *36*(6), 843–854. https://doi.org/10.1038/ijo.2011.223.
6. Avery, A., Langley-Evans, S. C., Harrington, M., & Swift, J. A. (2016). Setting targets leads to greater long-term weight losses and 'unrealistic' targets increase the effect in a large community-based commercial weight management group. *Journal of Human Nutrition and Dietetics*, *29*(6), 687–696. https://doi.org/10.1111/jhn.12393.

7. Bellicha, A., van Baak, M. A., Battista, F., et al. (2021). Effect of exercise training on weight loss, body composition changes, and weight maintenance in adults with overweight or obesity: An overview of 12 systematic reviews and 149 studies. *Obesity Reviews*, *22*(Suppl 4), e13256. https://doi.org/10.1111/obr.13256.

8. Ben Slama, F., Achour, A., Belhadj, O., Hsairi, M., Oueslati, M., & Achour, N. (2002). Obesity and lifestyle in a population of male school children aged 6 to 10 years in Ariana (Tunisia). *La Tunisie Médicale*, *80*(9), 542–547.

9. Brehm, B. J., Seeley, R. J., Daniels, S. R., & D'Alessio, D. A. (2003). A randomized trial comparing a very low carbohydrate diet and a calorie-restricted low-fat diet on body weight and cardiovascular risk factors in healthy women. *The Journal of Clinical Endocrinology and Metabolism*, *88*(4), 1617–1623. https://doi.org/10.1210/jc.2002-021480.

10. Bueno, N. B., Melo, I. S. V. d., Oliveira, S. L. d., & Ataide, T. d. R. (2013). Very-low-carbohydrate ketogenic diet vs. low-fat diet for long-term weight loss: A meta-analysis of randomized controlled trials. *British Journal of Nutrition*, *110*(7), 1178–1187. https://doi.org/10.1017/S0007114513000548.

11. Caprio, M., Infante, M., Moriconi, E., et al. (2019). Very-low-calorie ketogenic diet (VLCKD) in the management of metabolic diseases: A systematic review and consensus statement from the Italian Society of Endocrinology (SIE). *Journal of Endocrinological Investigation*, *42*(12), 1365–1386. https://doi.org/10.1007/s40618-019-01095-3.

12. Carraça, E., Encantado, J., Battista, F., et al. (2021). Effective behavior changes techniques to promote physical activity in adults with overweight or obesity: A systematic review and meta-analysis. *Obesity Reviews*, *22*(12), e13258. https://doi.org/10.1111/obr.13258.

13. Castellana, M., Conte, E., Cignarelli, A., et al. (2020). Efficacy and safety of very low-calorie ketogenic diet (VLCKD) in patients with overweight and obesity: A systematic review and meta-analysis. *Reviews in Endocrine & Metabolic Disorders*, *21*(1), 5–16. https://doi.org/10.1007/s11154-019-09525-7.

14. Castelnuovo, G., Pietrabissa, G., Manzoni, G. M., et al. (2017). Cognitive behavioral therapy to aid weight loss in obese patients: Current perspectives. *Psychology Research and Behavior Management*, *10*, 10. https://doi.org/10.2147/PRBM.S126312.

15. Chiu, C. H., Ko, M. C., Wu, L. S., et al. (2017). Benefits of different intensity of aerobic exercise in modulating body composition among obese young adults: A pilot randomized controlled trial. *Health and Quality of Life Outcomes*, *15*(1), 168. https://doi.org/10.1186/s12955-017-0761-4.

16. Corica, D., Aversa, T., Valenzise, M., et al. (2018). Does family history of obesity, cardiovascular, and metabolic diseases influence onset and severity of childhood obesity? *Frontiers in Endocrinology*, *9*, 187. https://doi.org/10.3389/fendo.2018.00187.

17. Dalle Grave, R., Calugi, S., Gavasso, I., El Ghoch, M., & Marchesini, G. (2013). A randomized trial of energy-restricted high-protein versus high-carbohydrate, low-fat diet in morbid obesity. *Obesity*, *21*(9), 1774–1781. https://doi.org/10.1002/oby.20442.

18. de Lannoy, L., Cowan, T., Fernandez, A., & Ross, R. (2021). Physical activity, diet, and weight loss in patients recruited from primary care settings: An update on obesity management interventions. *Obesity Science and Practice*, *7*(5), 619–628. https://doi.org/10.1002/osp4.548.

19. Ditschuneit, H. H., Flechtner-Mors, M., Johnson, T. D., & Adler, G. (1999). Metabolic and weight-loss effects of a long-term dietary intervention in obese patients. *The American Journal of Clinical Nutrition*, *69*(2), 198–204. https://doi.org/10.1093/ajcn/69.2.198.

20. Donnelly, J. E., Blair, S. N., Jakicic, J. M., et al. (2009). American College of Sports Medicine position stand. Appropriate physical activity intervention strategies for weight loss and prevention of weight regain for adults. *Medicine and Science in Sports and Exercise*, *41*(7), 459–471. https://doi.org/10.1249/MSS.0b013e318194a04c.

21. Donnelly, J. E., Honas, J. J., Smith, B. K., Mayo, M., et al. (2013). Aerobic exercise alone results in clinically significant weight loss for men and women: Midwest Exercise Trial 2. *Obesity*, *21*(2), E219–E228. https://doi.org/10.1002/oby.20273.

22. Donnelly, J. E., Jacobsen, D. J., Heelan, K. S., Seip, R., & Smith, S. (2000). The effects of 18 months of intermittent vs. continuous exercise on aerobic capacity, body weight and composition, and metabolic fitness in previously sedentary, moderately obese females. *International Journal of Obesity and Related Metabolic Disorders*, *24*(5), 566–572. https://doi.org/10.1038/sj.ijo.0801213.

23. Donnelly, J. E., Smith, B. K., Dunn, L., et al. (2007). Comparison of a phone vs clinic approach to achieve 10% weight loss. *International Journal of Obesity*, *31*(8), 1270–1276. https://doi.org/10.1038/sj.ijo.0803606.

24. Driscoll, S., Meyerowitz-Katz, G., Ahlenstiel, G., Reynolds, T., Reid, K., & Bishay, R. H. (2021). Efficacy of telephone health coaching integration with standard multidisciplinary care for adults with obesity attending a weight management service: A pilot study. *Nutrients*, *13*(12), 4078. https://doi.org/10.3390/nu13124078.

25. Duffey, K. J., Gordon-Larsen, P., Jacobs, D. R., Williams, O. D., & Popkin, B. M. (2007). Differential associations of fast food and restaurant food consumption with 3-year change in body mass index: The Coronary Artery Risk Development in Young Adults Study. *The American Journal of Clinical Nutrition*, *85*(1), 201–208. https://doi.org/10.1093/ajcn/85.1.201.

26. Fabricatore, A. N. (2007). Behavior therapy and cognitive-behavioral therapy of obesity: Is there a difference? *Journal of the American Dietetic Association*, *107*(1), 92–99. https://doi.org/10.1016/j.jada.2006.10.012.

27. Forgione, N., Deed, G., Kilov, G., & Rigas, G. (2018). Managing obesity in primary care: Breaking down the barriers. *Advances in Therapy*, *35*(2), 191–198. https://doi.org/10.1007/s12325-017-0651-7.

28. Foster, G. D., Wyatt, H. R., Hill, J. O., et al. (2010). Weight and metabolic outcomes after 2 years on a low-carbohydrate versus low-fat diet. *Annals of Internal Medicine*, *153*(3), 147–157. https://doi.org/10.7326/0003-4819-153-3-201008030-00004.

29. Franz, M. J., Boucher, J. L., Rutten-Ramos, S., & VanWormer, J. J. (2015). Lifestyle weight-loss intervention outcomes in overweight and obese adults with type 2 diabetes: A systematic review and meta-analysis of randomized clinical trials. *Journal of the Academy of Nutrition and Dietetics*, *115*(9), 1447–1463. https://doi.org/10.1016/j.jand.2015.05.007.

30. Gaesser, G. A., & Angadi, S. S. (2021). Obesity treatment: Weight loss versus increasing fitness and physical activity for reducing health risks. *iScience*, *24*(3), 102995. https://doi.org/10.1016/j.isci.2021.102995.

31. Gardner, C. D., Trepanowski, J. F., Del Gobbo, L. C., et al. (2018). Effect of low-fat vs low-carbohydrate diet on 12-month weight loss in overweight adults and the association with genotype pattern or insulin secretion: The DIETFITS randomized clinical trial. *Journal of the American Medical Association*, *319*(7), 667–679. https://doi.org/10.1001/jama.2018.0245.

32. Garvey, W. T., Mechanick, J. I., Brett, E. M., et al. (2016). American Association of Clinical Endocrinologists and American College of Endocrinology comprehensive clinical practice guidelines for medical care of patients with obesity. *Endocrine Practice*, *22*(Suppl. 3), 1–203. https://doi.org/10.4158/EP161365.GL.

33. Garvey, W. T., Ryan, D. H., Look, M., et al. (2012). Two-year sustained weight loss and metabolic benefits with controlled-release phentermine/topiramate in obese and overweight adults (SEQUEL): A randomized, placebo-controlled, phase 3 extension study. *The American Journal of Clinical Nutrition*, *95*(2), 297–308. https://doi.org/10.3945/ajcn.111.023158.

34. Ghachem, A., Prud'homme, D., Rabasa-Lhoret, R., & Brochu, M. (2017). Effects of a 6-month caloric restriction induced-weight loss program in obese postmenopausal women with and without the metabolic syndrome: A MONET study. *Menopause*, *24*(8), 908–915. https://doi.org/10.1097/GME.0000000000000887.

35. Goldstein, S. P., Goldstein, C. M., Bond, D. S., Raynor, H. A., Wing, R. R., & Thomas, J. G. (2019). Associations between self-monitoring and weight change in behavioral weight loss interventions. *Health Psychology*, *38*(12), 1128–1136. https://doi.org/10.1037/hea0000775.

36. Grant, P., Piya, M., McGowan, B., & Taheri, S. (2014). The bariatric physician. *Clinical Medicine*, *14*(1), 30–33. https://doi.org/10.7861/clinmedicine.14-1-30.

37. Greenway, F. L., Fujioka, K., Plodkowski, R. A., et al. (2010). Effect of naltrexone plus bupropion on weight loss in overweight and obese adults (COR-I): A multicenter, randomized, double-blind, placebo-controlled, phase 3 trial. *The Lancet*, *376*(9741), 595–605. https://doi.org/10.1016/S0140-6736(10)60712-2.

38. Gudzune, K. A., Doshi, R. S., Mehta, A. K., et al. (2015). Efficacy of commercial weight loss programs: An updated systematic review. *Annals of Internal Medicine*, *162*(7), 501–512. https://doi.org/10.7326/M14-2238.

39. Harvey-Berino, J., West, D., Krukowski, R., et al. (2010). Internet delivered behavioral obesity treatment. *Preventive Medicine*, *51*(2), 123–128. https://doi.org/10.1016/j.ypmed.2010.04.007.

40. Hayes, C., & Kriska, A. (2008). Role of physical activity in diabetes management and prevention. *Journal of the American Dietetic Association*, *108*(S1), S19–S23. https://doi.org/10.1016/j.jada.2008.09.021.

41. Ho, S. S., Dhaliwal, S. S., Hills, A. P., & Pal, S. (2012). The effect of 12 weeks of aerobic, resistance or combination exercise training on cardiovascular risk factors in the overweight and obese in a randomized trial. *BMC Public Health*, *12*, 704. https://doi.org/10.1186/1471-2458-12-704.

42. Hollander, P., Gupta, A. K., Plodkowski, R., et al. (2013). Effects of naltrexone sustained-release/bupropion sustained-release combination therapy on body weight and glycemic parameters in overweight and obese patients with type 2 diabetes. *Diabetes Care*, *36*(12), 4022–4029. https://doi.org/10.2337/dc13-0651.

43. Jacob, S., Rabbia, M., Meier, M. K., & Hauptman, J. (2009). Orlistat 120 mg improves glycaemic control in type 2 diabetic patients with or without concurrent weight loss. *Diabetes, Obesity & Metabolism*, *11*(4), 361–371. https://doi.org/10.1111/j.1463-1326.2008.01014.x.

44. Jensen, M. D., Ryan, D. H., Apovian, C. M., et al. (2014). 2013 AHA/ACC/TOS'S guideline for the management of overweight and obesity in adults: A report of the American College of Cardiology/American Heart Association Task Force on Practice Guidelines and The Obesity Society. *Circulation*, *129*(25_suppl_2), S102–S138. https://doi.org/10.1161/01.cir.0000437739.71477.ee.

45. Juchacz, K., Kłos, P., Dziedziejko, V., & Wójciak, R. W. (2021). The effectiveness of supportive psychotherapy in weight loss in a group of young overweight and obese women. *Nutrients*, *13*(2), 532. https://doi.org/10.3390/nu13020532.

46. Kannan, U., Vasudevan, K., Balasubramaniam, K., Yerrabelli, D., Shanmugavel, K., & John, N. A. (2014). Effect of exercise intensity on lipid profile in sedentary obese adults. *Journal of Clinical and Diagnostic Research*, *8*(7), BC08–BC10. https://doi.org/10.7860/JCDR/2014/7574.4582.

47. Kelley, C. P., Sbrocco, G., & Sbrocco, T. (2016). Behavioral modification for the management of obesity. *Primary Care*, *43*(1), 159–175. https://doi.org/10.1016/j.pop.2015.10.005.

48. Knowler, W. C., Barrett-Connor, E., et al. (2002). Reduction in the incidence of type 2 diabetes with lifestyle intervention or metformin. *The New England Journal of Medicine*, *346*(6), 393–403. https://doi.org/10.1056/NEJMoa012512.

49. Kuna, S. T., Reboussin, D. M., Strotmeyer, E. S., et al. (2021). Effects of weight loss on obstructive sleep apnea severity: Ten-year results of the Sleep AHEAD study. *American Journal of Respiratory and Critical Care Medicine*, *203*(2), 221–229. https://doi.org/10.1164/rccm.202007-2690OC.

50. Kushner, R. F. (2014). Weight loss strategies for treatment of obesity. *Progress in Cardiovascular Diseases*, *56*(4), 465–472. https://doi.org/10.1016/j.pcad.2014.01.003.

51. Kushner, R. F., Calanna, S., Davies, M., et al. (2020). Semaglutide 2.4 mg for the treatment of obesity: Key elements of the STEP trials 1 to 5. *Obesity*, *28*(6), 1050–1061. https://doi.org/10.1002/oby.22866.

52. Larsen, J. K., van Ramshorst, B., Geenen, R., et al. (2004). Binge eating and its relationship to outcome after laparoscopic adjustable gastric banding. *Obesity Surgery*, *14*(8), 1111–1117. https://doi.org/10.1381/0960892042423411.

53. Li, Z., Hong, K., Saltsman, P., et al. (2005). Long-term efficacy of soy-based meal replacements vs an individualized diet plan in obese type II DM patients: Relative effects on weight loss, metabolic parameters, and C-reactive protein. *European Journal of Clinical Nutrition*, *59*(4), 411–418. https://doi.org/10.1038/sj.ejcn.1602106.

54. Li, Z., Maglione, M., Tu, W., et al. (2005). Meta-analysis: Pharmacologic treatment of obesity. *Annals of Internal Medicine*, *142*(7), 532–546. https://doi.org/10.7326/0003-4819-142-7-200504050-00012.

55. Lichtman, S. W., Pisarska, K., Berman, E. R., et al. (1992). Discrepancy between self-reported and actual caloric intake and exercise in obese subjects. *The New England Journal of Medicine*, *327*(27), 1893–1898. https://doi.org/10.1056/NEJM199212313272701.

56. Lin, X., & Li, H. (2021). Obesity: Epidemiology, pathophysiology, and therapeutics. *Frontiers in Endocrinology, 12*, 706978. https://doi.org/10.3389/fendo.2021.706978.

57. Look AHEAD Research Group, Wing, R. R., Bolin, P., & Brancati, F. L. (2013). Cardiovascular effects of intensive lifestyle intervention in type 2 diabetes. *The New England Journal of Medicine, 369*(2), 145–154. https://doi.org/10.1056/NEJMoa1212914.

58. Look AHEAD Research Group. (2014). Eight-year weight losses with an intensive lifestyle intervention: The Look AHEAD study. *Obesity, 22*(1), 5–13. https://doi.org/10.1002/oby.20662.

59. Mansoor, N., Vinknes, K. J., Veierød, M. B., & Retterstøl, K. (2016). Effects of low-carbohydrate diets vs. low-fat diets on body weight and cardiovascular risk factors: A meta-analysis of randomised controlled trials. *The British Journal of Nutrition, 115*(3), 466–479. https://doi.org/10.1017/S0007114515004855.

60. Mb, N. A., Tronieri, J. S., & Wadden, T. A. (2000). Behavioral approaches to obesity management. In K. R. Feingold, B. Anawalt, A. Boyce, et al. (Eds.), *Endotext* [Internet]. South Dartmouth (MA): MDText.com, Inc. Available from: http://www.ncbi.nlm.nih.gov/books/NBK278952/ (accessed on 10 September 2024).

61. Min, J., Kim, S. Y., Shin, I. S., Park, Y. B., & Lim, Y. W. (2021). The effect of meal replacement on weight loss according to calorie-restriction type and proportion of energy intake: A systematic review and meta-analysis of randomized controlled trials. *Journal of the Academy of Nutrition and Dietetics, 121*(9), 1551–1564.e3. https://doi.org/10.1016/j.jand.2021.05.020.

62. Moraes, A. d. S., Padovani, R. d. C., La Scala Teixeira, C. V., et al. (2021). Cognitive behavioral approach to treat obesity: A randomized clinical trial. *Frontiers in Nutrition, 8*, 14. https://doi.org/10.3389/fnut.2021.618611.

63. Moriconi, E., Camajani, E., Fabbri, A., Lenzi, A., & Caprio, M. (2021). Very-low-calorie ketogenic diet as a safe and valuable tool for long-term glycemic management in patients with obesity and type 2 diabetes. *Nutrients, 13*(3), 758. https://doi.org/10.3390/nu13030758.

64. Murawski, M. E., Milsom, V. A., Ross, K. M., et al. (2009). Problem solving, treatment adherence, and weight-loss outcome among women participating in lifestyle treatment for obesity. *Eating Behaviors, 10*(3), 146–151. https://doi.org/10.1016/j.eatbeh.2009.02.001.

65. Muscogiuri, G., El Ghoch, M., Colao, A., et al. (2021). European guidelines for obesity management in adults with a very low-calorie ketogenic diet: A systematic review and meta-analysis. *Obesity Facts, 14*(3), 222–245. https://doi.org/10.1159/000518019.

66. Nicoll, R., & Henein, M. Y. (2018). Caloric restriction and its effect on blood pressure, heart rate variability, and arterial stiffness and dilatation: A review of the evidence. *International Journal of Molecular Sciences, 19*(3), 751. https://doi.org/10.3390/ijms19030751.

67. Nothwehr, F., & Yang, J. (2007). Goal setting frequency and the use of behavioral strategies related to diet and physical activity. *Health Education Research, 22*(4), 532–538. https://doi.org/10.1093/her/cyl122.

68. Paoli, A., Rubini, A., Volek, J. S., & Grimaldi, K. A. (2013). Beyond weight loss: A review of the therapeutic uses of very-low-carbohydrate (ketogenic) diets. *European Journal of Clinical Nutrition, 67*(8), 789–796. https://doi.org/10.1038/ejcn.2013.116.

69. Perri, M. G., Shankar, M. N., Daniels, M. J., et al. (2020). Effect of telehealth extended care for maintenance of weight loss in rural U.S. communities: A randomized clinical trial. *JAMA Network Open, 3*(11), e206764. https://doi.org/10.1001/jamanetworkopen.2020.6764.

70. Pi-Sunyer, X., Astrup, A., Fujioka, K., et al. (2015). A randomized, controlled trial of 3.0 mg of liraglutide in weight management. *The New England Journal of Medicine*, *373*(1), 11–22. https://doi.org/10.1056/NEJMoa1506225.

71. Ross, K. M., Qiu, P., You, L., & Wing, R. R. (2019). Week-to-week predictors of weight loss and regain. *Health Psychology*, *38*(12), 1150–1158. https://doi.org/10.1037/hea0000825.

72. Ross, R., Janssen, I., Dawson, J., et al. (2004). Exercise-induced reduction in obesity and insulin resistance in women: A randomized controlled trial. *Obesity Research*, *12*(5), 789–798. https://doi.org/10.1038/oby.2004.98.

73. Rubino, D., Abrahamsson, N., Davies, M., et al. (2021). Effect of continued weekly subcutaneous semaglutide vs placebo on weight loss maintenance in adults with overweight or obesity: The STEP 4 randomized clinical trial. *Journal of the American Medical Association*, *325*(14), 1414–1425. https://doi.org/10.1001/jama.2021.2735.

74. Ruggenenti, P., Abbate, M., Ruggiero, B., et al. (2017). Renal and systemic effects of calorie restriction in patients with type 2 diabetes with abdominal obesity: A randomized controlled trial. *Diabetes*, *66*(1), 75–86. https://doi.org/10.2337/db16-0792.

75. Sacks, F. M., Bray, G. A., Carey, V. J., et al. (2009). Comparison of weight-loss diets with different compositions of fat, protein, and carbohydrates. *The New England Journal of Medicine*, *360*(9), 859–873. https://doi.org/10.1056/NEJMoa0804748.

76. Sadeghirad, B., Duhaney, T., Motaghipisheh, S., Campbell, N. R. C., & Johnston, B. C. (2016). Influence of unhealthy food and beverage marketing on children's dietary intake and preference: A systematic review and meta-analysis of randomized trials. *Obesity Reviews*, *17*(10), 945–959. https://doi.org/10.1111/obr.12423.

77. Samaha, F. F., Iqbal, N., Seshadri, P., et al. (2003). A low-carbohydrate as compared with a low-fat diet in severe obesity. *The New England Journal of Medicine*, *348*(21), 2074–2081. https://doi.org/10.1056/NEJMoa022637.

78. Saunders, K. H., Umashanker, D., Igel, L. I., Kumar, R. B., & Aronne, L. J. (2018). Obesity pharmacotherapy. *The Medical Clinics of North America*, *102*(1), 135–148. https://doi.org/10.1016/j.mcna.2017.09.001.

79. Schwingshackl, L., & Hoffmann, G. (2013). Comparison of effects of long-term low-fat vs high-fat diets on blood lipid levels in overweight or obese patients: A systematic review and meta-analysis. *Journal of the Academy of Nutrition and Dietetics*, *113*(12), 1640–1661. https://doi.org/10.1016/j.jand.2013.08.007.

80. Shai, I., Schwarzfuchs, D., Henkin, Y., et al. (2008). Weight loss with a low-carbohydrate, Mediterranean, or low-fat diet. *The New England Journal of Medicine*, *359*(3), 229–241. https://doi.org/10.1056/NEJMoa0708681.

81. Sigal, R. J., Kenny, G. P., Wasserman, D. H., Castaneda-Sceppa, C., & White, R. D. (2006). Physical activity/exercise and type 2 diabetes: A consensus statement from the American Diabetes Association. *Diabetes Care, 29*(6), 1433–1438.

82. Singh, R. K., Kumar, P., & Mahalingam, K. (2017). Molecular genetics of human obesity: A comprehensive review. *Comptes Rendus Biologies, 340*(2), 87–108.

83. Smethers, A. D., & Rolls, B. J. (2018). Dietary management of obesity: Cornerstones of healthy eating patterns. *The Medical Clinics of North America, 102*(1), 107–124.

84. Son, J. W., & Kim, S. (2020). Comprehensive review of current and upcoming anti-obesity drugs. *Diabetes & Metabolism Journal, 44*(6), 802–818.

85. Stern, L., Iqbal, N., Seshadri, P., et al. (2004). The effects of low-carbohydrate versus conventional weight loss diets in severely obese adults: One-year follow-up of a randomized trial. *Annals of Internal Medicine, 140*(10), 778–785.

86. Sukkar, S. G., & Muscaritoli, M. (2021). A clinical perspective of low carbohydrate ketogenic diets: A narrative review. *Frontiers in Nutrition, 8*, 642628.

87. Svetkey, L. P., Batch, B. C., Lin, P. H., et al. (2015). Cell phone intervention for you (CITY): A randomized, controlled trial of behavioral weight loss intervention for young adults using mobile technology. *Obesity, 23*(10), 2133–2141.

88. Swift, D. L., Johannsen, N. M., Lavie, C. J., Earnest, C. P., Blair, S. N., & Church, T. S. (2016). Effects of clinically significant weight loss with exercise training on insulin resistance and cardiometabolic adaptations. *Obesity, 24*(4), 812–819.

89. Swinburn, B. A., Sacks, G., Hall, K. D., et al. (2011). The global obesity pandemic: Shaped by global drivers and local environments. *The Lancet, 378*(9793), 804–814.

90. Telles, S., Gangadhar, B. N., & Chandwani, K. D. (2016). Lifestyle modification in the prevention and management of obesity. *Journal of Obesity, 2016*, 5818601.

91. Torgerson, J. S., Hauptman, J., Boldrin, M. N., & Sjöström, L. (2004). XENical in the Prevention of Diabetes in Obese Subjects (XENDOS) Study: A randomized study of orlistat as an adjunct to lifestyle changes for the prevention of type 2 diabetes in obese patients. *Diabetes Care, 27*(1), 155–161.

92. Tragni, E., Vigna, L., Ruscica, M., et al. (2021). Reduction of cardio-metabolic risk and body weight through a multiphasic very-low calorie ketogenic diet program in women with overweight/obesity: A study in a real-world setting. *Nutrients, 13*(6), 1804.

93. Tudor-Locke, C., & Bassett, D. R. (2004). How many steps/days are enough? Preliminary pedometer indices for public health. *Sports Medicine, 34*(1), 1–8.

94. Veldhorst, M. A., Smeets, A. J., Soenen, S., et al. (2008). Protein-induced satiety: Effects and mechanisms of different proteins. *Physiology & Behavior, 94*(3), 300–307.

95. Vissers, D., Hens, W., Taeymans, J., Baeyens, J. P., Poortmans, J., & Van Gaal, L. (2013). The effect of exercise on visceral adipose tissue in overweight adults: A systematic review and meta-analysis. *PLoS ONE, 8*(2), e56415.

96. Voils, C. I., Olsen, M. K., Gierisch, J. M., et al. (2017). Maintenance of weight loss after initiation of nutrition training: A randomized trial. *Annals of Internal Medicine, 166*(7), 463–471.

97. Wadden, T. A., Hollander, P., Klein, S., et al. (2013). Weight maintenance and additional weight loss with liraglutide after low-calorie-diet-induced weight loss: The SCALE Maintenance randomized study. *International Journal of Obesity, 37*(10), 1443–1451.

98. Wadden, T. A., Webb, V. L., Moran, C. H., & Bailer, B. A. (2012). Lifestyle modification for obesity. *Circulation, 125*(9), 1157–1170.

99. Watson, P., Wiers, R. W., Hommel, B., Gerdes, V. E. A., & de Wit, S. (2017). Stimulus control over action for food in obese versus healthy-weight individuals. *Frontiers in Psychology, 8*, 580.

100. Wen, H., & Wang, L. (2017). Reducing effect of aerobic exercise on blood pressure of essential hypertensive patients. *Medicine (Baltimore), 96*(24), e6150.

101. Wilding, J. P. H., Batterham, R. L., Calanna, S., et al. (2021). Once-weekly semaglutide in adults with overweight or obesity. *The New England Journal of Medicine, 384*(10), 989–1002.

102. Willaing, I., Ladelund, S., Jørgensen, T., Simonsen, T., & Nielsen, L. M. (2004). Nutritional counselling in primary health care: A randomized comparison of an intervention by general practitioner or dietician. *European Journal of Cardiovascular Prevention and Rehabilitation, 11*(6), 513–520.

103. Willis, E. A., Creasy, S. A., Honas, J. J., Melanson, E. L., & Donnelly, J. E. (2020). The effects of exercise session timing on weight loss and components of energy balance: Midwest exercise trial 2. *International Journal of Obesity, 44*(1), 114–124.

104. Willis, L. H., Slentz, C. A., Bateman, L. A., et al. (2012). Effects of aerobic and/or resistance training on body mass and fat mass in overweight or obese adults. *Journal of Applied Physiology, 113*(12), 1831–1837.

105. Wing, R. R., Lang, W., Wadden, T. A., et al. (2011). Benefits of modest weight loss in improving cardiovascular risk factors in overweight and obese individuals with type 2 diabetes. *Diabetes Care, 34*(6), 1481–1486.

106. Wirth, A., Wabitsch, M., & Hauner, H. (2014). The prevention and treatment of obesity. *Dtsch Ärztebl International, 111*(40), 705–713.

107. Witham, M. D., & Avenell, A. (2010). Interventions to achieve long-term weight loss in obese older people: A systematic review and meta-analysis. *Age and Ageing, 39*(2), 176–184.

108. Zubrzycki, A., Cierpka-Kmiec, K., Kmiec, Z., & Wrońska, A. (2018). The role of low-calorie diets and intermittent fasting in the treatment of obesity and type-2 diabetes. *Journal of Physiology and Pharmacology, 69*(2), 163–172

INDEX

C

D

E

F

G

H

I

K

L

M

N

O

P

Kolibri 360 GmbH
Ferdinand-Jühlke-Straße 7
99095 Erfurt, Deutschland
produktsicherheit@kolibri360.de